Pediatric Otolaryngology

Editor

HAROLD S. PINE

PEDIATRIC CLINICS
OF NORTH AMERICA

www.pediatric.theclinics.com

August 2013 • Volume 60 • Number 4

ELSEVIER

1600 John F. Kennedy Boulevard • Suite 1800 • Philadelphia, Pennsylvania, 19103-2899

http://www.theclinics.com

THE PEDIATRIC CLINICS OF NORTH AMERICA Volume 60, Number 4
August 2013 ISSN 0031-3955, ISBN-13: 978-0-323-18614-8

Editor: Kerry Holland
Developmental Editor: Donald Mumford

The Pediatric Clinics of North America (ISSN 0031-3955) is published bimonthly by Elsevier Inc., 360 Park Avenue South, New York, NY 10010-1710. Months of issue are February, April, June, August, October, and December. Periodicals postage paid at New York, NY and additional mailing offices. Subscription prices are $191.00 per year (US individuals), $462.00 per year (US institutions), $259.00 per year (Canadian individuals), $614.00 per year (Canadian institutions), $308.00 per year (international individuals), $614.00 per year (international institutions), $93.00 per year (US students and residents), and $159.00 per year (international and Canadian residents and students). To receive students/resident rare, orders must be accompanied by name of affiliated institution, date of term, and the signature of program/residency coordinator on institution letterhead. Orders will be billed at individual rate until proof of status is received. Foreign air speed delivery is included in all *Clinics* subscription prices. All prices are subject to change without notice. **POSTMASTER:** Send address changes to *The Pediatric Clinics of North America*, Elsevier Health Sciences Division, Subscription Customer Service, 3251 Riverport Lane, Maryland Heights, MO 63043. **Customer Service: 1-800-654-2452 (US and Canada). From outside of the US and Canada: 1-314-447-8871. Fax: 1-314-447-8029. For print support, E-mail: JournalsCustomerService-usa@elsevier.com. For online support, E-mail: JournalsOnlineSupport-usa@elsevier.com.**

Reprints. For copies of 100 or more, of articles in this publication, please contact the Commercial Reprints Department, Elsevier Inc., 360 Park Avenue South, New York, NY 10010-1710. Tel.: 212-633-3812; Fax: 212-462-1935; E-mail: reprints@elsevier.com.

The Pediatric Clinics of North America is also published in Spanish by McGraw-Hill Inter-americana Editores S.A., Mexico City, Mexico; in Portuguese by Riechmann and Affonso Editores, Rua Comandante Coelho 1085, CEP 21250, Rio de Janeiro, Brazil; and in Greek by Althayia SA, Athens, Greece.

The Pediatric Clinics of North America is covered in *MEDLINE/PubMed (Index Medicus), Excerpta Medica, Current Contents, Current Contents/Clinical Medicine, Science Citation Index, ASCA, ISI/BIOMED,* and *BIOSIS*.

Printed in the United States of America.

PROGRAM OBJECTIVE
The goal of the *Pediatric Clinics of North America* is to keep practicing physicians and residents up to date with current clinical practice in pediatrics by providing timely articles reviewing the state-of-the-art in patient care.

TARGET AUDIENCE
All practicing pediatricians, physicians and healthcare professionals who provide patient care to pediatric patients.

LEARNING OBJECTIVES
Upon completion of this activity, participants will be able to:
1. Review pediatric cochlear implantation and its expanding applications and outcomes.
2. Describe chronic rhinosinusitis and chronic cough in children.
3. Recognize enlarged neck lymph nodes in children.

ACCREDITATION
The Elsevier Office of Continuing Medical Education (EOCME) is accredited by the Accreditation Council for Continuing Medical Education (ACCME) to provide continuing medical education for physicians.

The EOCME designates this journal-based CME activity for a maximum of 15 *AMA PRA Category 1 Credit*(s)™. Physicians should claim only the credit commensurate with the extent of their participation in the activity.

All other health care professionals completing continuing education credit for this activity will be issued a certificate of participation.

DISCLOSURE OF CONFLICTS OF INTEREST
The EOCME assesses conflict of interest with its instructors, faculty, planners, and other individuals who are in a position to control the content of CME activities. All relevant conflicts of interest that are identified are thoroughly vetted by EOCME for fair balance, scientific objectivity, and patient care recommendations. EOCME is committed to providing its learners with CME activities that promote improvements or quality in healthcare and not a specific proprietary business or a commercial interest.

The planning committee, staff, authors and editors listed below have identified no financial relationships or relationships to products or devices they or their spouse/life partner have with commercial interest related to the content of this CME activity:
Nathan S. Alexander, MD; Oren Cavel, MD; Nicole Congleton; Allison M. Dobbie, MD; Charles S. Ebert Jr, MD, MPH; Patrick Froehlich, MD; Chantal Giguere, MD; Benjamin Hartley, MBBS, BSc, FRCS (ORL-HNS); Chantal Hickey, MD; Kerry Holland; Kevin C. Huoh, MD; Sharon Hughes Gnagi, MD; Kedar Kakodkar, MD; Paul Krakovitz, MD; Indu Kumari; Elton M. Lambert, MD; Annie Lapointe, MD, MPH; Sandy Lavery; Arielle Levy, MD, MEd; Jill McNair; Shraddha Mukerji, MD; Harold S. Pine, MD; Victoria Possamai, MBChB, FRCS (ORL-HNS); Karthik Rajasekaran, MD; Sharon D. Ramos, MD; Kristina W. Rosbe, MD; Austin S. Rose, MD; Soham Roy, MD, FACS, FAAP; Joseph L. Russell, MD; Scott A. Schraff, MD; James W. Schroeder, Jr, MD; Brian D. Thorp, MD; Michael Underbrink, MD, MBA; Naren N. Venkatesan, MD; Johana B. Castro Wagner, MD; David R. White, MD; Dayton L. Young, MD; Francoise Yung, MD; Adam M. Zanation, MD.

UNAPPROVED/OFF-LABEL USE DISCLOSURE
The EOCME requires CME faculty to disclose to the participants:
1. When products or procedures being discussed are off-label, unlabelled, experimental, and/or investigational (not US Food and Drug Administration [FDA] approved); and
2. Any limitations on the information presented, such as data that are preliminary or that represent ongoing research, interim analyses, and/or unsupported opinions. Faculty may discuss information about pharmaceutical agents that is outside of FDA-approved labelling. This information is intended solely for CME and is not intended to promote off-label use of these medications. If you have any questions, contact the medical affairs department of the manufacturer for the most recent prescribing information.

TO ENROLL
To enroll in the *Pediatric Clinics of North America* Continuing Medical Education program, call customer service at 1-800-654-2452 or sign up online at http://www.theclinics.com/home/cme. The CME program is available to subscribers for an additional annual fee of USD 261.

METHOD OF PARTICIPATION
In order to claim credit, participants must complete the following:
1. Complete enrolment as indicated above.
2. Read the activity.
3. Complete the CME Test and Evaluation. Participants must achieve a score of 70% on the test. All CME Tests and Evaluations must be completed online.

CME INQUIRIES/SPECIAL NEEDS
For all CME inquiries or special needs, please contact elsevierCME@elsevier.com.

Contributors

EDITOR

HAROLD S. PINE, MD, FAAP, FACS
Associate Professor of Pediatric Otolaryngology, Department of Otolaryngology-Head and Neck Surgery, University of Texas Medical Branch, Galveston, Texas

AUTHORS

NATHAN S. ALEXANDER, MD
Clinical Instructor, Department of Otolaryngology, Northwestern University, Feinberg School of Medicine, Chicago, Illinois

OREN CAVEL, MD
Sainte-Justine Pediatric Airway Simulation Group, Department of Otorhinolaryngology, Sainte-Justine Mother and Child University Hospital, University of Montreal, Montreal, Quebec, Canada

ALLISON M. DOBBIE, MD
Clinical Fellow, Division of Pediatric Otolaryngology, Department of Otolaryngology-Head and Neck Surgery, Medical University of South Carolina, Charleston, South Carolina

CHARLES S. EBERT Jr, MD, MPH
Department of Otolaryngology-Head & Neck Surgery, University of North Carolina School of Medicine, Chapel Hill, North Carolina

PATRICK FROEHLICH, MD, PhD
Sainte-Justine Pediatric Airway Simulation Group, Department of Otorhinolaryngology, Sainte-Justine Mother and Child University Hospital, University of Montreal, Montreal, Quebec, Canada

CHANTAL GIGUERE, MD
Sainte-Justine Pediatric Airway Simulation Group, Department of Otorhinolaryngology, Sainte-Justine Mother and Child University Hospital, University of Montreal, Montreal, Quebec, Canada

SHARON H. GNAGI, MD
Department of Otolaryngology, Mayo Clinic Arizona, Phoenix, Arizona

BENJAMIN HARTLEY, MBBS, BSc, FRCS (ORL-HNS)
Consultant Paediatric Otolaryngologist – Head and Neck Surgeon, Department of ENT Surgery, Great Ormond Street Hospital for Children, London, United Kingdom

CHANTAL HICKEY, MD
Sainte-Justine Pediatric Airway Simulation Group, Department of Anesthesia, Sainte-Justine Mother and Child University Hospital, University of Montreal, Montreal, Quebec, Canada

KEVIN C. HUOH, MD
Fellow in Pediatric Otolaryngology, Department of Otolaryngology-Head and Neck
Surgery, Stanford University School of Medicine, Stanford, California

KEDAR KAKODKAR, MD
Clinical Instructor, Department of Otolaryngology, Northwestern University, Feinberg
School of Medicine, Chicago, Illinois

PAUL KRAKOVITZ, MD
Vice Chairman, Surgical Operations; Section Head, Pediatric Otolaryngology, Head and
Neck Institute, Assistant Professor, Lerner College of Medicine, Cleveland Clinic,
Cleveland, Ohio

ELTON LAMBERT, MD
Chief Resident, Department of Otorhinolaryngology, University of Texas-Houston School
of Medicine, Houston, Texas

ANNIE LAPOINTE, MD, MPH
Sainte-Justine Pediatric Airway Simulation Group, Department of Otorhinolaryngology,
Sainte-Justine Mother and Child University Hospital, University of Montreal, Montreal,
Quebec, Canada

ARIELLE LEVY, MD, MEd
Sainte-Justine Pediatric Airway Simulation Group, Department of Emergency Medicine,
Sainte-Justine Mother and Child University Hospital, University of Montreal, Montreal,
Quebec, Canada

SHRADDHA MUKERJI, MD
Department of Otolaryngology, University of Texas-Medical Branch at Galveston,
Galveston, Texas

HAROLD S. PINE, MD, FAAP, FACS
Associate Professor of Pediatric Otolaryngology, Department of Otolaryngology-Head
and Neck Surgery, University of Texas Medical Branch, Galveston, Texas

VICTORIA POSSAMAI, MBChB, FRCS (ORL-HNS)
Fellow in Paediatric Otolaryngology, Department of ENT Surgery, Great Ormond Street
Hospital for Children, London, United Kingdom

KARTHIK RAJASEKARAN, MD
Head and Neck Institute, Cleveland Clinic, Cleveland, Ohio

SHARON D. RAMOS, MD
Department of Otolaryngology, University of Texas-Medical Branch at Galveston,
Galveston, Texas

KRISTINA W. ROSBE, MD, FAAP, FACS
Professor of Otolaryngology and Pediatrics, Director, Division of Pediatric
Otolaryngology, Department of Otolaryngology-Head and Neck Surgery, University
of California, San Francisco, San Francisco, California

AUSTIN S. ROSE, MD
Department of Otolaryngology-Head & Neck Surgery, University of North Carolina School
of Medicine, Chapel Hill, North Carolina

SOHAM ROY, MD, FACS, FAAP
Associate Professor and Director of Pediatric Otolaryngology, Department of
Otorhinolaryngology, University of Texas-Houston School of Medicine, Houston, Texas

JOSEPH L. RUSSELL, MD
Otolaryngology Resident, Department of Otolaryngology-Head and Neck Surgery,
University of Texas Medical Branch, Galveston, Texas

SCOTT A. SCHRAFF, MD, FAAP
Chief, Division of Pediatric Otolaryngology, Department of Otolaryngology, Phoenix
Children's Hospital, Phoenix, Arizona

JAMES W. SCHROEDER Jr, MD, FACS, FAAP
Assistant Professor, Department of Otolaryngology, Northwestern University, Feinberg
School of Medicine, Chicago, Illinois

BRIAN D. THORP, MD
Department of Otolaryngology-Head & Neck Surgery, University of North Carolina School
of Medicine, Chapel Hill, North Carolina

MICHAEL UNDERBRINK, MD
Assistant Professor, Department of Otolaryngology-Head and Neck Surgery, University of
Texas Medical Branch, Galveston, Texas

NAREN N. VENKATESAN, MD
Department of Otolaryngology-Head and Neck Surgery, University of Texas Medical
Branch, Galveston, Texas

JOHANA B. CASTRO WAGNER, MD
Department of Pediatrics, University of Texas Medical Branch, Galveston, Texas

DAVID R. WHITE, MD
Associate Professor, Chief, Division of Pediatric Otolaryngology, Department of
Otolaryngology-Head and Neck Surgery, Medical University of South Carolina,
Charleston, South Carolina

DAYTON L. YOUNG, MD
Assistant Professor of Otolaryngology, Department of Otolaryngology-Head and Neck
Surgery, University of Texas Medical Branch, Galveston, Texas

FRANCOISE YUNG, MD
Sainte-Justine Pediatric Airway Simulation Group, Department of Anesthesia,
Sainte-Justine Mother and Child University Hospital, University of Montreal, Montreal,
Quebec, Canada

ADAM M. ZANATION, MD
Department of Otolaryngology-Head & Neck Surgery, University of North Carolina School
of Medicine, Chapel Hill, North Carolina

Contents

Preface: Pediatric Otolaryngology   xv

Harold S. Pine

Tonsillectomy and Adenoidectomy   793

Sharon D. Ramos, Shraddha Mukerji, and Harold S. Pine

> Adenotonsillectomy (AT) is one of the most common pediatric surgical
> procedures performed in the United States; more than 530,000 are per-
> formed annually in children younger than 15 years of age. AT was tradition-
> ally performed for recurrent tonsillitis and its sequelae but in recent times,
> sleep-disordered breathing/obstructive sleep apnea in children has
> emerged as the primary indication for surgical removal of adenoids and
> tonsils. The new guidelines used by clinicians to identify children who
> are appropriate candidates for AT address indications based primarily
> on obstructive and infectious causes.

Otitis Media and Ear Tubes   809

Elton Lambert and Soham Roy

> The placement of myringotomy tubes remains an effective treatment of
> recurrent acute otitis media and chronic otitis media with effusion. Infants
> and young children are prone to these entities because of their immature
> anatomy and immunology. Several host, pathogenic, and environmental
> factors contribute to the development of these conditions. The identifica-
> tion and modification of some these factors can preclude the need for
> intervention. The procedure continues to be one of the most common out-
> patient pediatric procedures. Close vigilance and identification of potential
> complications is of utmost importance in the ongoing management of the
> child with middle ear disease.

Pediatric Obstructive Sleep Apnea Syndrome   827

Nathan S. Alexander and James W. Schroeder Jr

> Pediatric obstructive sleep apnea syndrome (OSAS) is a common health
> problem diagnosed and managed by various medical specialists, including
> family practice physicians, pediatricians, pulmonologists, and general and
> pediatric otolaryngologists. If left untreated, the sequelae can be severe.
> Over the last decade, significant advancements have been made in the
> evidence-based management of pediatric OSAS. This article focuses on
> the current understanding of this disease, its management, and related
> clinical practice guidelines.

Pediatric Cochlear Implantation: Expanding Applications and Outcomes   841

Joseph L. Russell, Harold S. Pine, and Dayton L. Young

> Cochlear implantation is a revolutionary yet time-sensitive treatment for
> deaf children that must be performed within a critical window of time, in

early life, for a congenitally deafened child to receive maximum benefit. Potential candidates should therefore be referred for evaluation early. Primary reasons for delay of cochlear implantation include slow referrals for care, parental delays, and payer delays. It is vital that all newborn children undergo hearing screening to identify deaf children at birth, and for parents, health care providers, and health care payers to be educated about the indications, important benefits, and reasonable risks of cochlear implantation for deaf children.

Laryngopharyngeal Reflux Disease in Children   865

Naren N. Venkatesan, Harold S. Pine, and Michael Underbrink

Extraesophageal reflux disease, commonly called laryngopharyngeal reflux disease (LPRD), continues to be an entity with more questions than answers. Although the role of LPRD has been implicated in various pediatric diseases, it has been inadequately studied in others. LPRD is believed to contribute to failure to thrive, laryngomalacia, recurrent respiratory papillomatosis, chronic cough, hoarseness, esophagitis, and aspiration among other pathologies. Thus, LPRD should be considered as a chronic disease with a variety of presentations. High clinical suspicion along with consultation with an otolaryngologist, who can evaluate for laryngeal findings, is necessary to accurately diagnose LPRD.

Voice Disorders in Children   879

Victoria Possamai and Benjamin Hartley

This article reviews the management of voice disorders in children. We describe the relevant anatomy and development of the larynx throughout childhood, which affects voice. We consider the epidemiologic data to establish the size of the problem. The assessment of the patient in the clinic is described stepwise through the history, examination, laryngoscopy, and extra tests. We then review the common voice disorders encountered and their management, concluding with discussion of future directions, which may herald advances in this field.

Laryngomalacia   893

Allison M. Dobbie and David R. White

 Videos of flexible fiberoptic laryngoscopy and supraglottoplasty accompany this article

Laryngomalacia is the most common cause of stridor in infants. Stridor results from upper airway obstruction caused by collapse of supraglottic tissue into the airway. Most cases of laryngomalacia are mild and self-resolve, but severe symptoms require investigation and intervention. There is a strong association with gastroesophageal reflux disease in patients with laryngomalacia, and thus medical treatment with antireflux medications may be indicated. Supraglottoplasty is the preferred surgical treatment of laryngomalacia, reserved only for severe cases. Proper identification of those patients who require medical and surgical intervention is key to providing treatment with successful outcomes.

Nasal Obstruction in Newborns   903

Sharon H. Gnagi and Scott A. Schraff

> Nasal obstruction is a serious clinical scenario in the newborn infant with a large differential diagnosis. This article reviews the etiologies of nasal obstruction to aid the pediatrician in prompt evaluation, diagnosis, and treatment.

Enlarged Neck Lymph Nodes in Children   923

Karthik Rajasekaran and Paul Krakovitz

> Pediatric cervical lymphadenopathy is a challenging medical condition for the patient, family, and physician. There are a wide variety of causes for cervical lymphadenopathy and an understanding of these causes is paramount in determining the most appropriate workup and management. A thorough history and physical examination are important in narrowing the differential diagnosis. Diagnostic studies and imaging studies play an important role as well. This article reviews the common causes of lymphadenopathy, and presents a methodical approach to a patient with cervical lymphadenopathy.

Infantile Hemangiomas of the Head and Neck   937

Kevin C. Huoh and Kristina W. Rosbe

> Infantile hemangiomas (IHs) are benign vascular tumors. Clinical history and physical examination are the most important factors for diagnosis, with most IHs having a typical presentation. Treatment is required for some IHs that cause significant cosmetic deformity or functional compromise. Propranolol is the first-line treatment of most IHs. Ongoing research is increasing our understanding of the pathophysiology of these tumors and should help to identify future potential therapeutic targets.

Chronic Cough in Children   951

Johana B. Castro Wagner and Harold S. Pine

 Video of cough caused by *Bordetella pertussis* in a child accompanies this article

> The management of chronic cough, a common complaint in children, is challenging for most health care professionals. Millions of dollars are spent every year on unnecessary testing and treatment. A rational approach based on a detailed interview and a thorough physical examination guides further intervention and management. Inexpensive and simple homemade syrups based on dark honey have proved to be an effective measure when dealing with cough in children.

Pediatric Dysphagia   969

Kedar Kakodkar and James W. Schroeder Jr

> Feeding and swallowing disorders in the pediatric population are becoming more common, particularly in infants born prematurely and in children with chronic medical conditions. The normal swallowing mechanism is divided into 4 stages: the preparatory, the oral, the pharyngeal, and the

esophageal phases. Feeding disorders have multiple causes: medical, nutritional, behavioral, psychological, and environmental factors can all contribute. Pathologic conditions involving any of the anatomic sites associated with the phases of swallowing can negatively impact the coordination of these phases and lead to symptoms of dysphagia and feeding intolerance.

Chronic Rhinosinusitis in Children   979

Austin S. Rose, Brian D. Thorp, Adam M. Zanation, and Charles S. Ebert Jr

Chronic rhinosinusitis (CRS) affects nearly 37 million people in the United States each year and accounts for approximately $6 billion in direct and indirect health care costs. Despite its prevalence and significant impact, little is known about its exact cause and pathophysiology, and significant controversy remains regarding appropriate treatment options. Basic science research, however, has shown recent promise toward improving understanding of the innate and environmental factors underlying the pathophysiology of CRS. The hope is that this will also lead to advances in treatment for children adversely affected by this common yet complicated disease.

Training: Simulating Pediatric Airway   993

Oren Cavel, Chantal Giguere, Annie Lapointe, Arielle Levy, Francoise Yung, Chantal Hickey, and Patrick Froehlich

 Video of simulated pediatric airway performance accompanies this article

Training in the management of pediatric airway cases has been limited by the number of cases and by the involved risks to the child. Simulation is an alternative and accessible means to practice that complex psychomotor task in a safe and reproducible environment. A high-fidelity baby mannequin provides an acceptable airway anatomic resemblance combined with measurable respiratory and cardiovascular parameters, allowing practice to be interactive and challenging. The availability of simulation laboratories within hospitals and the development of pathology-inspired accessories for the mannequins will determine the rate of adherence of ENT departments to this evolving field of simulation-based education.

Index   1005

PEDIATRIC CLINICS OF NORTH AMERICA

FORTHCOMING ISSUES

October 2013
Pediatric Emergencies
Richard Lichenstein, MD, *Editor*

December 2013
Pediatric Hematology
Catherine Manno, MD, *Editor*

February 2014
Adolescent Cardiac Issues
Richard Humes, MD, and
Pooja Gupta, MD, *Editors*

RECENT ISSUES

June 2013
Critical Care of the Pediatric Patient
Derek S. Wheeler, MD, *Editor*

April 2013
**Advances in the Diagnosis and Treatment
of Pediatric Infectious Diseases**
Chandy C. John, MD, *Editor*

February 2013
Breastfeeding Updates for the Pediatrician
Ardythe L. Morrow, PhD, and
Caroline J. Chantry, MD, *Editors*

RELATED INTEREST

Otolaryngologic Clinics of North America June 2012 (Volume 45:3)
Pediatric Otolaryngology: Challenges in Multi-system Disease
Austin S. Rose, MD, *Editor*

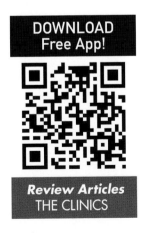

Preface

Pediatric Otolaryngology

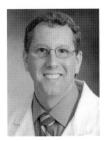

Harold S. Pine, MD, FAAP, FACS
Editor

The field of pediatric otolaryngology has a rich family tree. I have been fortunate enough to have met and been trained by some of those who make up the sturdy trunk of that tree. The authors of this issue represent the hardy branches from which the next generation of pediatric otolaryngologists is already blossoming. It is encouraging to see an ever-growing group of highly motivated individuals who have chosen to spend their professional careers working with children and their ear, nose, and throat problems. The list of members in both ASPO (American Society of Pediatric Otolaryngology) and ESPO (European Society of Pediatric Otolaryngology) continues to grow. There are approximately 20 institutions offering pediatric otolaryngology fellowships around the United States. Even in developing countries, there are dedicated individuals who spend much of their time helping children with otolaryngologic issues. My training and travels have afforded me eye-opening experiences and the chance to meet and work with surgeons from around the world. A special thanks to the team at Great Ormond Street in London, the dedicated otolaryngologists in Israel, and the amazingly gifted surgeons from Vietnam.

The articles have been written predominantly for the practicing pediatrician but I have no doubt there is worthwhile material for the general otolaryngologist as well as pediatric otolaryngologists. Those of us who take care of children are faced with the same routine kinds of cases but also a host of challenging perplexing problems eager for novel solutions.

Indications for surgery continue to evolve. There are new guidelines to review in the articles on "Tonsillectomy and Adenoidectomy" as well as "Otitis Media and Ear Tubes." We are learning more about the far-reaching implications of children with obstructive sleep apnea. Read the article on "Pediatric Obstructive Sleep Apnea Syndrome" for a great review. Have your families ever asked about the benefits of cochlear implants? Read the article on "Pediatric Cochlear Implantation: Expanding Applications and Outcomes" and you will be armed with the latest outcomes research and an easy way to organize the host of benefits of implanting deaf children besides just giving them back the miracle of hearing. Hardly a day goes by in the clinic where

Pediatr Clin N Am 60 (2013) xv–xvi
http://dx.doi.org/10.1016/j.pcl.2013.05.001
0031-3955/13/$ – see front matter © 2013 Published by Elsevier Inc.

reflux does not come up. "Laryngopharyngeal Reflux in Children" will get you up to speed on the latest information in this rapidly evolving topic. The world of laryngology and voice has traditionally been an adult topic but now, because of some really innovative people and smaller scopes, "Voice Disorders in Children" can be diagnosed and treated more effectively. Noisy breathing in the newborn can be a frightening symptom for parents and doctors alike. Take a look through "Laryngomalacia" as well as "Nasal Obstruction in Newborns" for detailed reviews and excellent ways to approach these common clinical problems.

"Enlarged Neck Lymph Nodes in Children" offers some great easy-to-read charts to help you formulate a broad differential diagnosis. What an exciting time for the parents of children who have Hemangiomas. The treatment of choice clearly has switched from high-dose steroids to propranolol. See this article, "Infantile Hemangiomas of the Head and Neck," for a review and proposed guidelines for initiating treatment. "Chronic Cough in Children" and "Pediatric Dysphagia" address 2 frustrating problems seen in the pediatric population. Are you curious how buckwheat honey can help? Sinus issues in children continue to be very common especially in the face of increasing daycare exposure. Are you uncertain when to use the diagnosis of acute sinusitis or how the treatment regimens have changed? Do you know when it is appropriate to refer children for surgery? The article "Chronic Rhinosinusitis in Children" can help clear things up. Finally, the last decade has seen a real increase in the use of simulation for both medical student education and residency training. See "Training for Simulating Pediatric Airway" for one method of teaching complicated airway endoscopy in a controlled setting.

The world of pediatric otolaryngology is changing rapidly. I suspect there will soon be subcertification to recognize those surgeons who possess that evolving body of knowledge. How we learn and study is also changing. Gone are the days of backpacks full of heavy textbooks and highlighters. Today, it's all about fancy tablets and instant access to almost anything. Be sure to check out the on-line version of this issue to take advantage of the cool videos within the individual articles. I certainly hope I can be involved with producing the first ever digital textbook of *Pediatric Otolaryngology*. A project like this will require the continued support and enthusiasm of all the wonderful authors who have contributed to this issue. I am thankful for their time and energy.

Finally, a word of thanks to some amazing people and mentors who have helped me along throughout the years. Thank you, Dr Amelia Drake, for introducing me to pediatric ENT and to Mr Martin Bailey in London, for showing me how to do things meticulously. Thank you, Dr Brent Senior, who brought me along to Vietnam, and the kind people at Resource Exchange International, who allow me to come back every year. Thank you, Dr Austin Rose, for standing by me through thick and thin and for remaining a great friend. Thank you to the whole team at UTMB Galveston. It is an honor to be on your team. And most of all, I want to thank my wife, Allie, and my 3 children, James, Nathan, and Sophie. You enrich me beyond measure and fuel the fire that allows me to get up every day and try to "take great care of kids." I am on all of your personal or professional family trees.

With my sincerest gratitude,
EXPECT EXCELLENCE

Harold S. Pine, MD, FAAP, FACS
Department of Otolaryngology—Head and Neck Surgery
301 University Boulevard
7.104 John Sealy Annex
Galveston, TX 77555, USA

E-mail address:
hspine@utmb.edu

Tonsillectomy and Adenoidectomy

Sharon D. Ramos, MD[a],*, Shraddha Mukerji, MD[b],
Harold S. Pine, MD[b]

KEYWORDS

- Adenotonsillectomy • Sleep-disordered breathing/Obstructive sleep apnea
- Clinical recurrent tonsillitis

KEY POINTS

- Adenotonsillectomy is the second most common procedure performed in children.
- Sleep-disordered breathing/obstructive sleep apnea is the most common indication for pediatric adenotonsillectomy.
- New stringent criteria (Paradise criteria) have been developed for consideration of tonsillectomy for recurrent tonsillitis.
- Tylenol Codeine should be used with caution for postoperative pain control.
- Parents need to be counseled regarding obesity, adenotonsillectomy, and postoperative cure rates and complications.
- No studies have shown adverse effects on immunity after adenotonsillectomy.

INTRODUCTION

Adenotonsillectomy (AT) is one of the most common pediatric surgical procedures performed in the United States; more than 530,000 are performed annually in children younger than 15 years of age.[1] AT was traditionally performed for recurrent tonsillitis and its sequelae but, in recent times, sleep-disordered breathing (SDB)/obstructive sleep apnea (OSA) in children has emerged as the primary indication for surgical removal of adenoids and tonsils.[2] The new guidelines used by clinicians to identify children who are appropriate candidates for AT address indications based primarily on obstructive and infectious causes.

---

[a] Department of Otolaryngology, University of Texas-Medical Branch at Galveston, 301 University Boulevard, JSA 7.104, Galveston, TX 77555-0521, USA; [b] Department of Otolaryngology, University of Texas-Medical Branch at Galveston, 301 University Boulevard, Galveston, TX 77555, USA
* Corresponding author.
E-mail address: sdramos@utmb.edu

Pediatr Clin N Am 60 (2013) 793–807
http://dx.doi.org/10.1016/j.pcl.2013.04.015
0031-3955/13/$ – see front matter © 2013 Elsevier Inc. All rights reserved.

pediatric.theclinics.com

ANATOMY

The Waldeyer ring of lymphoid tissue at the nasopharyngeal and oropharyngeal openings constitutes the first line of defense against ingested and inhaled pathogens. The lingual tonsils, the palatine tonsils, and the nasopharyngeal tonsils (adenoids) constitute the Waldeyer tonsillar ring.[3,4]

The palatine tonsils are located at the junction of the oral cavity and the oropharynx. The tonsillar fossa is composed of 3 muscles: the palatoglossus, which forms the anterior tonsillar pillar; the palatopharyngeus, which is the posterior tonsillar pillar; and the superior constrictor muscle of the pharynx, which forms the tonsillar bed. The tonsil lies between the palatoglossus and palatopharyngeal muscles. The tonsillar fossa is innervated by the tonsillar branches of the glossopharyngeal nerve and branches of the lesser palatine nerves. The blood supply to the tonsil enters primarily at the lower pole through the tonsillar branch of the dorsal lingual artery and the tonsillar branch of the facial artery.[5] The ascending pharyngeal artery and the lesser palatine artery supply the tonsil via its upper pole. Venous blood drains into the internal jugular vein. The efferent lymphatic drainage is via the upper deep cervical nodes (jugulodigastric or tonsillar nodes) behind the angle of the mandible.[5]

The palatine tonsil differs from the lingual and nasopharyngeal tonsils (adenoids) in that it has a thin capsule on the deep surface. This capsule is a portion of the pharyngobasilar fascia and extends into the tonsil to form septa that conduct nerves, blood vessels, and lymphatic vessels. The surface of the tonsil is lined by stratified squamous epithelium, which extends deep into the tissue forming tonsillar crypts.

The nasopharyngeal tonsils (adenoids) are located with the apex pointing toward the nasal septum and the base toward the roof and posterior wall of the nasopharynx. Adenoids are fully developed during the seventh month of gestation and continue to grow until the fifth year of life.[5,6] Adenoid tissue is lined by respiratory epithelium; its exposed surface is covered by stratified and pseudostratified ciliated columnar epithelium. Unlike the palatine tonsils, there is no capsule surrounding the adenoids. The blood supply to the adenoids is from the ascending pharyngeal artery, the ascending palatine artery, the pharyngeal branch of the maxillary artery, the artery of the pterygoid canal, and the tonsillar branch of the facial artery.[5] Venous drainage occurs via the internal jugular and facial veins. The pharyngeal plexus provides the nerve supply to the adenoids. The lymphatic drainage is to the retropharyngeal and pharyngomaxillary space lymph nodes.[5]

IMMUNOLOGY OF THE ADENOIDS AND TONSILS

The adenoids and tonsils are strategically positioned to serve as secondary lymphoid organs. They initiate an immune response against airborne antigens entering the body through the nose and mouth. Both contain predominantly B-cell lymphocytes (50%–65%); they also contain T-cell lymphocytes (40%) and mature plasma cells (3%). Both are involved in inducing secretory immunity and regulating secretory immunoglobulin production.[5] The tonsils are immunologically most active between the ages of 3 and 10 years.[5,7] In patients with chronic or recurrent tonsillitis, the process of antigen presentation within the tonsil and adenoids is altered, which results in reduced activation of local B cells and decreased antibody production.[5,7]

There are conflicting studies regarding the effects of AT on immunity. One study showed that in children previously immunized with live polio vaccine, there was a 3- to 4-fold decrease in the level of IgA antibody in their nasopharyngeal secretions.[3,4] The study also showed a delay and a lowered nasopharyngeal secretory immune response in seronegative children who had undergone AT and subsequent live oral polio vaccine administration.[3,5] Another study has shown better neutrophil chemotaxis after tonsillectomy and another demonstrated increased IgG and IgM production.[5] Overall, there are no studies that indicate a significant clinical impact on the immune system after AT.[3,4]

INDICATIONS FOR TONSILLECTOMY AND ADENOIDECTOMY

Recurrent throat infections and chronic adenotonsillar hypertrophy associated with airway obstruction are the most common indications for AT.

SDB/OSA

SBD is characterized by recurrent or complete upper obstruction during sleep, resulting in disruption of normal ventilation and sleep patterns. OSA is diagnosed when SDB is present in combination with an abnormal sleep study showing obstructive events.[6,7] A sleep study or polysomnography (PSG) is considered the gold standard for diagnosing and assessing the severity of OSA but it is not necessary in every child with suspected sleep apnea.[7] PSG is discussed in detail later in this article.

In otherwise healthy children, adenotonsillar hypertrophy is the major cause of SDB. There are several grading systems for assessing tonsillar size. The most commonly used grading scale for tonsillar hypertrophy was described by Brodsky. The Brodsky grading scale (**Table 1**) from 0 to 4 is based on the percentage of oropharyngeal airway occupied by the tonsils.[8] The oropharyngeal airway is designated by the linear distance between the 2 anterior tonsillar pillars.[8] Tonsillar hypertrophy is defined as 3+ or 4+ (**Fig. 1**). Tonsils need not be kissing to be graded as 4+. Although this grading system is easy to understand and follow, many studies have shown that the volume of the adenoids and tonsils relative to the oropharynx is a better determinant of the severity of SDB/OSA.[9,10] Both SDB and OSA have been known to increase the risk of behavioral problems such as irritability, aggression, and depression and may exacerbate symptoms of attention-deficit hyperactivity disorder. Patients may have poor school performance because of daytime sleepiness, and problems with memory and attention. Children with severe SDB may also suffer from morning headaches, failure to thrive, and enuresis.[4,7,11] These symptoms have been shown to improve or resolve after tonsillectomy for SDB/OSA. However, SDB is often multifactorial and may persist after tonsillectomy, particularly in children with other comorbid conditions, especially obesity.

Table 1 The Brodsky grading scale for tonsil size	
Grade	**Description**
0	Tonsils within the tonsillar fossa
1	Tonsils just outside the tonsillar fossa and occupy ≤25% of the oropharyngeal width
2	Tonsils occupy 26%–50% of oropharyngeal width
3	Tonsils occupy 51%–75% of oropharyngeal width
4	Tonsils occupy >75% of the oropharyngeal width

Data from Ng S, Lee D, Martin A, et al. Reproducibility of clinical grading of tonsillar size. Arch Otolaryngol Head Neck Surg 2010;136:159–62.

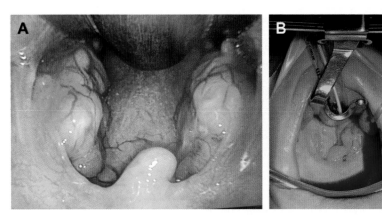

Fig. 1. (*A*) Patient with OSA and tonsillar hypertrophy (3+ tonsils). (*B*) Patient with 4+ tonsils causing significant pharyngeal obstruction (kissing tonsils).

Obesity and AT

The prevalence of OSA/SDB in obese children is 25% to 40%.[6,12] Factors that contribute to SDB/OSA in obese children include adenotonsillar hypertrophy, altered neuromuscular tone resulting in greater upper airway collapsibility during sleep, central adiposity, and an excess mechanical load on the chest wall resulting in increased work of breathing.[12] AT can reduce the severity of OSA/SDB in obese children but is usually curative in only about 10% to 25% compared with 80% in children of normal weight, other parameters being comparable.[6,12–14] Obese children are also more likely to have respiratory complications after AT.[6] Obese children should be counseled regarding weight loss and the future need for use of positive airway pressure techniques.[12]

Tonsillar asymmetry may raise concern for tumor or lymphoma of the larger tonsil. However, the presence of tonsillar asymmetry alone is not an indication for tonsillectomy.[15,16] A thorough clinical assessment including history, physical examination, and appropriate laboratory testing is indicated.

Recurrent Tonsillitis

Viral infections are the most common cause of acute tonsillitis/pharyngitis; adenovirus is the most common cause of nonstreptococcal tonsillitis.[17] Group A β-hemolytic streptococcus is the most common bacterial cause of acute pharyngitis; its peak incidence occurs in children 5 to 6 years of age during the winter and spring.[17,18] The most common viruses and bacteria causing recurrent tonsillitis are outlined in **Box 1**.

Patients with acute tonsillitis may present with malaise, fever, fullness of throat, odynophagia, dysphagia, otalgia, headache, body aches, cervical lymphadenopathy, and shivering. It is important for clinicians to accurately document acute episodes of throat infections, including body temperature, pharyngeal/tonsillar erythema, tonsil size, tonsillar exudate, cervical adenopathy (presence, size, and tenderness), and the results of microbiological testing (throat cultures, rapid strep test) for group A β-hemolytic streptococci.[17]

Clinical Practice Guidelines

New guidelines recommend watchful waiting for a 12-month period for recurrent throat infections in children not meeting the Paradise criteria (**Box 2**).[7] However,

Box 1
Common causes of recurrent tonsillitis

Viral

- Adenovirus
- Rhinovirus
- Corona
- Influenza virus
- Epstein-Barr virus

Bacterial

- Group A β-hemolytic streptococcus
- *Moraxella catarrhalis*
- *Haemophilus influenzae*

Data from Regoli M, Chiappini E, Bonsignori F, et al. Update on the management of acute pharyngitis in children. Ital J Pediatr 2011;37:10. http://dx.doi.org/10.1186/1824-7288-37-10.

patients with a history of recurrent severe infections requiring hospitalization, or those who have had sequelae such as peritonsillar abscess or Lemierre syndrome may be considered for AT before the end of the 12-month observation period even if they do not meet the frequency criteria.[7] Patients who significantly benefit from a

Box 2
Paradise criteria for tonsillectomy

Criterion definition

- Minimum frequency of sore throat episodes 7 or more episodes in the preceding year, OR
- 5 or more episodes in each of the preceding 2 years, OR
- 3 or more episodes in each of the preceding 3 years

Clinical features (sore throat plus the presence of 1 or more qualifies as a counting episode)

- Temperature >38.3°C, OR
- Cervical lymphadenopathy (tender lymph nodes or >2 cm), OR
- Tonsillar exudate, OR
- Positive culture for group A β-hemolytic streptococcus

Treatment

- Antibiotics administered in conventional dosage for proved or suspected streptococcal episodes

Documentation

- Each episode and its qualifying features substantiated by contemporaneous notation in a clinical record, OR
- If not fully documented, subsequent observance by the clinician of 2 episodes of throat infection with patterns of frequency and clinical features consistent with the initial history

Data from Baugh RF, Archer SM, Mitchell RB. Clinical practice guidelines: tonsillectomy in children. Otolaryngol Head Neck Surg 2010;144(Suppl 1):S1–30.

tonsillectomy are those with proper documentation of the severity and frequency of the illness.[19–21] Such children will see a reduction in the number and severity of subsequent infections for at least 2 years.[7]

In addition, tonsillectomy may be considered in children with recurrent tonsillitis and multiple antibiotic allergies, specific syndromes such as PFAPA (periodic fever, aphthous stomatitis, pharyngitis, and adenitis) and associated tonsillitis even if they do not meet Paradise criteria. Poorly validated indications for tonsillectomy include halitosis, dysphagia, muffled speech, febrile seizures, and malocclusion.[7]

INDICATION FOR ADENOIDECTOMY (ADENOID REMOVAL) ALONE

Adenoid hypertrophy (**Fig. 2**) is associated with upper airway obstruction, OSA, recurrent otitis media, chronic otitis media with effusion, chronic adenoiditis, and chronic rhinosinusitis.[22,23] It was initially believed that adenoid size led to mechanical obstruction of the eustachian tube resulting in middle ear effusion.[5,24] However, studies have shown that biofilms of bacteria in adenoid tissue cause inflammation and mucosal edema leading to eustachian tube dysfunction and development of otitis media.[24,25] Several studies have demonstrated that adenoid removal in patients with otitis media reduces the incidence of future episodes of otitis media and reduces the need for subsequent ventilation tubes. Therefore, adenoidectomy should be considered in patients who require a second set of ventilation tubes or those patients undergoing their first set of ventilation tubes who have symptoms of chronic nasal obstruction.[5] Indications for adenoidectomy are summarized in **Box 3**.

Studies have also shown that bacterial biofilms are prominent in the adenoids of patients with chronic sinusitis and patients may benefit initially from an adenoidectomy rather than extensive sinus surgery.[5] Similarly, children with chronic purulent rhinitis secondary to chronic adenoiditis who are unresponsive to medical management may also benefit from adenoidectomy.

POLYSOMNOGRAPHY AND SDB

Polysomnography (PSG) is commonly referred to as a sleep study; it is the gold standard for objectively diagnosing and quantifying the severity of SDB in children and allows for preoperative planning.[6] A clinical diagnosis of SDB in children is known to be a poor predictor of disease severity.[2,6,26] PSG can differentiate OSA from primary

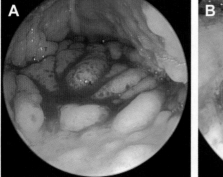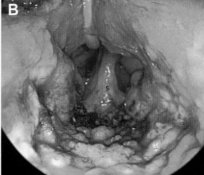

Fig. 2. (*A*) Patient with significant adenoid hypertrophy causing almost complete choanal obstruction (A, adenoid bed; T, torus tubaris). (*B*) After adenoidectomy (S, nasal septum).

Box 3
Indications for adenoidectomy

- Along with tonsillectomy for SDB/OSA
- Chronic otitis media with effusion and eustachian tube dysfunction
- Recurrent acute sinusitis with failure of medical treatment

---

snoring and can rule out other sleep disorders such as periodic limb movements, narcolepsy, and nocturnal seizures as well as document central apneas and hypoventilatory efforts.[6] PSG electrographically records simultaneous physiologic parameters during sleep. These include gas exchange, respiratory effort, airflow, snoring, sleep stage, body position, limb movement, and heart rhythm. Sleep studies maybe performed in a sleep laboratory with continuous attendance (gold standard) or at home with a portable device, unattended. The latter typically only measures respiratory effort, airflow, heart rate, and arterial oxygen saturation via pulse oximetry, resulting in a limited study.[6,27]

In an attended sleep study, children typically spend the night with their parent or guardian in the sleep laboratory but the child is required to sleep alone on the bed. Several electrodes and sensors are placed on the patient (**Fig. 3**) to measure the following: electroencephalogram (EEG) is measured by placing occipital, cranial, and frontal leads; electrooculogram (EOG) measures eye movement; electromyograms (EMG) of the chin and anterior tibilias monitor movement; electrocardiogram (ECG) measures cardiac rate and rhythm; airflow through the nose and mouth are measured by a nasal air pressure transducer and oronasal thermosensor, respectively; respiratory effort is measured by chest and abdominal movement; arterial oxygenation is measured by pulse oxymetry; and in some laboratories the patient may be monitored during sleep using an infrared video camera; snoring can be

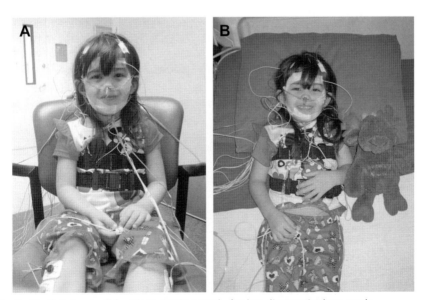

Fig. 3. (*A, B*) A 5-year-old patient getting ready for her diagnostic sleep study.

recorded using a microphone secured to the neck (**Fig. 4**).[1,28] The EEG, EMG, and EOG are used to trace the stages of sleep. The study is then scored in accordance with the American Academy of Sleep Medicine guidelines and a report is generated.[28]

There are no standardized criteria for interpreting sleep studies in children; adult OSA criteria are not applicable to children.[6,7] The following terms/indices are important when interpreting sleep study results in children[29]:

- Apnea: a decrease in the oronasal thermal sensor of 90% or more from baseline for the duration of 2 baseline breaths
- Hypopnea: decrease nasal air pressure by 50% or more from baseline lasting for 2 breaths and must be associated with oxygen desaturation of 3% or greater or an arousal/awakening
- Obstructive apnea: apneic event associated with an increase in respiratory effort during the event
- Central apnea: apneas without associated respiratory effort; the event must last at least 20 seconds *or* 2 missed breaths with an arousal/awakening or with oxygen desaturation of 3% or more
- Mixed apnea: apneic event that begins with an absent respiratory effort (central apnea) but effort resumes in the last portion of the event
- Respiratory effort-related arousal (RERA): an arousal that is preceded by a respiratory effort that does not meet the criteria for apnea or hypopnea; Nasal air pressure flattens and decreases in amplitude but not more than 50% and is associated with snoring, noisy breathing, increased work of breathing, or increase in end-tidal or transcutaneous P_{CO_2}.
  - Apnea index (AI): measures apneas per hour
  - Apnea-hypopnea index (AHI): measures apneas and hypopneas per hour
  - Respiratory distress index (RDI): measures apneas, hypopneas, and RERAs per hour

Although there is no general consensus in interpreting or defining the severity of OSA in children, most sleep specialists consider PSG in a child to be abnormal if there are pulse oximetry levels less than 92% or an AHI greater than 1 (more than 1 apneic or hypopneic event in 2 or more consecutive breaths per hour) or both.[1,7] Children may have significant oxygen desaturation levels (<85%) with a low AHI, therefore the interpretation of oxygen desaturation is as important as the AHI in assessing the severity of OSA and the need for treatment.[7] An AHI greater than 5 is considered to be clinically

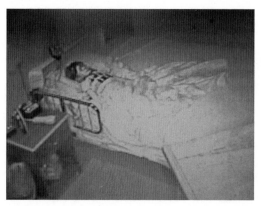

Fig. 4. Patient being monitored during her sleep study using an infrared video camera.

significant and is considered by many to warrant tonsillectomy.[7,28] Patients who undergo a tonsillectomy with or without adenoidectomy for OSA benefit from inpatient hospital admission and monitoring after surgery if they are less than 3 years old or have severe OSA, defined as having an AHI of 10 or more obstructive events per hour or an oxygen saturation nadir less than 80%.[6] Children younger than 3 years of age with SDB symptoms are at increased risk of respiratory compromise after tonsillectomy compared with older children.[6]

PSG is indicated for the following children[7]:

- Obese children (body mass index, calculated as weight in kilograms divided by the square of height in meters ≥95th percentile) with suspected OSA
- Children with associated comorbidities: Down syndrome, craniofacial abnormalities (Alpert, Crouzon, Pfeiffer, Treacher Collins, and Nager syndromes), neuromuscular disorders, sickle cell disease, and mucopolysaccharidoses
- Children in whom there is a discordance between tonsillar size, physical examination, and the reported severity of sleep apnea
- Parents requesting a sleep study to make a decision regarding surgery

SURGICAL TECHNIQUES

Tonsillectomy with/without adenoidectomy is the second most common surgical procedure performed in the pediatric population. Tonsillectomy is defined as a surgical procedure that completely removes the tonsil, including its capsule, by dissecting the peritonsillar space between the tonsil capsule and the muscular wall.[7] Tonsillotomy is subtotal removal of the tonsils without violating the tonsil capsule.[30] The various techniques currently used are as follows:

- Cold dissection (scalpel, guillotine, and snare) has been the traditional method used for tonsillectomies. The tonsil and its capsule are separated from the surrounding tissues using metal instruments and hemostasis is obtained through ligature of the blood vessels.
- Electrocautery (monopolar) is one of the most common techniques used in pediatric tonsillectomies. Electrocautery applies electric energy, generating temperatures of 400°C to 600°C, directly to the tonsillar area and separates the tonsil from the underlying pharyngeal muscle. It also has the ability to coagulate blood vessels and achieve hemostasis during the dissection. Electrocautery (**Fig. 5**) reduces intraoperative blood loss and the risk of immediate postoperative

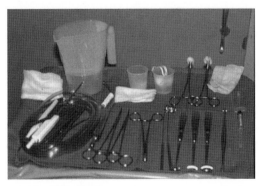

Fig. 5. Electrocautery and suction Bovie.

hemorrhage but increases the risk of secondary hemorrhage compared with cold dissection AT.[7,31] Although rare, airway fire and other fire-related injuries are a potential risk of using electrocautery in an oxygen-rich environment.[32]

- Coblation (ArthroCare Corporation, Sunnyvale, CA) was first used in orthopedic surgery in 1997 and was then approved by the US Food and Drug Administration (FDA) for tonsillectomy in 2001.[32] Coblation (**Fig. 6**) uses bipolar radiofrequency energy, rather than heat, to remove tissue.[33] This technique ablates and coagulates soft tissue by generating a high-energy plasma field.[32,33] The ionized plasma field is generated by a radiofrequency current that passes through a normal saline medium between the device tip (electrode) and the tissue. The ionized field of sodium molecules breaks molecular bonds and produces a melting tissue effect. The coblation device works at a much lower temperature of 40°C to 70°C compared with electrocautery.[32,33] Some studies suggest that the lower temperature used in coblation results in reduced thermal damage to surrounding tissue and muscle, which in turn results in less postoperative pain.[34] Other studies report that there is less postoperative pain than with electrocautery only on the day of surgery (day 0).[31] There is also less risk of fire-related injuries compared with electrocautery because coblation uses bipolar energy for coagulation and the electrodes of the device are bathed in saline solution.[32]

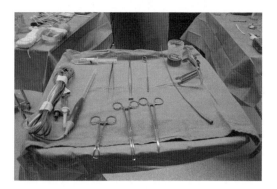

Fig. 6. Coblation.

- The microdebrider can be used to perform intracapsular tonsillectomies. This technique removes about 90% of the tonsillar tissue with a rapidly rotating blade that suctions out excised tissue while preserving the tonsillar capsule. This technique is not commonly used because of the possibility of tonsillar regrowth leading to recurrence of SDB/OSA and tonsillitis.[35] Microdebrider tonsillectomy is associated with decreased postoperative morbidity but greater intraoperative blood loss compared with electrocautery tonsillectomies. Similar intraoperative blood loss was seen when comparing the use of the microdebrider for adenoidectomies with the adenoid curette.

COMPLICATIONS

AT is a relatively safe procedure but complications do occur. These include postoperative hemorrhage, anesthetic and airway risks, aspiration, pulmonary edema, atlantoaxial subluxation, mandible dislocation, eustachian tube injury, nasopharyngeal stenosis, velopharyngeal insufficiency, and psychological trauma.[36] Mortality rates for tonsillectomy have been estimated to be between 1 in 16,000 to 1 in 35,000 and these deaths are attributed to bleeding, aspiration, cardiopulmonary failure, electrolyte imbalance, or anesthetic complications.[37] Complications are more common in patients with craniofacial disorders, Down syndrome, cerebral palsy, major heart disease, or bleeding disorders and in children younger than 3 years old with proven OSA.[7] Postoperative complaints include odynophagia, nausea, vomiting, referred otalgia, fever, and dehydration.[36] Referred otalgia and loss of taste over the posterior third of the tongue is commonly seen after tonsillectomy secondary to temporary injury to the glossopharyngeal nerve.[5]

Postoperative Pain

Oropharyngeal pain is significant and near universal regardless of the method used for surgery. It can lead to poor oral intake and dehydration.[30] It can also delay discharge from the hospital or readmission for pain control and intravenous fluids until the patient can maintain adequate fluid intake. Patients are usually sent home on oral analgesics; these include acetaminophen with codeine, acetaminophen alone, and/or nonsteroidal antiinflammatory drugs (NSAIDs). A new boxed warning by the FDA will be added to codeine-containing products about the risk of codeine for postoperative pain management after AT.[38] This is attributed to the genetic variation of the cytochrome 450 enzyme CYP2D6 and its association with ultrarapid metabolism of codeine, leading to increased levels of its active metabolite, morphine.[39,40] These increased levels of morphine can cause respiratory depression and death; currently only a small number of cases have been reported.[39,40] For other patients, acetaminophen with codeine is ineffective because they are poor metabolizers of codeine and almost no morphine is produced.[39] The use of NSAIDs has been controversial because of their effect on platelet function and increased risk for postoperative bleeding.[7,41] Several studies suggest, however, that NSAIDs, with the exception of ketorolac, can be safely used for pain relief after tonsillectomy.[7,41,42]

Postoperative Hemorrhage

Postoperative hemorrhage is one of the most common complications associated with AT. Postoperative hemorrhage rates range from 0.5% to 10%.[5] Posttonsillectomy hemorrhage is divided into 2 categories: primary hemorrhage, occurring less than 24 hours after surgery and secondary hemorrhage occurring after 24 hours, most commonly on postoperative days 5 to 10.[43] The cause of primary hemorrhage is generally attributed to inadequate hemostasis during the procedure.[44,45] Secondary (delayed) hemorrhage is believed to be a result of the sloughing of the superficial eschar from the tonsillar fossa and/or infection.[43] Postoperative hemorrhage after tonsillectomy may or may not require hemostasis in the operating room. Immediate postoperative bleeding after adenoidectomy can be controlled initially with topical nasal decongestant drops. However, patients with significant bleeding should be taken back to the operating room for examination of the nasopharynx and hemostasis.[5]

Postoperative Edema

Postoperative edema of the tongue, nasopharynx, and palate can cause upper airway obstruction. A nasal trumpet and/or intravenous corticosteroid therapy may be necessary to relieve obstruction. Postoperative pulmonary edema can occur in patients with a history of OSA and cor pulmonale secondary to adenotonsillar hypertrophy. These patients require close observation postoperatively and continuous pulse oximetry.[5]

Hypernasal Speech and Velopharyngeal Insufficiency

Hypernasal speech immediately after surgery is common. This occurs secondary to pain, which in turn limits the movement of the tonsillar pillars and soft palate. This is usually transient and resolves within several weeks.[5] Velopharyngeal insufficiency (VPI) is an unusual complication related to adenoidectomy. Patients present with hypernasal speech and reflux of fluids through the nose. Patients may require evaluation and management by speech pathology. Children with a history of cleft palate or submucosal cleft should not undergo an adenoidectomy to prevent this complication. Patients with bifid uvula without any evidence of hypernasal speech or submucus cleft at the time of surgery can undergo complete adenoidectomy without increased risk of VPI. If there is any doubt about the function/structure of the palate, a modified adenoidectomy or limited adenoidectomy is performed where only the choanal part of the adenoid tissue is removed. This helps to relieve adenoid obstruction and at the same time helps to preserve palatal function. Surgical intervention for VPI is reserved for patients who do not respond to speech therapy for at least 1 year.[5]

Nasopharyngeal Stenosis

Nasopharyngeal stenosis is a rare complication after AT and in almost all cases it occurs because of aggressive cauterization at the time of surgery. Patients with nasopharyngeal stenosis have scarring of the uvula down to the posterior pharyngeal wall secondary to excessive cauterization with extensive mucosal destruction.[5] The posterior tonsillar pillars and soft palate adhere to the posterior pharyngeal wall resulting in partial or complete obstruction of the nasopharyngeal airway. Care must be taken when removing lymphoid tissue from the torus tubaris and lateral nasopharynx during an adenoidectomy. Treatment depends on the location and severity of stenosis and surgical intervention is usually required for resolution.[5]

Atlantoaxial Subluxation (Grisel Syndrome)

Atlantoaxial subluxation (Grisel syndrome) is a rare complication of AT, resulting from decalcification of the anterior arch of the atlas and laxity of the anterior transverse ligament between the atlas and axis in the cervical spine.[44] Patients present with a stiff neck, spasms of the sternocleidomastoid or deep cervical muscle. Patients typically hold their head to one side with slight rotation toward the opposite side. Radiographic evaluation of the anteroposterior and lateral cervical spine with flexion-extension may aid in the diagnosis. In severe cases, computed tomography or magnetic resonance imaging may be necessary. Most cases of atlantoaxial instability are secondary to infection or trauma.[44] Management may require intravenous antibiotics and possible cervical traction.[5,44] Patients with Down syndrome are more susceptible to traumatic atlantoaxial subluxation after an AT. Thus, great care is taken with cervical spine manipulation during surgery in patients with Down syndrome. Cervical flexion/extension films are not indicated in these patients if the neurologic examination is normal before surgery.

SUMMARY

- SDB/OSA is the most common current indication for pediatric AT.
- Children with even moderately severe recurrent tonsillitis (except those meeting the Paradise criteria) may derive benefit from watchful waiting for a period of 1 year.
- AT is not curative in obese children with OSA; it may be associated with increased risk of postoperative respiratory complications.
- Surgical techniques are safe and the risk of complications is low in properly selected patients.

REFERENCES

1. Trager N, Schultz B, Pollock AN, et al. Polysomnographic values in children 2-9 years old: additional data and review of the literature. Pediatr Pulmonol 2005; 40:22–30.
2. Mitchell RB, Pereira KD, Friedman NR. Sleep-disordered breathing in children: survey of current practice. Laryngoscope 2006;116:956–8.
3. Brandzaeg P. Immune function of nasopharyngeal tissue. Adv Otorhinolaryngol 2011;72:20–4.
4. Brandtzaeg P. Immunology of tonsils and adenoids: everything the ENT surgeon needs to know. Int J Pediatr Otorhinolaryngol 2003;67:S69–76.
5. Shirley WP, Woolley AL, Wiatrak BJ. Pharyngitis and adenotonsillar disease. In: Flint PW, Haughey BH, Lund VJ, et al, editors. Cummings Otolaryngology - head and neck surgery, vol. 3. Philadelphia: Mosby Elsevier; 2010. p. 2783–5, 2795–96, 2799–801.
6. Rolans S, Rosenfeld R, Brooks L, et al. Clinical guidelines: polysomnography for sleep-disordered breathing prior to tonsillectomy in children. Otolaryngol Head Neck Surg 2011;145(Suppl 1):S1–15.
7. Baugh RF, Archer SM, Mitchell RB. Clinical practice guidelines: tonsillectomy in children. Otolaryngol Head Neck Surg 2010;144(Suppl 1):S1–30.
8. Ng S, Lee D, Martin A, et al. Reproducibility of clinical grading of tonsillar size. Arch Otolaryngol Head Neck Surg 2010;136:159–62.
9. Arens R, McDonough JM, Corbin AM, et al. Upper airway size analysis by magnetic resonance imaging of children with obstructive sleep apnea syndrome. Am J Respir Crit Care Med 2003;167:65–70.
10. Arens R, McDough JM, Cosatrino AT, et al. Magnetic resonance imaging of upper airway structure of children with obstructive sleep apnea syndrome. Am J Respir Crit Care Med 2001;164:698–703.
11. Basha S, Bialowas C, Ende K, et al. Effectiveness of adenotonsillectomy in the resolution of nocturnal enuresis secondary to obstructive sleep apnea. Laryngoscope 2005;115:1101–3.
12. Narang I, Mathew JL. Childhood obesity and obstructive sleep apnea. J Nutr Metab 2012;2012:134202. http://dx.doi.org/10.1155/2012/134202.
13. Mitchell RB. Adenotonsillectomy for obstructive sleep apnea in children: outcome evaluated by pre- and postoperative polysomnography. Laryngoscope 2007;117: 1844–54.
14. Costa DJ, Mitchell R. Adenotonsillectomy for obstructive sleep apnea in obese children: a meta-analysis. Otolaryngol Head Neck Surg 2009;140:455–60.
15. Puttasiddaiah P, Kumar M, Gopalan P, et al. Tonsillectomy and biopsy for asymptomatic asymmetric tonsillar enlargement: are we right? J Otolaryngol 2007;36: 161–3.
16. Sunkaraneni VS, Jones SE, Prasai A, et al. Is unilateral tonsillar enlargement alone an indication for tonsillectomy? J Laryngol Otol 2006;120:E21.
17. Chiappini E, Principi N, Mansi N, et al. Management of acute pharyngitis in children: summary of the Italian National Institute of Health Sciences. Clin Ther 2012; 34:1442–58.e2.
18. Regoli M, Chiappini E, Bonsignori F, et al. Update on the management of acute pharyngitis in children. Ital J Pediatr 2011;37:10. http://dx.doi.org/10.1186/1824-7288-37-10.
19. Paradise JL, Bluestone CD, Colborn DK, et al. Tonsillectomy and adenoidectomy for recurrent throat infection in moderately affected children. Pediatrics 2002;110:7–15.

20. van Staaij BK, van der Akker EH, Rovers MM, et al. Effectiveness of adenotonsillectomy in children with mild symptoms of throat infections or adenotonsillar hypertrophy: open, randomized controlled trial. BMJ 2004;329:651.

21. Burton MJ, Glasziou PP. Tonsillectomy or adenotonsillectomy versus non surgical treatment for chronic/recurrent acute tonsillitis. Cochrane Database Syst Rev 2009;(1):CD001802.

22. Grindle CR, Murray RC, Chennupati SK, et al. Incidence of revision adenoidectomy in children. Laryngoscope 2011;121:2128–30.

23. Joshua B, Bahar G, Sulkes J, et al. Adenoidectomy: long-term follow-up. Otolaryngol Head Neck Surg 2006;135:576–80.

24. Andreoli SM, Schlosser RJ, Wang LF, et al. Adenoid ciliostimulation in children with chronic otitis media. Otolaryngol Head Neck Surg 2013;148(1):135–9.

25. Saafan ME, Ibrahim WS, Tomoum MO. Role of adenoid biofilm in chronic otitis media with effusion in children. Eur Arch Otorhinolaryngol 2012. http://dx.doi.org/10.1007/s00405-012-2259-1.

26. Brietzke SE, Katz ES, Roberson DW. Can history and physical examination reliably diagnose pediatric obstructive sleep apnea/hypopnea syndrome? A systemic review of the literature. Otolaryngol Head Neck Surg 2004;131(6): 827–32.

27. Kahlke PE, Witmans MB, Alabdoulsalam T, et al. Full-night versus 4 hour evening polysomnography in children less than 2 years of age. Sleep Med 2013;14(2): 177–82.

28. Chang L, Wu J, Cao L. Combination of symptoms and oxygen desaturation index in predicting childhood obstructive sleep apnea. Int J Pediatr Otorhinolaryngol 2012. http://dx.doi.org/10.1016/j.ijporl.2012.11.028.

29. Takashima M. Sleep medicine and sleep apnea surgery. In: Pasha R, Golub JS, editors. Otolaryngology: head and neck surgery: clinical reference guide. San Diego (CA): Plural Publishing; 2011. p. 163, 67.

30. Tunkel DE, Hotchkiss KS, Carson K, et al. Efficacy of powered intracapsular tonsillectomy and adenoidectomy. Laryngoscope 2008;118:1295–302.

31. Jones D, Kenna M, Guidi J, et al. Comparison of postoperative pain in pediatric patients undergoing coblation tonsillectomy versus cautery tonsillectomy. Otolaryngol Head Neck Surg 2011;144(6):972–7.

32. Walner DL, Miller SP, Villines D, et al. Coblation tonsillectomy in children: incidence of bleeding. Laryngoscope 2012;122:2330–6.

33. Alexiou V, Salazar-Silvia M, Jervis PN, et al. Modern technology-assisted vs conventional tonsillectomy, a meta-analysis of randomized controlled trials. Arch Otolaryngol Head Neck Surg 2011;137(6):558–70.

34. Heidemann C, Wallen M, Aakesson M, et al. Post-tonsillectomy hemorrhage: assessment of risk factors with special attention to introduction of coblation technique. Eur Arch Otorhinolaryngol 2009;266:1011–5.

35. Stansifer K, Szramowski M, Barazsu L, et al. Microdebrider tonsillectomy associated with more intraoperative blood loss than electrocautery. Int J Pediatr Otorhinolaryngol 2012;76:1437–41.

36. Gallagher T, Wilcox L, McGuire E, et al. Analyzing factors associated with major complications after adenotonsillectomy in 4776 patients: comparing three tonsillectomy techniques. Otolaryngol Head Neck Surg 2011;142:886–92.

37. Stevenson A, Myer C, Shuler M, et al. Complications and legal outcomes of tonsillectomy malpractice claims. Laryngoscope 2012;122:71–4.

38. FDA Drug Safety Communication. Safety review update of codeine use in children; new boxed warning and contraindication on use after tonsillectomy and/or

adenoidectomy. Available at: www.fda.gov/Drugs/drugssafety/ucm339112.htm. Accessed February 20, 2013.

39. Kelly L, Rieder M, Anker J, et al. More codeine fatalities after tonsillectomy in North American children. Pediatrics 2012;129:e1343. http://dx.doi.org/10.1542/peds.2011-2538. Accessed February 20, 2013.

40. Ciszkowski C, Madadi P, Phillips MS, et al. Codeine, ultrarapid-metabolism genotype, and post operative death. N Engl J Med 2009;361:827–8.

41. Krishna S, Hughes L, Lin S. Postoperative hemorrhage with non-steroidal anti-inflammatory drug use after tonsillectomy. Arch Otolaryngol Head Neck Surg 2003;129:1086–9.

42. Cardwell ME, Sivister G, Smith AF. Non-steroidal anti-inflammatory drugs and perioperative bleeding in paediatric tonsillectomy. Cochrane Database Syst Rev 2005;(2):CD003591.

43. Ozkiris M, Kapusuz Z, Yildirim YS, et al. The effect of paracetamol, metamizole sodium and ibuprofen on postoperative hemorrhage following pediatric tonsillectomy. Int J Pediatr Otorhinolaryngol 2012;76:1027–9.

44. Collison P, Mettler B. Factors associated with post-tonsillectomy hemorrhage. Ear Nose Throat J 2000;79(8):640–2, 644, 646.

45. Bocciolini C, Dall'Olio D, Cunsolo E, et al. Grisel's syndrome: a rare complication following adenoidectomy. Acta Otorhinolaryngol Ital 2005;25(4):245–9.

Otitis Media and Ear Tubes

Elton Lambert, MD, Soham Roy, MD*

KEYWORDS

- Otitis • Ear infection • Tubes • Otorrhea • Effusion

KEY POINTS

- Myringotomy tube insertion is one of the most common pediatric ambulatory procedures performed in the United States and is used in the treatment of recurrent acute otitis media (RAOM) and chronic otitis media with effusion (COME).
- Several anatomic, genetic, environmental, and pathogenic factors contribute to the development of RAOM and COME and should be identified when considering placement of a myringotomy tube.
- Preoperative evaluation includes a good history and physical examination with adjunctive tests such as audiometry.
- Myringotomy tubes are usually placed in children with more than 3 episodes of acute otitis media in 6 months or 4 in a year, or persistent otitis media with effusion for at least 3 months.
- Both otolaryngologists and primary care physicians should observe a child closely for complications and adverse events of myringotomy tubes including tube otorrhea, early tube extrusion, retained tubes, refractory middle ear disease, and other suppurative or otologic sequelae of chronic middle ear disease.

INTRODUCTION

The placement of myringotomy tubes is one of the most common procedures performed in children. In 2006, more than 667,000 procedures were performed in the Unites States in patients younger than 15 years.[1] Recurrent acute otitis media (RAOM), chronic otitis media with effusion (COME), and their associated suppurative and otologic complications are commonly managed with the procedure. Eighty percent of infants experience at least 1 episode of acute otitis media (AOM), with 40% having 6 or more recurrences by the age of 7 years. The significance of the disease entity cannot be overstated.[2,3] COME is one of the most important causes of preventable, acquired hearing loss in children, making optimal management of the condition vital.[4]

Disclosures: None.
Department of Otorhinolaryngology, University of Texas-Houston School of Medicine, 6431 Fannin Street, MSB 5.036, Houston, TX 77030, USA
* Corresponding author.
E-mail address: Soham.Roy@uth.tmc.edu

In 2007, there were some 11 million primary care visits for AOM.[5] The critical issue for any primary care provider surrounds the decision for subspecialty referral. Failure to offer myringotomy tubes in the patient with RAOM or COME can have grave sequelae. Hearing loss, speech delay, poor school performance, and decreased quality of life are significant factors in the development of a child.[6] Inadequately managed AOM can also lead to suppurative complications, including cholesteatoma, labyrinthitis, meningitis, and sigmoid sinus thrombosis. Primary care providers should identify those patients who should be evaluated for placement of myringotomy tubes as early as possible.

In this article, the relevant developmental anatomy that predisposes the young child to middle ear disease, the clinical spectrum of diseases that can be managed effectively with myringotomy tube placement, and the indications and basic steps for the procedure are reviewed. The primary care provider plays an integral role in postoperative surveillance, and thus, we also cover some of the more common complications and issues surrounding postoperative care.

DEVELOPMENT AND ANATOMY OF THE MIDDLE EAR AND EUSTACHIAN TUBE

The tympanic membrane (TM) is a trilaminar structure that is important in converting sound pressure waves into mechanical vibrations. The outer epithelial layer is derived from ectoderm and has migratory properties that are important in the pathophysiology of cholesteatoma. The central fibrous layer is mesodermally derived, with collagen fibers arranged within the lamina propia. The inner lamina is a mucosal layer that is a continuation of the lining of the middle ear.

Fig. 1 shows the surface anatomy of the TM. The color, mobility, integrity, and translucence of the ear drum should be assessed during the physical examination. Mobility should be assessed by pneumatic otoscopy. A normally concave TM moves easily with the application of negative and positive pressure. Disruption of this pattern could indicate eustachian tube dysfunction.

The eustachian tube is the pressure regulator of the middle ear. A negative pressure normally develops in the middle ear because of an imbalance in the atmospheric air delivered via the eustachian tube and the passive transmucosal absorption of nitrogen

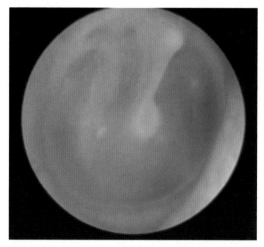

Fig. 1. Normal TM.

by the middle ear mucosa.[7] The eustachian tube periodically opens, which reestablishes the pressure gradient. The eustachian tube also clears middle ear secretions and protects the middle ear from nasopharyngeal secretions. Eustachian tube dysfunction is dependent on its relationship to the tensor veli palatini muscle, which facilitates its opening, and how it relates to the skull base. The eustachian tube is shorter, wider, and in a more horizontal position in the young child and lies within a more adult configuration by age 7 years.[8] This situation contributes to the increased prevalence of otitis media in younger children.[9] Bylander and colleagues[10] showed that even normal pediatric patients had higher prevalence of negative middle ear pressures when compared with adults, and studies have shown that children prone to ear infections had poorer eustachian tube function than age controls.[11]

CLINICAL MANIFESTATIONS
AOM

The diagnosis of AOM is contingent on the presence of ear pain, evidence of middle ear inflammation (redness, bulging), and a middle ear effusion.[12] An example is shown in **Fig. 2**. Cases of uncomplicated AOM can be managed with antibiotics; although a period of observation in children older than 6 months is appropriate in some cases.[13] *Streptococcus pneumoniae* and *Haemophilus influenzae* continue to be the most prevalent bacteria associated with AOM.[14] Although antibiotic resistance continues to be a concern in the management of the disease, amoxicillin is still first choice of antibiotics in AOM.[13]

Most children experience 1 episode of AOM by age 3 years, with studies showing that between 40% and 80% of young children experience at least 1 episode of AOM in the first few years of life.[15,16] A subset of these children develop recalcitrant AOM and RAOM that require further medical therapy or consideration of surgical therapy.

Otitis Media with Effusion

Eustachian tube dysfunction leads to negative middle ear pressure, which leads to the accumulation of mucosal secretions within the middle ear. Otitis media with effusion (OME) (middle ear fluid) occurs when fluid occurs behind an intact TM without the

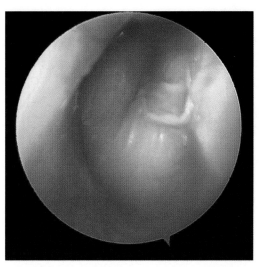

Fig. 2. AOM. Note the bulging of the TM and the purulence in the middle ear.

presence of acute inflammation.[17] On physical examination, a serous effusion can often be distinguished from a mucoid one (**Fig. 3**). Serous otitis media seems to be more responsive to medical treatment. Mucoid effusions have been shown to have higher levels of mucin, lysozyme, secretory immunoglobulin A, and interleukin 8 and have a higher viscosity, which may make the effusion harder to treat.[18] The pathophysiologic factors that lead to the formation of each type of effusion have not been fully elucidated.

More than 50% of children experience an episode of OME within the first year of life with upwards of 60% having had an effusion by age 2.[19] Many of these effusions resolve, but persistent OME can cause hearing loss, with associated detriment to the social and language development of a child. An observation of 3 months is acceptable except in children who are likely to fail conservative management (eg, those with craniofacial abnormalities or immune deficiencies).

Retractions of the TM

The TM is divided into the pars tensa and the pars flaccida. Retractions of the TM often occur after long-standing hypoventilation of the eustachian tube and subsequent negative middle ear pressure. The parts of the ear drum may lie in a medial position over structures such as the incudostapedial joint and cochlear promontory. The ear drum can become inherently weak and form fibrotic scar within the middle ear (**Fig. 4**).[20]

Although retractions can be caused by multiple ear infections or long-standing OME, neither middle ear inflammation nor persistent middle ear secretions need be present. Retractions that are not managed effectively can lead to conductive hearing loss, chronic infections, polyps, and ossicular chain erosion. Long-standing retraction pockets may be lead to cholesteatoma formation, especially with pars flaccida retractions.[21] Serious complications such as labyrinthine fistula have also been reported.[22]

CAUSES OF PEDIATRIC MIDDLE EAR DISEASE

Consideration must be given to the causes that may lead to RAOM, OME, and retractions of the TM. Understanding and identifying these factors may lead one to avoid

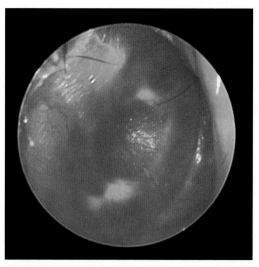

Fig. 3. COME. Note the dull nature of the TM.

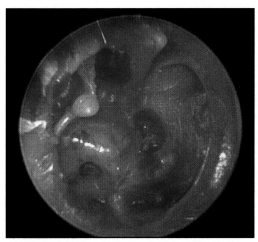

Fig. 4. Severely retracted TM. The incudostapedial joint and promontory of the cochlea are readily visible.

surgical therapy or pursue more urgent therapy if indicated. These factors may be dependent on the host, the environment, or any of the offending organisms that may lead to these disease processes. A summary of these factors is shown in **Table 1**.

Host Factors

As stated earlier, the young child is more susceptible to otitis as a consequence of the anatomic differences in the configuration of the eustachian tube compared with that of an adult. The immaturity of the immune system may also have significance. Although most children between the ages of 6 and 11 months have at least 1 episode of AOM, COME and RAOM are more likely when the first episode occurs when the child is less than 6 months.[23] There have been mixed results as to the significance of gender as it plays a role the development of chronic ear disese.[24,25]

The importance of host defenses cannot be overstated. Children with primary immune deficiencies often present with AOM. This finding is especially true in entities like IgG2 deficiency, which leaves the individual especially susceptible to encapsulated bacteria.[26] Clinical judgment is needed to determine the need for further

Table 1	
Factors associated with the development of middle ear disease in children	
Host	Pathogen
Age	Bacterial
Immunology	Antimicrobial resistance
Acquired immunity	Biofilms
Innate immunity	Nasopharyngeal colonization
Allergic disease/atopy	(adenoid pad)
Genetic	Viruses
Ciliary motility (eg, Kartagener syndrome)	Environment
Craniofacial disorders (eg, craniosynostoses)	Smoking
Cleft lip/palate	Day care/siblings
	Breastfeeding
	Pacifier use

immunologic screening, when patients with RAOM present with atypical courses that may point to an immunologic deficiency.[27]

Although immunologic deficiencies are obvious avenues for the development of RAOM and OME, subtle differences in immunocompetence may contribute as well. Children with RAOM have been shown to have decreased IgA levels (important for mucosal defenses) when compared with children without RAOM.[28] IgG levels within the adenoids tend to increase as a child grows, which may also contribute to the decreasing prevalence of ear infections as a child gets older. Patients with OME tend to show a slower increase in these levels when compared with children not prone to OME.[28] Children with OME have also been shown to have an immune response that is biased toward a Th2 cytokine profile, which has been linked to other chronic inflammatory states such as chronic rhinosinusitis.[29]

The innate immunity also plays a role in the defenses against otitis media. Epithelial cells, dendritic cells of the middle ear, and nasopharynx express pattern recognition receptors that are important for recognizing offending pathogens. Defects in toll-like receptors can lead to difficulty in the clearance of middle ear effusions and the phagocytosis and intracellular killing of organisms.[30] Molecules such as human defensins, cathelicidins, lysozyme, bacteriocins, surfactant proteins, cationic peptides, halocidin, and xylitol also contribute to the innate immunity to both viral and bacterial otitis media.[30]

A recently defined entity within the realm of middle ear disease is eosinophilic otitis media (EOM), which is characterized by tenacious, viscous yellow effusion that is exquisitely difficult to treat. Higher levels of IgE are found in effusions of EOM when compared with common OME, and the entity may be immunologically related to diseases such as allergic fungal sinusitis and allergic bronchopulmonary aspergillosis.[31]

A multitude of genetically based disorders can also lead to persistent or recurrent ear infections. Disorders of ciliary motility, like Kartagener syndrome and primary ciliary dyskinesia (PCD), interfere with the effective clearance of secretions of the upper respiratory tract, including the middle ear. PCD is autosomal recessive and affects both sexes equally, with an incidence that ranges from 1 in 15,000 births to 1 in 40,000 births.[32] Fifty percent of PCD is associated with Kartagener syndrome, which encompasses a triad including recurrent sinusitis, bronchiectasis, and situs inversus. Although conservative treatment can be pursued for RAOM and OME for these patients, myringotomy tube insertion is more often than not the most viable option in managing the disease. Patients with PCD have a high rate of persistent otorrhea (10%–50%) after placement of ear tubes.[33,34]

The presence of craniofacial abnormalities may also influence the development of chronic ear issues. The middle ear, ossicles, and eustachian tube are formed by a complex interaction between the first and second branchial arches and the first branchial pouch. Disorders that affect these embryologic structures can lead to eustachian tube dysfunction with ensuing middle ear disease.

Intact paratubal musculature is also paramount to eustachian tube dysfunction. The levator veli palatini arises from the petrous apex and the medial lamina of the eustachian tube cartilage and its fibers extending downward and medially to the midline of the palate, interdigitating with the contralateral muscle. The tensor veli palatini originates from the medial pterygoid plate, with its tendon hooking around the pterygoid hamulus, with subsequent insertion on the palatine aponeurosis. The levator muscle assists in eustachian tube opening via isotonic contraction, which hinges on an intact sling along the soft palate, whereas the tensor causes direct opening via its interaction with the tubal cartilage. Disruption of normal palatal anatomy (as seen in cleft palate) results in ineffective eustachian tube opening because of isometric contraction of the levator muscle and ineffective shortening of the tensor muscle.[35] OME in patients with cleft palate is almost universal, with a prevalence of 90%.[36] There are mixed results as to whether cleft palate surgery with restoration of a palatal sling improved middle ear function.[37,38]

Pierre-Robin sequence (and its associated cleft palate), Treacher-Collins syndrome, Apert syndrome and other syndromes associated with craniosynostosis, Down syndrome, and velocardiofacial syndrome are associated with an increased risk for the development of chronic ear problems.[39–42] These children should be carefully monitored for the development of RAOM and OME. The developmental and speech delays found in these patients would be confounded by unrecognized hearing loss caused by middle ear disease, and they often require multiple ear tube insertions.

Pathogen Factors

Otitis media is an infection that is significantly influenced by the synergistic effect between bacteria and viruses. The most common upper respiratory viruses include influenza A, respiratory syncytial virus (RSV), adenovirus, and rhinovirus. The bacteria present are those that commonly colonize the nasopharynx, including *Streptococcus pneumonia,* nontypeable *Haemophilus influenzae*, and *Moraxella catarrhalis*.[43] The universal pneumococcal vaccination of children has led to an increased prevalence of *H influenzae* isolates.[43]

Seasonal variations in the prevalence of otitis media match the seasonal variation of common viral illnesses.[44] These viruses alter eustachian tube function via mechanisms including decreased mucociliary action, altered mucus secretion, and a change in the cytokine profile. Children can have transient OME with an upper respiratory infection without superimposed bacterial infection. Twenty percent to 73% of viral upper respiratory infections are accompanied by OME, with RSV showing the greatest prevalence.[44] The natural history of most virally mediated sterile OME is that of resolution, so a period of observation is warranted before any intervention is undertaken.

Bacterial otitis media is a polymicrobial infection. Most patients are treated easily with antibiotics, but this is becoming a more complicated issue. Bacteria have developed fascinating ways to combat eradication. Bacteria can be embedded in biofilms (polymeric matrices attached to a living surface) as opposed to planktonic state. Bacteria within biofilms are characterized by a slow rate of metabolism and tolerance to high concentrations of antibiotics.[45] Biofilms within the adenoids may contribute as a reservoir for infection in both RAOM and OME, which may necessitate removal in patients who continue to have chronic ear problems despite ear tube insertion.[46]

Although *Streptococcus pneumonia,* nontypeable *H influenzae*, and *Moraxella catarrhalis* are the most important bacteria in acute infections, organisms including *Pseudomonas aeruginosa*, coagulase-negative *Staphylococcus* and methicillin-resistant *Staphylococcus aureus* become more prevalent in chronic infections, making treatment more problematic.[47] Antimicrobial resistance will continue to be an emerging problem. Careful selection of patients who will benefit from antibiotic treatment should be the mainstay of management.

Environmental Factors

Many environmental factors contribute to diseases of the upper aerodigestive tract, including otitis media. Parental smoking can concur a 2-fold increased risk of developing otitis media,[48] and a dose-response relationship is evident.[49] Tobacco smoke has many effects that can lead to increased middle ear disease in children, including damage to the respiratory mucosa, decreased mucociliary transport, increased virulence of bacteria, changes to the innate immunity, and an enhanced Th2 immunologic profile.[50]

Breast milk has many antimicrobial, immunomodulatory, and antiinflammatory properties that compensate for the immature immune system of the growing infant.[51] Breast milk helps to modulate the IgG profile of the infant to fight the organisms most commonly associated with otitis media. Breastfed babies have significantly lower rates of AOM and OME when compared with formula-fed infants.[52,53] At least partial breastfeeding for 6 months may lead to an 80% reduction on rates of middle ear disease.[54] There is evidence that the strong tongue-palate relationship associated with breastfeeding may help with middle ear aeration. The supine position used in bottle feeding can also lead to reflux of secretions into the middle ear.[55]

Children attending day care and those with siblings are exposed to a large array of viral and bacterial pathogens. Day care contributes to increasing the risk of otitis media because of the large numbers of children and close person-to-person contact. Frequent exposure can also lead to the exchange of antimicrobial-resistant bacteria.[56] Attendance in day care may be associated with up to a 30% increase in the risk of AOM, with an apparent relationship found between the number of children at the center and the burden of disease.[57]

Pacifier use,[58] obesity,[59] ethnicity, and socioeconomic status[60] have also been studied as risk factors for the development of middle ear disease, but their contributions to the development RAOM and OME require further research.

MYRINGOTOMY TUBE INSERTION
Indications

The American Academy of Pediatricians, the American Academy of Family Physicians, and the American Academy of Otolaryngology have put forward guidelines for the effective management of RAOM and OME. Children who have had more than 3 episodes of AOM in a 6-month period and more than 4 episodes in a 1-year period should be considered for insertion of tympanostomy tubes.[13] When managing these patients, those patients who are at an increased risk of speech and language delay should be identified for early intervention; those not at high risk should be managed with observation for at least 3 months, and a hearing evaluation should be obtained in patients with OME for at least 3 months.[61] Children with eustachian tube dysfunction without middle ear inflammation can be considered for the procedure when complications such as hearing loss, disequilibrium/vertigo, tinnitus, autophony, and severe retraction pockets are present. Tympanostomy tubes can also be inserted as a part of the management of the suppurative complications of AOM, including mastoiditis.

History and Physical Examination

The history of a child in whom tympanostomy tube insertion is being considered should detail the number of ear infections and severity and laterality of ear infections. A history of duration and type of antibiotic treatment should also be reviewed with the family. Concerns about a child's hearing loss should be elicited from the parents. An investigation into the host, pathogenic, and environmental factors (as described earlier) that may contribute to middle ear disease should also be sought. This strategy is especially important because tympanostomy tube insertion can often be avoided if some of these risk factors are modified (eg, removing a child from day care). A carefully taken family, past medical, and birth history may also be helpful. A history of any tympanostomy tube insertions, adenoidectomy, and mastoid and TM/ossiculoplasty procedures should be noted.

Signs of AOM and OME can be found on physical examination. The features of the TM including scarring, monomeric segments (from previous tympanostomy tube insertions), retractions, and perforations give important clues to the presence of middle ear disease not only in the affected ear but in the contralateral ear. The presence of craniofacial abnormalities with or without associated cleft palate may lead one to pursue intervention at an earlier time. Subtle findings such as a submucosal cleft shown by a bifid uvula or notched soft palate of the zona pellucida (indicating a dehiscence in soft palate musculature) should be sought. Adenoidectomy may be deferred in the patient with a submucosal cleft because of the increased risk of velopharyngeal insufficiency. The importance of behavioral observations during the physical examinations cannot be overstated. Developmental and speech delays can be assessed at this time. Inappropriate responses to voices can point to hearing loss even before audiometric data are obtained.

Adjunctive Tests

Computed tomography and magnetic resonance imaging are not routinely obtained before insertion of tympanostomy tubes. These modalities are useful in cases of suspected cholesteatoma, mastoiditis, or intracranial sequelae of AOM, but not in uncomplicated RAOM or OME. Lateral neck radiographs may be obtained for suspicion of adenoid hypertrophy.

Any child being considered for insertion of a myringotomy tube should have an audiometric evaluation by an experienced audiologist. Visual reinforcement audiology can be used in patients who are ages 6 months to 2 years and involves observing a child in a sound field for reactions to a sound stimulus. Play audiometry can be used in children aged 2 to 5 years and is similar to conventional audiometry, which can be performed in most children aged 5 years and older. Tympanometry is an objective measure of middle ear function. It is obtained by placing a small probe in the ear canal and obtained by plotting the acoustic energy of a reflected tone as a function of pressure in the ear canal. It is a measure of TM compliance. The peak of the tympanogram gives valuable information. A peak at more than –200 daPa indicates normal middle ear functions. Values between –200 and –400 daPa indicate negative middle ear pressure, whereas a flat tympanogram with normal ear canal volume indicates an effusion. A flat tympanogram with large ear canal volume may indicate a perforation or a patent ear tube.[62]

Most patients with OME have a moderate conductive hearing loss on audiometry and type B curve on tympanometry.[63] Patients with RAOM may have normal audiograms between episodes, but hearing should be documented in the preoperative setting. Otoacoustic emissions, a test of functionality of hair cells of the inner ear, can also prove helpful, especially in patients who are younger than 6 months or in whom audiometry is precluded for other reasons. Otoacoustic emissions are absent in most patients with OME.[64] Auditory brain stem response (ABR) is a neurophysiologic test that can be used as an adjunct in infants with hearing loss. Conductive hearing loss can be shown via this modality. When clinically indicated, intraoperative ABR can be performed in conjunction with myringotomy tube insertion in order to investigate cases of sensorineural and mixed hearing loss.[65] These objective measures of hearing should be repeated after myringotomy tube insertion.

Alternative Treatments

In RAOM, parents may choose to continue observation with conservative treatment and antibiotics. This strategy does risk the development of antibiotic resistance and permanent damage to the hearing mechanisms. The American Academy of Pediatrics in a recent practice guideline recommended against repeated antibiotics for RAOM.[13] Children with OME should undergo a 3-month observation period before intervention. This strategy may not be appropriate in cases complicated by cleft palate, immunologic deficiencies, and other craniofacial abnormalities. Conservative treatments for OME have historically included the optimization of allergic disease, use of antihistamines, and nasal steroid sprays. However these treatments are now considered to be ineffective and are no longer recommended.[61]

Rationale

Myringotomy tubes serve to equalize the middle ear pressure with atmospheric pressure, assisting or bypassing the eustachian tube in this regard. They allow more precise monitoring for the development of ear infections and allow for administration of topical antibiotics.

Procedure

Myringotomy with tube insertion is normally performed in the outpatient setting under monitored anesthesia care. Inhalant or intravenous anesthetics can be used for the procedure. Supplementation with nitrous oxide can be used for severe retractions of the TM. Nitrous oxide diffuses along a concentration gradient into the middle ear, often causing retractions to lift from the middle ear mucosa. The largest ear speculum, which can be comfortably placed in the ear canal and allow for adequate visualization, should be used. Cerumen should be gently removed from the ear canal to improve visualization, and prevent clogging of the ear tube postoperatively. Cerumen is removed with curettes, suction, or alligator forceps with care not to damage the lining of the ear canal. The TM should be inspected closely. If indicated, an incision is made in the TM. There are many variations, but we most commonly perform a radial incision centered between the umbo and the annulus within the anterior-inferior quadrant of the ear drum. Middle ear effusions should be meticulously aspirated (**Box 1**).

The myringotomy tube is atraumatically placed through the incision, and positioned so that the middle ear mucosa can be viewed through the lumen of the tube (**Fig. 5**). There are a variety of tubes that can be inserted, but they are generally of 2 types: smaller diameter/length tubes that naturally extrude by 1 to 2 years after insertion (eg, grommet tubes) and those with large diameters and lengths (eg, T tubes), which are intended to remain in the TM for longer periods.[66] Tympanostomy tubes can be made of a variety of materials, including silicone, thermoplastic elastomers, titanium, and silver impregnated materials. Topical antibiotics are placed at the end of the procedure to minimize the risk of persistent otorrhea.

Postoperative Care

Children can usually return to normal activity after myringotomy tube insertion. Analgesic medicine is generally not required after insertion. Some physicians encourage dry ear precautions, because liquid in the middle ear can lead to an acute infection or persistent otorrhea. While the children are showering and swimming, parents may use a cotton ball impregnated with petroleum jelly or fitted ear plugs to prevent the introduction of fluid into the middle ear.

Outcomes

Myringotomy tubes have been shown to improve hearing levels in patients with OME.[67,68] This improvement is especially seen in the first 6 to 9 months when compared with children whose OME is observed. Myringotomy with tube insertion

Box 1
Summary of practice model for myringotomy tube placement

Myringotomy Tube Insertion

Preoperative

- Confirm history and physical examination findings and determine candidacy for procedure
- Audiometry for evaluation of hearing
- Discuss the risk, benefits, and alternatives with the family members
- Discuss the expectant postoperative course, with special attention to most common complications that can occur

Perioperative

- Revisit indications for procedure with the parents before operation
- Discuss anesthetic plan with anesthesiologist
- Be sure to take special measures to appropriately decrease anxiety of child

Operative Technique

- Ensure adequate induction of anesthesia (monitored anesthesia care vs general depending on preference or synchronous procedures)
- Appropriate ear speculum chosen to visualize ear canal
- Atraumatic removal of cerumen
- Inspect the TM for effusions, retractions, monomeric segments
- Incise the TM (anterior-inferior quadrant used in our practice)
- Evacuate middle ear secretions
- Place myringotomy tubes
- Ear drops placed

Immediate Postoperative Period

- Assess child for postanesthesia complications
- Assess analgesic needs
- Reinforce expected postoperative course for child
- Give instructions as necessary, including dry ear precautions

Follow-Up

- Assess tube patency and position
- Inquire about and document any subjective improvement in child's hearing or quality of life
- Note any early complications
- Repeat audiometry
- Visits at 6-monthly to yearly intervals
- Earlier visits for complications such as persistent tube otorrhea, worsening hearing status, or return of recurrent infections

has been shown to improve hearing to a greater extent than myringotomy alone.[69] Patients with OME can expect a 4-dB to 15-dB improvement in hearing after placement.[67,68,70] This improvement in hearing is often maintained years after the procedure, with most experiencing no long-term hearing loss.[71]

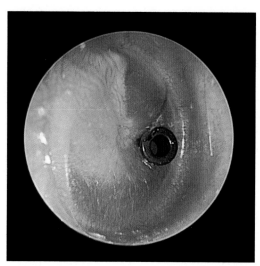

Fig. 5. Tympanostomy tube in place. Note the middle ear mucosa visible through the lumen of the tube.

Myringotomy tubes are effective in decreasing the number of infections in RAOM. After myringotomy tube insertion, children with RAOM can often expect a significant decrease in the number of infections every year.[70] In addition, episodes of AOM can be easily managed with topical antibiotics.[72]

The nature of recurrent infections and associated hearing loss can affect the quality of life of the child and the family. Myringotomy tube insertion has consistently been shown to have positive effects on quality of life in the domains of physical suffering, hearing loss, speech impairment, emotional well-being, limitations of activity, and caregiver distress.[73–75] A few patients (less than 5%) may have a lower quality of life, especially those with persistent tube otorrhea.[74] Anecdotally, it has been shown that patients with OME show some speech and developmental delay.[76] However, there have been many studies that question the long-term advantages of prompt tube insertion on speech/language development in otherwise normal children,[77–79] with clearer advantages present for patients who are considered higher risk for developmental delays.[80]

Complications

Monitoring for complications after myringotomy tube insertions is the responsibility of both the primary care provider and otolaryngologist. In a recent survey by the American Academy of Otolaryngology-Head and Neck Surgery Pediatric Otolaryngology Committee,[81] persistent otorrhea (7.8%), retained tube for more than 2 years (2.7%), granulation tissue or foreign body reaction (2.2%), atelectasis or monomeric TM (1.8%), perforation after extrusion (1.7%), tympanosclerosis (1.4%), and cholesteatoma caused by epithelial migration of ear canal lining through myringotomy tube (0.4%) were the most commonly encountered complications associated with myringotomy tube insertion.

Persistent otorrhea can be the result of a chronic infection and may be associated with microbial biofilm formation on the tube.[82] This finding highlights the need for strict dry ear precautions in some patients with ear tubes. Treatment of tube otorrhea includes topical antibiotics and, in some cases, a trial of systemic antibiotics. Removal of the tube may be necessary.

Early tube extrusion may occur in less than 5% of cases.[83] In this circumstance, the child can often be observed, and if ear problems persist, then consideration can be given to replacing the tube. Retaining a tube for more than 2 years increases the risk of perforation. Longer-term tubes also increase this risk. Myringoplasty with a variety of materials including fat graft, paper patch, and gelfoam can be performed for a persistent perforation after tube extrusion or at the time a retained tube is removed. Failure of these procedures may necessitate a formal tympanoplasty. Care must be taken in those children who continue to have eustachian tube dysfunction in whom attempts at perforation repair have lower success rates.

Up to 30% of patients require repeat tube insertions because of ongoing middle ear disease.[84] This number is increased in patients with cleft palate and immunologic disorders. Adenoidectomy is recommended if a repeat procedure is planned. The adenoids can become a reservoir for bacteria, especially with biofilm formation, or can physically obstruct the eustachian tube, thus contributing to middle ear disease. Adjunctive adenoidectomy is not recommended with primary tube insertion unless there is another clinical indication such as chronic rhinorrhea, sleep-disordered breathing, or chronic adenoiditis.[71,85,86] Some patients may also require longer-duration tube types during revision procedures.

SUMMARY

The placement of myringotomy tubes remains an effective treatment of RAOM and COME. Infants and young children are prone to these entities because of their immature anatomy and immunology. Several host, pathogenic, and environmental factors can contribute to the development of these conditions. The identification and modification of some these factors can preclude the need for intervention. The procedure continues to be one of the most common outpatient pediatric procedures performed in the United States. Close vigilance and identification of potential complications by pediatricians and otolaryngologists is of utmost importance in the ongoing management of the child with middle ear disease.

REFERENCES

1. Cullen KA, Hall MJ, Golosinskiy A. Ambulatory surgery in the United States, 2006. National Health Statistics Report No. 11. Hyattsville (MD): National Center for Health Statistics; 2009.
2. Teele DW, Klein JO, Rosner B. Epidemiology of otitis media during the first seven years of life in children in greater Boston: a prospective, cohort study. J Infect Dis 1989;160(1):83–94.
3. Vergison A, Dagan R, Arguedas A, et al. Otitis media and its consequences: beyond the earache. Lancet Infect Dis 2010;10(3):195–203.
4. Berman S. Otitis media in developing countries. Pediatrics 1995;96(1 Pt 1): 126–31.
5. Schappert SM, Rechtsteiner EA. Ambulatory medical care utilization estimates for 2007. Vital Health Stat 13 2011;(169):1–38.
6. Timmerman AA, Meesters CM, Speyer R, et al. Psychometric qualities of questionnaires for the assessment of otitis media impact. Clin Otolaryngol 2007; 32(6):429–39.
7. Bluestone CD. Pathogenesis of otitis media: role of eustachian tube. Pediatr Infect Dis J 1996;15(4):281–91.

8. Doyle WJ, Swarts JD. Eustachian tube-tensor veli palatini muscle-cranial base relationships in children and adults: an osteological study. Int J Pediatr Otorhinolaryngol 2010;74(9):986–90.

9. Sadler-Kimes D, Siegel MI, Todhunter JS. Age-related morphologic differences in the components of the eustachian tube/middle ear system. Ann Otol Rhinol Laryngol 1989;98(11):854–8.

10. Bylander A, Ivarsson A, Tjernstrom O. Eustachian tube function in normal children and adults. Acta Otolaryngol 1981;92(5–6):481–91.

11. Stenstrom C, Bylander-Groth A, Ingvarsson L. Eustachian tube function in otitis-prone and healthy children. Int J Pediatr Otorhinolaryngol 1991;21(2):127–38.

12. Karma PH, Penttila MA, Sipila MM, et al. Otoscopic diagnosis of middle ear effusion in acute and non-acute otitis media. I. The value of different otoscopic findings. Int J Pediatr Otorhinolaryngol 1989;17(1):37–49.

13. Lieberthal AS, Carroll AE, Chonmaitree T, et al. The diagnosis and management of acute otitis media. Pediatrics 2013;131(3):e964–99.

14. Casey JR, Pichichero ME. Changes in frequency and pathogens causing acute otitis media in 1995-2003. Pediatr Infect Dis J 2004;23(9):824–8.

15. Alho OP, Koivu M, Sorri M, et al. The occurrence of acute otitis media in infants. A life-table analysis. Int J Pediatr Otorhinolaryngol 1991;21(1):7–14.

16. Daly KA, Brown JE, Lindgren BR, et al. Epidemiology of otitis media onset by six months of age. Pediatrics 1999;103(6 Pt 1):1158–66.

17. van Zon A, van der Heijden GJ, van Dongen TM, et al. Antibiotics for otitis media with effusion in children. Cochrane Database Syst Rev 2012;(9):CD009163.

18. Chung MH, Choi JY, Lee WS, et al. Compositional difference in middle ear effusion: mucous versus serous. Laryngoscope 2002;112(1):152–5.

19. Daly KA, Hoffman HJ, Kvaerner KJ, et al. Epidemiology, natural history, and risk factors: panel report from the Ninth International Research Conference on Otitis Media. Int J Pediatr Otorhinolaryngol 2010;74(3):231–40.

20. Cassano M, Cassano P. Retraction pockets of pars tensa in pediatric patients: clinical evolution and treatment. Int J Pediatr Otorhinolaryngol 2010;74(2):178–82.

21. Karmody CS, Northrop C. The pathogenesis of acquired cholesteatoma of the human middle ear: support for the migration hypothesis. Otol Neurotol 2012;33(1):42–7.

22. Couloigner V, Molony N, Viala P, et al. Cartilage tympanoplasty for posterosuperior retraction pockets of the pars tensa in children. Otol Neurotol 2003;24(2):264–9.

23. Marchant CD, Shurin PA, Turczyk VA, et al. Course and outcome of otitis media in early infancy: a prospective study. J Pediatr 1984;104(6):826–31.

24. Karevold G, Kvestad E, Nafstad P, et al. Respiratory infections in schoolchildren: co-morbidity and risk factors. Arch Dis Child 2006;91(5):391–5.

25. Paradise JL, Rockette HE, Colborn DK, et al. Otitis media in 2253 Pittsburgh-area infants: prevalence and risk factors during the first two years of life. Pediatrics 1997;99(3):318–33.

26. Wilson NW, Hogan MB. Otitis media as a presenting complaint in childhood immunodeficiency diseases. Curr Allergy Asthma Rep 2008;8(6):519–24.

27. Wiertsema SP, Veenhoven RH, Sanders EA, et al. Immunologic screening of children with recurrent otitis media. Curr Allergy Asthma Rep 2005;5(4):302–7.

28. Eun YG, Park DC, Kim SG, et al. Immunoglobulins and transcription factors in adenoids of children with otitis media with effusion and chronic rhinosinusitis. Int J Pediatr Otorhinolaryngol 2009;73(10):1412–6.

29. Johnston BN, Preciado DA, Ondrey FG, et al. Presence of otitis media with effusion and its risk factors affect serum cytokine profile in children. Int J Pediatr Otorhinolaryngol 2008;72(2):209–14.

30. Underwood M, Bakaletz L. Innate immunity and the role of defensins in otitis media. Curr Allergy Asthma Rep 2011;11(6):499–507.

31. Iino Y. Role of IgE in eosinophilic otitis media. Allergol Int 2010;59(3):233–8.

32. Campbell RG, Birman CS, Morgan L. Management of otitis media with effusion in children with primary ciliary dyskinesia: a literature review. Int J Pediatr Otorhinolaryngol 2009;73(12):1630–8.

33. Kay DJ, Nelson M, Rosenfeld RM. Meta-analysis of tympanostomy tube sequelae. Otolaryngol Head Neck Surg 2001;124(4):374–80.

34. Vaile L, Williamson T, Waddell A, et al. Interventions for ear discharge associated with grommets (ventilation tubes). Cochrane Database Syst Rev 2006;(2): CD001933.

35. Huang MH, Lee ST, Rajendran K. A fresh cadaveric study of the paratubal muscles: implications for eustachian tube function in cleft palate. Plast Reconstr Surg 1997;100(4):833–42.

36. Klockars T, Rautio J. Early placement of ventilation tubes in cleft lip and palate patients: does palatal closure affect tube occlusion and short-term outcome? Int J Pediatr Otorhinolaryngol 2012;76(10):1481–4.

37. Dhillon RS. The middle ear in cleft palate children pre and post palatal closure. J R Soc Med 1988;81(12):710–3.

38. Xing X, Li B, Liu J. The effect of palate repair on middle ear function. Lin Chuang Er Bi Yan Hou Ke Za Zhi 1998;12(4):162–3 [in Chinese].

39. Makishima T, King K, Brewer CC, et al. Otolaryngologic markers for the early diagnosis of Turner syndrome. Int J Pediatr Otorhinolaryngol 2009;73(11): 1564–7.

40. Park AH, Wilson MA, Stevens PT, et al. Identification of hearing loss in pediatric patients with Down syndrome. Otolaryngol Head Neck Surg 2012;146(1): 135–40.

41. Rajenderkumar D, Bamiou D, Sirimanna T. Management of hearing loss in Apert syndrome. J Laryngol Otol 2005;119(5):385–90.

42. Reyes MR, LeBlanc EM, Bassila MK. Hearing loss and otitis media in velocardio-facial syndrome. Int J Pediatr Otorhinolaryngol 1999;47(3):227–33.

43. Murphy TF, Bakaletz LO, Smeesters PR. Microbial interactions in the respiratory tract. Pediatr Infect Dis J 2009;28(Suppl 10):S121–6.

44. Stockmann C, Ampofo K, Hersh AL, et al. Seasonality of acute otitis media and the role of respiratory viral activity in children. Pediatr Infect Dis J 2013;32(4): 314–9.

45. Bakaletz LO. Bacterial biofilms in the upper airway–evidence for role in pathology and implications for treatment of otitis media. Paediatr Respir Rev 2012; 13(3):154–9.

46. Saafan ME, Ibrahim WS, Tomoum MO. Role of adenoid biofilm in chronic otitis media with effusion in children. Eur Arch Otorhinolaryngol 2012. [Epub ahead of print].

47. Jung H, Lee SK, Cha SH, et al. Current bacteriology of chronic otitis media with effusion: high rate of nosocomial infection and decreased antibiotic sensitivity. J Infect 2009;59(5):308–16.

48. Csakanyi Z, Czinner A, Spangler J, et al. Relationship of environmental tobacco smoke to otitis media (OM) in children. Int J Pediatr Otorhinolaryngol 2012;76(7): 989–93.

49. Adair-Bischoff CE, Sauve RS. Environmental tobacco smoke and middle ear disease in preschool-age children. Arch Pediatr Adolesc Med 1998;152(2):127–33.

50. Yilmaz G, Caylan ND, Karacan CD. Effects of active and passive smoking on ear infections. Curr Infect Dis Rep 2012;14(2):166–74.

51. Labbok MH, Clark D, Goldman AS. Breastfeeding: maintaining an irreplaceable immunological resource. Nat Rev Immunol 2004;4(7):565–72.

52. Duffy LC, Faden H, Wasielewski R, et al. Exclusive breastfeeding protects against bacterial colonization and day care exposure to otitis media. Pediatrics 1997;100(4):E7.

53. Sabirov A, Casey JR, Murphy TF, et al. Breast-feeding is associated with a reduced frequency of acute otitis media and high serum antibody levels against NTHi and outer membrane protein vaccine antigen candidate P6. Pediatr Res 2009;66(5):565–70.

54. Hatakka K, Piirainen L, Pohjavuori S, et al. Factors associated with acute respiratory illness in day care children. Scand J Infect Dis 2010;42(9):704–11.

55. Tully SB, Bar-Haim Y, Bradley RL. Abnormal tympanography after supine bottle feeding. J Pediatr 1995;126(6):S105–11.

56. Greenberg D, Hoffman S, Leibovitz E, et al. Acute otitis media in children: association with day care centers–antibacterial resistance, treatment, and prevention. Paediatr Drugs 2008;10(2):75–83.

57. Dewey C, Midgeley E, Maw R. The relationship between otitis media with effusion and contact with other children in a British cohort studied from 8 months to 3 ½ years. The ALSPAC Study Team. Avon Longitudinal Study of Pregnancy and Childhood. Int J Pediatr Otorhinolaryngol 2000;55(1):33–45.

58. Niemela M, Uhari M, Mottonen M. A pacifier increases the risk of recurrent acute otitis media in children in day care centers. Pediatrics 1995;96(5 Pt 1):884–8.

59. Kuhle S, Kirk SF, Ohinmaa A, et al. The association between childhood overweight and obesity and otitis media. Pediatr Obes 2012;7(2):151–7.

60. Smith DF, Boss EF. Racial/ethnic and socioeconomic disparities in the prevalence and treatment of otitis media in children in the United States. Laryngoscope 2010;120(11):2306–12.

61. American Academy of Family Physicians, American Academy of Otolaryngology-Head and Neck Surgery, American Academy of Pediatrics Subcommittee on Otitis Media With Effusion. Otitis media with effusion. Pediatrics 2004;113(5):1412–29.

62. Onusko E. Tympanometry. Am Fam Physician 2004;70(9):1713–20.

63. Abdullah B, Hassan S, Sidek D. Clinical and audiological profiles in children with chronic otitis media with effusion requiring surgical intervention. Malays J Med Sci 2007;14(2):22–7.

64. Balatsouras DG, Koukoutsis G, Ganelis P, et al. Transiently evoked otoacoustic emissions in children with otitis media with effusion. Int J Otolaryngol 2012;2012: 269203.

65. Dornan B, Fligor B, Whittemore K, et al. Pediatric hearing assessment by auditory brainstem response in the operating room. Int J Pediatr Otorhinolaryngol 2011;75(7):935–8.

66. Morris MS. Tympanostomy tubes: types, indications, techniques, and complications. Otolaryngol Clin North Am 1999;32(3):385–90.

67. Medical Research Council Multicentre Otitis Media Study Group. Surgery for persistent otitis media with effusion: generalizability of results from the UK trial (TARGET). Trial of Alternative Regimens in Glue Ear Treatment. Clin Otolaryngol Allied Sci 2001;26(5):417–24.

68. MRC Multicentre Otitis Media Study Group. The role of ventilation tube status in the hearing levels in children managed for bilateral persistent otitis media with effusion. Clin Otolaryngol Allied Sci 2003;28(2):146–53.
69. Caye-Thomasen P, Stangerup SE, Jorgensen G, et al. Myringotomy versus ventilation tubes in secretory otitis media: eardrum pathology, hearing, and eustachian tube function 25 years after treatment. Otol Neurotol 2008;29(5): 649–57.
70. Franklin JH, Marck PA. Outcome analysis of children receiving tympanostomy tubes. J Otolaryngol 1998;27(5):293–7.
71. Popova D, Varbanova S, Popov TM. Comparison between myringotomy and tympanostomy tubes in combination with adenoidectomy in 3-7-year-old children with otitis media with effusion. Int J Pediatr Otorhinolaryngol 2010;74(7): 777–80.
72. Dohar J, Giles W, Roland P, et al. Choosing the best practice: evidence to support fluoroquinolone drops for acute otitis media through tympanostomy tubes. Pediatrics 2007;120(1):245–7 [author reply: 247].
73. Chow Y, Wabnitz DA, Ling J. Quality of life outcomes after ventilating tube insertion for otitis media in an Australian population. Int J Pediatr Otorhinolaryngol 2007;71(10):1543–7.
74. Rosenfeld RM, Bhaya MH, Bower CM, et al. Impact of tympanostomy tubes on child quality of life. Arch Otolaryngol Head Neck Surg 2000;126(5):585–92.
75. Witsell DL, Stewart MG, Monsell EM, et al. The Cooperative Outcomes Group for ENT: a multicenter prospective cohort study on the outcomes of tympanostomy tubes for children with otitis media. Otolaryngol Head Neck Surg 2005;132(2): 180–8.
76. Klausen O, Moller P, Holmefjord A, et al. Lasting effects of otitis media with effusion on language skills and listening performance. Acta Otolaryngol Suppl 2000;543:73–6.
77. Paradise JL, Dollaghan CA, Campbell TF, et al. Otitis media and tympanostomy tube insertion during the first three years of life: developmental outcomes at the age of four years. Pediatrics 2003;112(2):265–77.
78. Paradise JL, Feldman HM, Campbell TF, et al. Effect of early or delayed insertion of tympanostomy tubes for persistent otitis media on developmental outcomes at the age of three years. N Engl J Med 2001;344(16):1179–87.
79. Paradise JL, Feldman HM, Campbell TF, et al. Tympanostomy tubes and developmental outcomes at 9 to 11 years of age. N Engl J Med 2007;356(3):248–61.
80. Rosenfeld RM, Jang DW, Tarashansky K. Tympanostomy tube outcomes in children at-risk and not at-risk for developmental delays. Int J Pediatr Otorhinolaryngol 2011;75(2):190–5.
81. Derkay CS, Carron JD, Wiatrak BJ, et al. Postsurgical follow-up of children with tympanostomy tubes: results of the American Academy of Otolaryngology-Head and Neck Surgery Pediatric Otolaryngology Committee National Survey. Otolaryngol Head Neck Surg 2000;122(3):313–8.
82. Barakate M, Beckenham E, Curotta J, et al. Bacterial biofilm adherence to middle-ear ventilation tubes: scanning electron micrograph images and literature review. J Laryngol Otol 2007;121(10):993–7.
83. Erdoglija M, Sotirovic J, Baletic N. Early postoperative complications in children with secretory otitis media after tympanostomy tube insertion in the Military Medical Academy during 2000-2009. Vojnosanit Pregl 2012;69(5):409–13.
84. MRC Multicentre Otitis Media Study Group. Adjuvant adenoidectomy in persistent bilateral otitis media with effusion: hearing and revision surgery outcomes

through 2 years in the TARGET randomised trial. Clin Otolaryngol 2012;37(2): 107–16.

85. Hammaren-Malmi S, Saxen H, Tarkkanen J, et al. Adenoidectomy does not significantly reduce the incidence of otitis media in conjunction with the insertion of tympanostomy tubes in children who are younger than 4 years: a randomized trial. Pediatrics 2005;116(1):185–9.

86. Mattila PS, Hammaren-Malmi S, Saxen H, et al. Adenoidectomy and nasopharyngeal carriage of *Streptococcus pneumoniae* in young children. Arch Dis Child 2010;95(9):696–702.

Pediatric Obstructive Sleep Apnea Syndrome

Nathan S. Alexander, MD, James W. Schroeder Jr, MD*

KEYWORDS

- Obstructive sleep apnea • Pediatric • Management • Clinical practice guidelines
- OSAS

KEY POINTS

- Pediatric obstructive sleep apnea syndrome (OSAS) is a common health problem, which if left untreated, may have a deleterious impact on neurocognitive and behavioral outcomes, physical development, and cardiovascular health.
- Nocturnal polysomnography (PSG) is the gold standard method for diagnosing pediatric OSAS, however its performance and interpretation in the pediatric population has not been well standardized.
- The first-line treatment for pediatric OSAS is adenotonsillectomy. Reduced efficacy rates are seen in obese children. Persistent OSAS postoperatively must be investigated, and other levels of airway obstruction should be addressed.
- Patients at high risk for respiratory complications after adenotonsillectomy should undergo preoperative PSG, and those less than 3 years of age and those with severe OSAS should be considered for postoperative admission.

INTRODUCTION

Pediatric obstructive sleep apnea syndrome (OSAS) is a common health problem diagnosed and managed by various medical specialists, including family practice physicians, pediatricians, pulmonologists, and general and pediatric otolaryngologists. If left untreated, the sequelae can be severe. In the last decade, significant advancements have been made in the evidence-based management of pediatric OSAS. This article focuses on the current understanding of this disease and its management, and related clinical practice guidelines.

TERMINOLOGY

Sleep-disordered breathing (SDB) is characterized by an abnormal respiratory pattern during sleep and includes snoring, mouth breathing, and pauses in breathing.[1] SDB is

Division of Pediatric Otolaryngology, Ann & Robert H. Lurie Children's Hospital of Chicago, 225 East Chicago Avenue, Box 25, Chicago, IL 60611-2605, USA
* Corresponding author.
E-mail address: jschroeder@luriechildrens.org

Pediatr Clin N Am 60 (2013) 827–840
http://dx.doi.org/10.1016/j.pcl.2013.04.009
0031-3955/13/$ – see front matter © 2013 Elsevier Inc. All rights reserved.

the most common indication for tonsillectomy with or without adenoidectomy; 530,000 such procedures are performed annually in the United States on children younger than 15 years of age.[1,2] SDB is a clinical diagnosis and encompasses the spectrum of disorders ranging in severity from primary snoring (PS) to upper airway resistance syndrome (UARS) to OSAS. It is estimated that 3% to 12% of children have PS, which is characterized by snoring without associated apneas, gas exchange abnormalities, or arousals on polysomnography (PSG).[3–5] UARS is characterized by snoring associated with repetitive occurrences of respiratory effort-related arousals (RERAs) without oxygen desaturations. It is hypothesized that UARS can lead to daytime symptoms resembling OSAS.[6] The diagnosis of UARS requires the use of an esophageal pressure monitor during overnight PSG. This is not routine in most centers, thus its prevalence is not well known in the pediatric population.[4,7] There is some variability in the exact definition of the term OSAS. The American Academy of Pediatrics (AAP) clinical practice guideline on the diagnosis and management of childhood OSAS defines OSAS in children as a disorder of breathing during sleep characterized by prolonged partial upper airway obstruction and/or intermittent complete obstruction that disrupts normal ventilation during sleep and normal sleep patterns accompanied by associated signs and symptoms characteristic of the disorder.[8] The American Academy of Otolaryngology Head and Neck Surgery (AAOHNS) clinical practice guideline on PSG for SDB before tonsillectomy in children states that OSAS is diagnosed when SDB (clinically) is accompanied by an abnormal PSG with obstructive events.[1] The prevalence of OSAS in children is believed to range from 1% to 10%.[3,9–11]

MORBIDITY
Signs/Symptoms

The signs and symptoms of pediatric OSAS are variable and are often dependent on age. Some daytime symptoms are more apparent in the older child. Nocturnal symptoms are often the most obvious to the parents of the child, and these often prompt the initial evaluation. Snoring is the most common associated symptom seen in children with SDB and OSAS. Some of the additional signs and symptoms are listed in **Table 1**. Excessive daytime sleepiness is seen more frequently in adolescents and/or obese children, but hyperactivity and inattention are more characteristic of pediatric OSAS. One way to measure sleepiness is by applying the Epworth Sleepiness Scale (ESS). Melendres and colleagues[12] compared 108 children with suspected SDB with 72 controls using a modified ESS and the Conners Abbreviated Symptom Questionnaire. They demonstrated that the children with suspected SDB were both sleepier and more hyperactive than the control patients. They found only weak correlation with the ESS and the PSG data obtained on the children with suspected SDB. Attempts to correlate physical examination findings to sleep apnea severity have also been made. The tonsils are typically graded on a clinically subjective scale from 0 to 4+, describing the amount of space occupied between the tonsillar pillars in the oropharynx (0, tonsils within fossa; 1+, <25%; 2+, >50%; 3+, >75%; 4+, >75%), Nolan and Brietzke[13] recently demonstrated in a systematic literature review that the association between subjective tonsil size and objective OSAS severity is weak at best.[14]

Academic/Behavioral

The association of SDB and OSAS with impaired neurocognitive and behavioral development has been well studied in the past decade. Untreated OSAS has been

Table 1
Symptoms and signs of pediatric OSAS

Nocturnal Symptoms	Daytime Symptoms	Signs/Findings
Snoring	Difficulty waking	Tonsil hypertrophy
Gasping	Unrefreshed on waking	High/large tongue position
Noisy breathing (typically inspiratory)	Excessive sleepiness	Growth disturbance
Paradoxic breathing	Hyperactivity	Obesity
Retractions (cervical or costal)	Aggression/moodiness	Failure to thrive
Witnessed apneas	Mouth breathing	Pulmonary hypertension
Restless sleep	Poor appetite	Systemic hypertension
Neck hyperextension	Dysphagia	Craniofacial abnormalities
Mouth breathing	Difficulty in school	Laryngomalacia
Nocturnal sweating		Nasal airway obstruction
Enuresis (after 6 mo continence)		Hypotonia
Parasomnia (walking, talking, terrors)		Gastroesophageal reflux
Bruxism		
Mouth breathing		

associated with poor learning, lower achievement, and attention deficit/hyperactivity disorder. Recent studies further delineate the association. For example, Gottlieb and colleagues[15] found significantly lower performance on measures of memory, executive function, and general intelligence in 5-year-old children with symptoms of SDB than in asymptomatic children.[16] In addition, Gozal and colleagues[17] demonstrated that children with lower academic performance in middle school (lower 25% of their class) were more likely to have snored during early childhood and to have required adenotonsillectomy (T&A) for snoring compared with their schoolmates in the top 25% of the class. Other studies have shown improved attention, executive functioning, analytical thinking, verbal functioning, memory, and academic progress at 6 to 12 months after T&A, suggesting a reversible effect of the neurocognitive morbidity incurred from SDB and obstructive sleep apnea (OSA).[4,14–20] Gozal[17] was the first to suggest that "learning debt" created by a delay in treatment or untreated SDB may only be partially reversible. Early sleep fragmentation may adversely affect future academic performance.[17] These studies also suggest that snoring may not be as benign as once believed.[18]

Behavioral problems such as social withdrawal and aggression have also been described in children with OSAS.[19] The prevalence of attention deficit/hyperactivity (ADHD) in the school-age population is 8% to 10%, whereas 20% to 30% of children with snoring and/or OSAS have significant problems with inattention and hyperactivity.[19–21] This connection is theorized to be secondary to the effect of fragmented, non-restorative sleep with intermittent hypoxia on the development of the prefrontal cortex, which is believed to be responsible for working memory, behavioral control, analysis, organization, and self-regulation of motivation.[19,22,23]

Medical

Failure to thrive and growth failure are believed to be slightly more common in children with OSAS.[24,25] This may be a result of increased energy consumption from increased work of breathing, decreased oral intake, and alterations of nocturnal growth hormone secretion patterns.[19,25] Growth spurt or some associated weight gain after T&A is often reported. A recent study by Smith and colleagues[26] demonstrated that aged 6 years or younger at the time of T&A was significantly predictive of having postoperative weight gain.

Cardiovascular morbidity in children with OSAS includes systemic hypertension, pulmonary hypertension, and cor pulmonale with heart failure. Intermittent airway obstruction may lead to alterations in intrathoracic pressure, sustained changes in systemic blood pressure and endothelial function, associated oxidative stress, and increased sympathetic tone.[19,27,28] Several studies have shown significant improvement of ambulatory blood pressure measurements, both systolic and diastolic, after treatment of OSAS with T&A. Tezer and colleagues[29] conducted a prospective noncontrolled study on 21 children with OSA diagnosed clinically and with lateral neck radiography and no reported cardiovascular disease. Using transthoracic echocardiography, they demonstrated abnormal ventricular diastolic functions, and subsequent normalization 3 months after T&A. Tal and colleagues[30] used radionucleotide vetriculography in 27 children clinically diagnosed with OSA, with no known preoperative cardiovascular disease. They demonstrated that 35% had a reduced right ventricular ejection fraction, and 67% had a wall motion abnormality preoperatively; both of these variables were markedly improved in 11 of the 27 children after T&A.

Systemic inflammation, as assessed by C-reactive protein (CRP) is notably higher in children with OSAS, which may place them at risk for substantial end-organ damage. Recent studies have shown that T&A significantly reduced the CRP levels in these children.[31]

DIAGNOSIS

The AAP published clinical practice guidelines for the diagnosis and management of childhood OSAS in 2002, and updated the guidelines in 2012. PSG is the gold standard method for diagnosing OSAS.[8] However, because of a shortage of sleep laboratories with pediatric expertise, alternative diagnostic tests, such as videotaping, nocturnal pulse oximetry, and daytime nap PSG, may be helpful adjuncts to the clinical history and physical examination. The drawback is that these alternative tests have weaker positive and negative predictive values than PSG.[1,8] The action statements from the AAP are listed in **Box 1**, and those patients considered to be at high risk (and therefore require postoperative observation) are listed in **Box 2**.[8]

The designation of PSG as the gold standard method for diagnosing OSAS in children highlights that the subjective clinical history and physical examination have poor sensitivity in distinguishing OSAS from PS.[4,32–34] Goldstein and colleagues[33] prospectively evaluated 30 children with obstructive symptoms by standard history, physical examination, and tape-recorded breathing during sleep. Only 55% of patients predicted clinically to have definite OSAS had a positive nocturnal PSG. Sixteen percent of the patients thought to be unlikely to have OSAS had a positive nocturnal PSG.

The diagnostic PSG parameters for pediatric OSAS are different from those for adult OSAS. OSAS in adults is defined as a respiratory pause lasting more than 10 seconds; the higher respiratory rate in children portends that shorter intervals of apnea are likely to be clinically significant.[3] The parameters that are primarily used in evaluating OSAS are the apnea-hypopnea index (AHI), RERAs, respiratory disturbance index (RDI), lowest oxygen saturation, and percentage of time with an end tidal CO_2 level greater than 50 mm Hg. In children, apnea is defined as a complete interruption of air flow lasting at least 2 breath periods, whereas hypopnea is defined as a reduction in air flow of 50% or more with associated arousal, awakening, or desaturation of 3% or more for the same duration using a nasal cannula pressure transducer.[19,35] RERAs are defined as a sequence of at least 2 breath periods that does not meet the requirements for apnea or hypopnea but results in increased respiratory effort and subsequent arousal from sleep. The AHI and RERAs may be combined to give the RDI.

Box 1
Key action statements by the AAP for diagnosis and management of pediatric OSA

As part of routine health maintenance, the clinician should inquire if the child snores. If yes, or if the child presents with signs/symptoms of OSAS, the clinician should perform a more focused examination.

If the child snores on a regular basis and has signs/symptoms of OSAS, the clinician should either (1) obtain PSG or (2) refer the patient to a sleep specialist or otolaryngologist for more extensive evaluation.

If PSG is not available, the clinician may order alternative diagnostic tests, such as nocturnal video recording, nocturnal pulse oximetry, daytime nap PSG, or ambulatory PSG.

If the child has OSAS with adenotonsillar hypertrophy, adenotonsillectomy is recommended as first-line treatment. If the child has OSAS without adenotonsillar hypertrophy, other treatments should be considered.

Clinicians should monitor high-risk (see **Box 2**) patients undergoing adenotonsillectomy as inpatients postoperatively.

Clinicians should clinically reassess all patients with OSAS for persisting signs/symptoms after therapy to determine if further therapy is required.

Clinicians should reevaluate high-risk patients for persistent OSAS after adenotonsillectomy, including those who had a significantly abnormal baseline PSG, have sequelae of OSAS, are obese or remain symptomatic after treatment, with an objective test or referral to a sleep specialist.

Clinicians should refer patients for continuous positive airway pressure management if symptoms/signs or objective evidence of OSAS persists after adenotonsillectomy or if adenotonsillectomy is not performed.

Clinicians should recommend weight loss in addition to other therapy if a child with OSAS is overweight or obese.

Clinicians may prescribe topical intranasal corticosteroids for children with mild OSAS in whom adenotonsillectomy is contraindicated or for children with mild postoperative OSAS (apnea-hypopnea index <5/h).

Adapted from Marcus CL, Brooks LJ, Draper KA, et al. Diagnosis and management of childhood obstructive sleep apnea syndrome. Pediatrics 2012;130:576–84; and *From* Roland PS, Rosenfeld RM, Brooks LJ, et al. Clinical practice guideline: polysomnography for sleep-disordered breathing prior to tonsillectomy in children. Otolaryngol Head Neck Surg 2011;145:S1–15; with permission.

The performance and interpretation of pediatric nocturnal PSG have not been well standardized.[5,19] There is controversy as to what constitutes an abnormal threshold in pediatric PSG. The American Academy of Sleep Medicine (AASM) published guidelines for the diagnosis of pediatric OSAS in 2007. The AASM guidelines incorporate caregiver reporting as well as PSG data. AHI of 1 or more per hour, frequent arousals from sleep associated with increased respiratory effort, arterial oxygen desaturation in association with apneic episodes, hypercapnea during sleep, and markedly negative esophageal pressure swings are all considered abnormal. Several other studies associate AHI of 1 or more as the threshold diagnostic for OSAS.[35–40] In addition, most sleep specialists consider a pulse oximetry level less than 92% to be abnormal (in adults, an oximetry level <85 is abnormal).[2,40] However, some consider an AHI greater than 5 to be more representative of the abnormal threshold and more diagnostic of pediatric OSAS.[41–43] Many would consider that an AHI greater than 5 warrants T&A; however, because there is no evidence-based cutoff value, some children with AHI less than 5 may still be symptomatic and require intervention.[2] Although there is no

---

Box 2
Risk factors for postoperative respiratory complications in children with OSAS undergoing adenotonsillectomy

Younger than 3 years of age

Severe OSAS on PSG (apnea-hypopnea index $\geq$10 and/or oxygen saturation nadir $\leq$80%)

Cardiac complications of OSAS

Failure to thrive

Obesity

Craniofacial anomalies

Neuromuscular disorders

Current respiratory infection

Adapted from Marcus CL, Brooks LJ, Draper KA, et al. Diagnosis and management of childhood obstructive sleep apnea syndrome. Pediatrics 2012;130:576–84; and *From* Roland PS, Rosenfeld RM, Brooks LJ, et al. Clinical practice guideline: polysomnography for sleep-disordered breathing prior to tonsillectomy in children. Otolaryngol Head Neck Surg 2011;145:S1–15; with permission.

---

general consensus on defining the level of severity of SDB in children based on AHI, the American Society of Anesthesiologists guideline defines severe OSA as AHI of 10 or more.[2,44]

Every child with SDB and suspected OSAS does not need overnight PSG before treatment (T&A). AAOHNS published clinical practice guidelines advocating the use of PSG before tonsillectomy in children with SDB if they exhibit any of the following: obesity, Down syndrome, craniofacial abnormalities, neuromuscular disorders, sickle cell disease, or mucopolysaccharidoses. In addition, it was recommended that the clinician advocate for PSG before tonsillectomy for SDB in children without any of these comorbidities for whom the need for surgery is uncertain or when there is discordance between tonsillar size on physical examination and the reported severity of SDB.[1]

TREATMENT
T&A

The first-line treatment of pediatric OSAS is T&A. Anatomically, the palatine tonsils and adenoids are the most common areas of hypertrophy contributing to a loss of patency of the upper airway during sleep. A literature review and meta-analysis by Brietzke and Gallagher[45] examined the overall success rate of T&A comparing PSG data before and after surgery. The report demonstrated that T&A was effective in treating OSAS in uncomplicated patients, with an average reduction in AHI of 13 events per hour; the overall treatment success was estimated at around 82%. These data reveal that T&A is not universally curative as initially presumed. However, some of the studies using preoperative and postoperative objective measuring using PSG targeted a clinical population treated at a tertiary care hospital, which may have included patients with more comorbidities and subsequently more severe OSA than is seen in the general pediatric population.[34] The efficacy of T&A may be better than 80%, especially in otherwise healthy nonobese children. In a recent meta-analysis, Friedman and colleagues[46] demonstrated an improvement in SDB after T&A in most children but a resolution in SDB was seen in only 60% to 70% of children after tonsillectomy; improvement versus resolution was dependent on the degree of overweight/obesity.[2] Obesity significantly reduces the success of T&A. In a meta-analysis of 4 studies, resolution of SDB in obese children after tonsillectomy occurred in 10% to 25% of patients.[2,47]

These reports revealing reduced efficacy of T&A highlight the importance of the AAP Key Action statements (see **Box 1**) regarding the reassessment of patients with persistent signs and symptoms after T&A, and reevaluation of those who are obese and/or had a significantly abnormal baseline PSG. The guidelines suggest that this should be done with an objective test (such as PSG at least 6–8 weeks after surgical therapy) or referral to a sleep specialist.[8]

Morbidity

The risks of T&A have been well described and include minor risks such as pain and potential dehydration, as well as more major risks such as upper airway obstruction, postoperative respiratory compromise, postoperative hemorrhage, velopharyngeal incompetence, nasopharyngeal stenosis, and death.[8] The complication rate after T&A in children reported in several series ranges from 0% to 32% with airway compromise representing 0% to 16%.[48–51] Obesity increases the postoperative risk of respiratory complications with an overall odds ratio of 7.[52] Several reports have shown an RDI of greater than 10 to be a risk factor for postoperative desaturation to less than 70% or postoperative hypercapnea to more than 45 mm Hg.[53] Most respiratory complications occur with induction of anesthesia or emergence from anesthesia postoperatively. Although both the AAP and AAOHNS guidelines make general recommendations for the postoperative admission of children younger than 3 years of age, several reports demonstrate no postoperative hemorrhage or airway distress in the patient population aged from 12 to 35 months.[5,8,54,55] Other risk factors for perioperative complications are listed in **Box 2**.

Adjunctive Medical Therapy

Although continuous positive airway pressure (CPAP) is the gold standard therapy for adult OSAS, it should only be considered as a second-line treatment in pediatric patients with OSAS because of the high success rate of surgery. Home nasal CPAP has been used in infants, prepubertal children, and pubertal children.[56] Several studies have demonstrated its use and efficacy.[56–59] Most studies highlight the importance of family training and using the appropriate nasal interface, which needs to be addressed regularly in the first 3 months of use, and every 6 months or annually thereafter given the rate of craniofacial growth.[56] Regular follow-up avoids associated complications, such as local discomfort, eye irritation, conjunctivitis, and skin ulceration.[4]

Weight loss is recommended in the AAP guidelines for children with OSAS who are obese. The efficacy of weight loss as measured by improvement in PSG parameters in the pediatric population is not well known. A meta-analysis of 342 adults after weight-loss surgery saw that a decrease in body mass index (calculated as weight in kilograms divided by the square of height in meters) of 57 to 37 kg/m^2 correlated to a reduction in the AHI from 54.7 to 15.8 events per hour.[60] Similar studies have not been done in children. Most data has been published in the adult literature, but 2 other studies in the pediatric literature showed that weight loss improved OSAS, but the degree of weight loss required has not been determined.[8,61,62]

Nasal patency is a crucial area to be addressed in children with OSAS. Hypertrophic inferior nasal turbinates can often cause nasal airway obstruction similar to that caused by adenoid hypertrophy. Failure to address nasal obstruction from turbinate hypertrophy at the time of T&A has been found to have a negative impact on the outcome.[63] Surgical reduction in the form of radiofrequency ablation or submucosal resection may be warranted. Nasal corticosteroids may also be effective if the cause of the mucosal hypertrophy seems to be allergic in nature. Brouillette and colleagues[64] demonstrated that by using a 6-week course of nasal fluticasone in 25 patients, the RDI was reduced from 11 to 6 events per hour.

Persistent OSAS

The breadth of surgical management options for treating persistent pediatric OSAS is beyond the scope of this article, but the recent literature describes improved understanding of the management of these patients, both diagnostically and therapeutically.

Drug-induced sleep endoscopy (DISE) is a tool that has been developed to evaluate multiple levels of upper airway during spontaneous ventilation while the patient is induced pharmacologically into unconscious sedation simulating sleep.[65,66] Several studies in the adult literature have shown DISE to be a valid and reliable method for determining the site of partial and complete upper airway obstruction (eg, nasal cavity, velum/palate, oropharyngeal walls, tongue base, epiglottis/supraglottis) viewed dynamically.[66–71] In a retrospective study, Truong and colleagues[72] demonstrated that in children with persistent OSAS after T&A and in children with OSAS naive to previous surgery, DISE was an effective diagnostic tool for identifying the sites of obstruction. DISE has identified the contribution of lingual tonsillar hypertrophy and occult laryngomalacia in pediatric OSAS. Laryngomalacia is the most common congenital laryngeal anomaly in infants and children, and is typically associated with inspiratory stridor.[73,74] Laryngomalacia contributes to SDB in children and adults and may not be associated with stridor. Thevasagayam and colleagues[75] estimated the prevalence of laryngomalacia in children presenting with SDB to be 3.9%. Several reports have shown marked improvements in PSG parameters after supraglottoplasty as a treatment of clinically significant laryngomalacia.[76–80]

When T&A fails to resolve OSAS, other surgical options exist. Palatal surgery, such as uvulopalatopharyngoplasty (UPPP), has been used to treat complicated OSAS in obese children, children with cerebral palsy, children with Down syndrome, as well as children with other neurologic impairments or craniofacial anomalies. In a study of 15 patients with neurologic impairments, Kershner and colleagues[81] showed that although there was a modest improvement in the oxygen saturation nadir on PSG, nearly 23% required additional intervention within the following 10 years. Tongue base obstruction may be present and contribute to OSA in children with conditions such as Beckwith-Wiedemann syndrome and Down syndrome. Genioglossal advancement, radiofrequency ablation of the tongue, partial midline glossectomy, lingual tonsillectomy are all surgical options that are aimed at improving oropharyngeal and hypopharyngeal obstruction with varying degrees of reported success.[82–87]

Rapid maxillary expansion devices have been described in prepubertal children in an effort to widen the hard palate and enlarge the nasal cavity. Villa and colleagues[88,89] reported that, in 14 children, a mean expansion of 3.7 mm for the intercanine distance and 5.0 mm for the interpremolar distance led to an improvement in AHI from 5.8 to 1.5 events per hour, a reduction in snoring, and a reduction in daytime symptoms; this improvement was found to be persistent at 24-month follow-up PSG.

Other craniofacial procedures such as distraction osteogenesis and mandibular distraction are options for children with mandibular hypoplasia or retrognathia, which can be seen in hemifacial microsomia, Treacher-Collins syndrome, or in Pierre Robin sequence. These procedures can often be done in infants in an effort to avoid a tracheostomy.[4,90–92]

Tracheostomy is the definitive surgical treatment of upper airway obstruction. It should be reserved for the treatment of severe OSAS in children who have failed other measures of medical and surgical therapy, in those who have associated anatomic or neuromotor issues, and in those who are not likely to gain any benefit from other treatment modalities.[3,4]

SUMMARY

Pediatric OSAS is a common medical problem seen in children of all ages. If left undiagnosed and/or untreated, OSAS can cause severe sequelae. The clinical practice guidelines from multiple medical specialties highlight the importance of screening for symptoms of SDB and subsequent appropriate diagnostic testing and referral for surgical or medical management. Nocturnal PSG is the gold standard test used to diagnose OSAS in children. However, it is not required in all cases. T&A remains the first-line treatment of pediatric OSAS. Given the increase in pediatric obesity and the known reduced efficacy of T&A in obese patients, additional therapy may be indicated in this population. Persistence of SDB symptoms after T&A necessitates further diagnostic testing.

REFERENCES

1. Roland PS, Rosenfeld RM, Brooks LJ, et al. Clinical practice guideline: polysomnography for sleep-disordered breathing prior to tonsillectomy in children. Otolaryngol Head Neck Surg 2011;145:S1–15.
2. Baugh RF, Archer SM, Mitchell RB, et al. Clinical practice guideline: tonsillectomy in children. Otolaryngol Head Neck Surg 2011;144:S1–30.
3. Chan J, Edman JC, Koltai PJ. Obstructive sleep apnea in children. Am Fam Physician 2004;69:1147–54.
4. Sterni LM, Tunkel DE. Obstructive sleep apnea in children: an update. Pediatr Clin North Am 2003;50:427–43.
5. Section on Pediatric Pulmonology, Subcommittee on Obstructive Sleep Apnea Syndrome, American Academy of Pediatrics. Clinical practice guideline: diagnosis and management of childhood obstructive sleep apnea syndrome. Pediatrics 2002;109:704–12.
6. Pepin JL, Guillot M, Tamisier R, et al. The upper airway resistance syndrome. Respiration 2012;83:559–66.
7. Goldstein NA, Pugazhendhi V, Rao SM, et al. Clinical assessment of pediatric obstructive sleep apnea. Pediatrics 2004;114:33–43.
8. Marcus CL, Brooks LJ, Draper KA, et al. Diagnosis and management of childhood obstructive sleep apnea syndrome. Pediatrics 2012;130:576–84.
9. Ferreira AM, Clemente V, Gozal D, et al. Snoring in Portuguese primary school children. Pediatrics 2000;106:E64.
10. Hultcrantz E, Lofstrand-Tidestrom B, Ahlquist-Rastad J. The epidemiology of sleep related breathing disorder in children. Int J Pediatr Otorhinolaryngol 1995;32(Suppl):S63–6.
11. Owen GO, Canter RJ, Robinson A. Overnight pulse oximetry in snoring and non-snoring children. Clin Otolaryngol Allied Sci 1995;20:402–6.
12. Melendres MC, Lutz JM, Rubin ED, et al. Daytime sleepiness and hyperactivity in children with suspected sleep-disordered breathing. Pediatrics 2004;114:768–75.
13. Nolan J, Brietzke SE. Systematic review of pediatric tonsil size and polysomnogram-measured obstructive sleep apnea severity. Otolaryngol Head Neck Surg 2011;144:844–50.
14. Brodsky L. Modern assessment of tonsils and adenoids. Pediatr Clin North Am 1989;36:1551–69.

15. Gottlieb DJ, Chase C, Vezina RM, et al. Sleep-disordered breathing symptoms are associated with poorer cognitive function in 5-year-old children. J Pediatr 2004;145:458–64.

16. Halbower AC, Degaonkar M, Barker PB, et al. Childhood obstructive sleep apnea associates with neuropsychological deficits and neuronal brain injury. PLoS Med 2006;3:e301.

17. Gozal D, Pope DW Jr. Snoring during early childhood and academic performance at ages thirteen to fourteen years. Pediatrics 2001;107:1394–9.

18. Kennedy JD, Blunden S, Hirte C, et al. Reduced neurocognition in children who snore. Pediatr Pulmonol 2004;37:330–7.

19. Chang SJ, Chae KY. Obstructive sleep apnea syndrome in children: epidemiology, pathophysiology, diagnosis and sequelae. Korean J Pediatr 2010;53:863–71.

20. Clinical practice guideline: diagnosis and evaluation of the child with attention-deficit/hyperactivity disorder. American Academy of Pediatrics. Pediatrics 2000; 105:1158–70.

21. Ali NJ, Pitson D, Stradling JR. Sleep disordered breathing: effects of adenotonsillectomy on behaviour and psychological functioning. Eur J Pediatr 1996;155: 56–62.

22. Beebe DW, Gozal D. Obstructive sleep apnea and the prefrontal cortex: towards a comprehensive model linking nocturnal upper airway obstruction to daytime cognitive and behavioral deficits. J Sleep Res 2002;11:1–16.

23. Chervin RD, Dillon JE, Bassetti C, et al. Symptoms of sleep disorders, inattention, and hyperactivity in children. Sleep 1997;20:1185–92.

24. Lind MG, Lundell BP. Tonsillar hyperplasia in children. A cause of obstructive sleep apneas, CO_2 retention, and retarded growth. Arch Otolaryngol 1982; 108:650–4.

25. Bonuck K, Parikh S, Bassila M. Growth failure and sleep disordered breathing: a review of the literature. Int J Pediatr Otorhinolaryngol 2006;70:769–78.

26. Smith DF, Vikani AR, Benke JR, et al. Weight gain after adenotonsillectomy is more common in young children. Otolaryngol Head Neck Surg 2013;148(3): 488–93.

27. Kwok KL, Ng DK, Cheung YF. BP and arterial distensibility in children with primary snoring. Chest 2003;123:1561–6.

28. Marcus CL, Greene MG, Carroll JL. Blood pressure in children with obstructive sleep apnea. Am J Respir Crit Care Med 1998;157:1098–103.

29. Tezer MS, Karanfil A, Aktas D. Association between adenoidal-nasopharyngeal ratio and right ventricular diastolic functions in children with adenoid hypertrophy causing upper airway obstruction. Int J Pediatr Otorhinolaryngol 2005;69: 1169–73.

30. Tal A, Leiberman A, Margulis G, et al. Ventricular dysfunction in children with obstructive sleep apnea: radionuclide assessment. Pediatr Pulmonol 1988;4: 139–43.

31. Ingram DG, Matthews CK. Effect of adenotonsillectomy on C-reactive protein levels in children with obstructive sleep apnea: a meta-analysis. Sleep Med 2013;14(2):172–6.

32. Carroll JL, McColley SA, Marcus CL, et al. Inability of clinical history to distinguish primary snoring from obstructive sleep apnea syndrome in children. Chest 1995;108:610–8.

33. Goldstein NA, Sculerati N, Walsleben JA, et al. Clinical diagnosis of pediatric obstructive sleep apnea validated by polysomnography. Otolaryngol Head Neck Surg 1994;111:611–7.

34. Rosen CL. Obstructive sleep apnea syndrome in children: controversies in diagnosis and treatment. Pediatr Clin North Am 2004;51:153–67, vii.
35. Berry RB, Budhiraja R, Gottlieb DJ, et al. Rules for scoring respiratory events in sleep: update of the 2007 AASM Manual for the Scoring of Sleep and Associated Events. Deliberations of the Sleep Apnea Definitions Task Force of the American Academy of Sleep Medicine. J Clin Sleep Med 2012;8:597–619.
36. Bixler EO, Vgontzas AN, Lin HM, et al. Sleep disordered breathing in children in a general population sample: prevalence and risk factors. Sleep 2009;32:731–6.
37. Huang YS, Guilleminault C, Li HY, et al. Attention-deficit/hyperactivity disorder with obstructive sleep apnea: a treatment outcome study. Sleep Med 2007;8:18–30.
38. Kheirandish L, Goldbart AD, Gozal D. Intranasal steroids and oral leukotriene modifier therapy in residual sleep-disordered breathing after tonsillectomy and adenoidectomy in children. Pediatrics 2006;117:e61–6.
39. O'Brien LM, Serpero LD, Tauman R, et al. Plasma adhesion molecules in children with sleep-disordered breathing. Chest 2006;129:947–53.
40. Traeger N, Schultz B, Pollock AN, et al. Polysomnographic values in children 2-9 years old: additional data and review of the literature. Pediatr Pulmonol 2005;40: 22–30.
41. Emancipator JL, Storfer-Isser A, Taylor HG, et al. Variation of cognition and achievement with sleep-disordered breathing in full-term and preterm children. Arch Pediatr Adolesc Med 2006;160:203–10.
42. O'Brien LM, Holbrook CR, Mervis CB, et al. Sleep and neurobehavioral characteristics of 5- to 7-year-old children with parentally reported symptoms of attention-deficit/hyperactivity disorder. Pediatrics 2003;111:554–63.
43. Rosen CL, Storfer-Isser A, Taylor HG, et al. Increased behavioral morbidity in school-aged children with sleep-disordered breathing. Pediatrics 2004;114: 1640–8.
44. Gross JB, Bachenberg KL, Benumof JL, et al. Practice guidelines for the perioperative management of patients with obstructive sleep apnea: a report by the American Society of Anesthesiologists Task Force on Perioperative Management of patients with obstructive sleep apnea. Anesthesiology 2006;104: 1081–93 [quiz: 117–8].
45. Brietzke SE, Gallagher D. The effectiveness of tonsillectomy and adenoidectomy in the treatment of pediatric obstructive sleep apnea/hypopnea syndrome: a meta-analysis. Otolaryngol Head Neck Surg 2006;134:979–84.
46. Friedman M, Wilson M, Lin HC, et al. Updated systematic review of tonsillectomy and adenoidectomy for treatment of pediatric obstructive sleep apnea/hypopnea syndrome. Otolaryngol Head Neck Surg 2009;140:800–8.
47. Costa DJ, Mitchell R. Adenotonsillectomy for obstructive sleep apnea in obese children: a meta-analysis. Otolaryngol Head Neck Surg 2009;140:455–60.
48. Berkowitz RG, Zalzal GH. Tonsillectomy in children under 3 years of age. Arch Otolaryngol Head Neck Surg 1990;116:685–6.
49. Postma DS, Folsom F. The case for an outpatient "approach" for all pediatric tonsillectomies and/or adenoidectomies: a 4-year review of 1419 cases at a community hospital. Otolaryngol Head Neck Surg 2002;127:101–8.
50. Rieder AA, Flanary V. The effect of polysomnography on pediatric adenotonsillectomy postoperative management. Otolaryngol Head Neck Surg 2005;132: 263–7.
51. Slovik Y, Tal A, Shapira Y, et al. Complications of adenotonsillectomy in children with OSAS younger than 2 years of age. Int J Pediatr Otorhinolaryngol 2003;67: 847–51.

52. Fung E, Cave D, Witmans M, et al. Postoperative respiratory complications and recovery in obese children following adenotonsillectomy for sleep-disordered breathing: a case-control study. Otolaryngol Head Neck Surg 2010;142: 898–905.

53. Sanders JC, King MA, Mitchell RB, et al. Perioperative complications of adenotonsillectomy in children with obstructive sleep apnea syndrome. Anesth Analg 2006;103:1115–21.

54. Mitchell RB, Pereira KD, Friedman NR, et al. Outpatient adenotonsillectomy. Is it safe in children younger than 3 years? Arch Otolaryngol Head Neck Surg 1997; 123:681–3.

55. Spencer DJ, Jones JE. Complications of adenotonsillectomy in patients younger than 3 years. Arch Otolaryngol Head Neck Surg 2012;138:335–9.

56. Guilleminault C, Lee JH, Chan A. Pediatric obstructive sleep apnea syndrome. Arch Pediatr Adolesc Med 2005;159:775–85.

57. Downey R 3rd, Perkin RM, MacQuarrie J. Nasal continuous positive airway pressure use in children with obstructive sleep apnea younger than 2 years of age. Chest 2000;117:1608–12.

58. Guilleminault C, Pelayo R, Clerk A, et al. Home nasal continuous positive airway pressure in infants with sleep-disordered breathing. J Pediatr 1995;127:905–12.

59. Waters KA, Everett FM, Bruderer JW, et al. Obstructive sleep apnea: the use of nasal CPAP in 80 children. Am J Respir Crit Care Med 1995;152:780–5.

60. Greenburg DL, Lettieri CJ, Eliasson AH. Effects of surgical weight loss on measures of obstructive sleep apnea: a meta-analysis. Am J Med 2009;122:535–42.

61. Kalra M, Inge T. Effect of bariatric surgery on obstructive sleep apnoea in adolescents. Paediatr Respir Rev 2006;7:260–7.

62. Verhulst SL, Franckx H, Van Gaal L, et al. The effect of weight loss on sleep-disordered breathing in obese teenagers. Obesity (Silver Spring) 2009;17: 1178–83.

63. Guilleminault C, Li KK, Khramtsov A, et al. Sleep disordered breathing: surgical outcomes in prepubertal children. Laryngoscope 2004;114:132–7.

64. Brouillette RT, Manoukian JJ, Ducharme FM, et al. Efficacy of fluticasone nasal spray for pediatric obstructive sleep apnea. J Pediatr 2001;138:838–44.

65. Croft CB, Pringle M. Sleep nasendoscopy: a technique of assessment in snoring and obstructive sleep apnoea. Clin Otolaryngol Allied Sci 1991;16:504–9.

66. Ulualp SO, Szmuk P. Drug-induced sleep endoscopy for upper airway evaluation in children with obstructive sleep apnea. Laryngoscope 2013;123: 292–7.

67. Berry S, Roblin G, Williams A, et al. Validity of sleep nasendoscopy in the investigation of sleep related breathing disorders. Laryngoscope 2005;115:538–40.

68. Rabelo FA, Braga A, Kupper DS, et al. Propofol-induced sleep: polysomnographic evaluation of patients with obstructive sleep apnea and controls. Otolaryngol Head Neck Surg 2010;142:218–24.

69. Rodriguez-Bruno K, Goldberg AN, McCulloch CE, et al. Test-retest reliability of drug-induced sleep endoscopy. Otolaryngol Head Neck Surg 2009;140: 646–51.

70. Sadaoka T, Kakitsuba N, Fujiwara Y, et al. The value of sleep nasendoscopy in the evaluation of patients with suspected sleep-related breathing disorders. Clin Otolaryngol Allied Sci 1996;21:485–9.

71. Steinhart H, Kuhn-Lohmann J, Gewalt K, et al. Upper airway collapsibility in habitual snorers and sleep apneics: evaluation with drug-induced sleep endoscopy. Acta Otolaryngol 2000;120:990–4.

72. Truong MT, Woo VG, Koltai PJ. Sleep Endoscopy as a diagnostic tool in pediatric obstructive sleep apnea. Int J Pediatr Otohinolaryngol 2012;76(5): 722–7.
73. Holinger LD. Etiology of stridor in the neonate, infant and child. Ann Otol Rhinol Laryngol 1980;89:397–400.
74. Zoumalan R, Maddalozzo J, Holinger LD. Etiology of stridor in infants. Ann Otol Rhinol Laryngol 2007;116:329–34.
75. Thevasagayam M, Rodger K, Cave D, et al. Prevalence of laryngomalacia in children presenting with sleep-disordered breathing. Laryngoscope 2010;120: 1662–6.
76. Chan DK, Truong MT, Koltai PJ. Supraglottoplasty for occult laryngomalacia to improve obstructive sleep apnea syndrome. Arch Otolaryngol Head Neck Surg 2012;138:50–4.
77. Digoy GP, Shukry M, Stoner JA. Sleep apnea in children with laryngomalacia: diagnosis via sedated endoscopy and objective outcomes after supraglotto-plasty. Otolaryngol Head Neck Surg 2012;147:544–50.
78. Powitzky R, Stoner J, Fisher T, et al. Changes in sleep apnea after supraglotto-plasty in infants with laryngomalacia. Int J Pediatr Otorhinolaryngol 2011;75: 1234–9.
79. Valera FC, Tamashiro E, de Araujo MM, et al. Evaluation of the efficacy of supra-glottoplasty in obstructive sleep apnea syndrome associated with severe lar-yngomalacia. Arch Otolaryngol Head Neck Surg 2006;132:489–93.
80. Zafereo ME, Taylor RJ, Pereira KD. Supraglottoplasty for laryngomalacia with obstructive sleep apnea. Laryngoscope 2008;118:1873–7.
81. Kerschner JE, Lynch JB, Kleiner H, et al. Uvulopalatopharyngoplasty with ton-sillectomy and adenoidectomy as a treatment for obstructive sleep apnea in neurologically impaired children. Int J Pediatr Otorhinolaryngol 2002;62: 229–35.
82. Miller FR, Watson D, Boseley M. The role of the Genial Bone Advancement Trephine system in conjunction with uvulopalatopharyngoplasty in the multilevel management of obstructive sleep apnea. Otolaryngol Head Neck Surg 2004; 130:73–9.
83. Farrar J, Ryan J, Oliver E, et al. Radiofrequency ablation for the treatment of obstructive sleep apnea: a meta-analysis. Laryngoscope 2008;118:1878–83.
84. Friedman M, Soans R, Gurpinar B, et al. Evaluation of submucosal minimally invasive lingual excision technique for treatment of obstructive sleep apnea/hypopnea syndrome. Otolaryngol Head Neck Surg 2008;139:378–84 [discus-sion: 85].
85. Lin AC, Koltai PJ. Persistent pediatric obstructive sleep apnea and lingual ton-sillectomy. Otolaryngol Head Neck Surg 2009;141:81–5.
86. Maturo SC, Mair EA. Coblation lingual tonsillectomy. Otolaryngol Head Neck Surg 2006;135:487–8.
87. Maturo SC, Mair EA. Submucosal minimally invasive lingual excision: an effec-tive, novel surgery for pediatric tongue base reduction. Ann Otol Rhinol Laryngol 2006;115:624–30.
88. Villa MP, Malagola C, Pagani J, et al. Rapid maxillary expansion in children with obstructive sleep apnea syndrome: 12-month follow-up. Sleep Med 2007;8: 128–34.
89. Villa MP, Rizzoli A, Miano S, et al. Efficacy of rapid maxillary expansion in chil-dren with obstructive sleep apnea syndrome: 36 months of follow-up. Sleep Breath 2011;15:179–84.

90. Cohen SR, Simms C, Burstein FD. Mandibular distraction osteogenesis in the treatment of upper airway obstruction in children with craniofacial deformities. Plast Reconstr Surg 1998;101:312–8.

91. Monasterio FO, Drucker M, Molina F, et al. Distraction osteogenesis in Pierre Robin sequence and related respiratory problems in children. J Craniofac Surg 2002;13:79–83 [discussion: 84].

92. Williams JK, Maull D, Grayson BH, et al. Early decannulation with bilateral mandibular distraction for tracheostomy-dependent patients. Plast Reconstr Surg 1999;103:48–57 [discussion: 58–9].

Pediatric Cochlear Implantation
Expanding Applications and Outcomes

Joseph L. Russell, MD, Harold S. Pine, MD, Dayton L. Young, MD*

KEYWORDS

- Cochlear • Implant • Implantation • Pediatric • Deafness • Hearing loss
- Outcomes

KEY POINTS

- Cochlear implants have revolutionized the treatment and quality of life of children born with severe to profound sensorineural hearing loss.
- Of the children born with profound hearing loss in the United States, 50% now receive at least 1 cochlear implant; bilateral implantation is becoming increasingly more common.
- The surgery to place a cochlear implant is straightforward in most cases and children can usually go home the same day.
- Congenitally deafened children who are implanted within a critical window of time, early in life, have better outcomes than those implanted at older ages.
- The benefits of cochlear implantation are far reaching and include not only improved hearing and speech but also improved quality of life, better educational opportunities, and increased earning potential.

INTRODUCTION

Cochlear implants are small surgically implanted electronic devices, about the size of a pacemaker, that are designed to restore a sense of sound to individuals with severe to profound deafness. Although the first cochlear implants, developed more than 30 years ago, did little more than provide a sense of awareness of sounds and cadences,[1] modern cochlear implant systems have become highly effective at providing the ability for patients to perceive and understand speech. They have become so effective at providing speech perception ability that cochlear implants are now considered to be standard of care in the treatment of children with severe to profound sensorineural hearing loss (SNHL).[2–5]

Department of Otolaryngology—Head and Neck Surgery, University of Texas Medical Branch, 301 University Boulevard, Route 0521, Galveston, TX 77555, USA
* Corresponding author.
E-mail address: dlyoung@utmb.edu

Pediatr Clin N Am 60 (2013) 841–863
http://dx.doi.org/10.1016/j.pcl.2013.04.008
0031-3955/13/$ – see front matter © 2013 Elsevier Inc. All rights reserved.

BACKGROUND

In the United States, 1 out of every 1000 children is born with profound, bilateral SNHL.[6] Until the advent of cochlear implantation in children through research trials in the 1980s and US Food and Drug Administration (FDA) approval in 1990, these patients were destined to live in a world without sound, one fraught with severe challenges. Compared with other disabled persons, those with severe to profound deafness have historically had the lowest median education achievement level, the lowest median annual family income, the lowest rate of participation in the labor force, the lowest rate of persons in professional and technical jobs, and the poorest self-rated general health.[7] Forty-four percent of profoundly deaf children do not graduate high school, compared with 19% of the general population, and only 5% of deaf children graduate college, compared with 13% of the general population. Of those who do successfully graduate high schools for the deaf, the average reading ability is at the third-grade level and the average computational ability is at the fourth-grade level.[8,9] The loss of work productivity and cost of special education, medical services, and assistive devices yields an estimated cost to society of more that 1 million dollars over the lifetime of an individual who is born with profound hearing loss.[10]

Cochlear implantation has radically changed the outlook for congenitally deafened children. At the time of this writing, more than 50% of children with profound SNHL in the United States receive at least 1 cochlear implant.[11] Of these children, 75% are able to attend mainstream schools by high school age and only 5% require full-time special education services.[12] Furthermore, 50% exhibit age-appropriate vocabulary scores by kindergarten.[13] Although these statistics are impressive, it is expected that the current trend toward implanting children at younger ages and more recent advances in cochlear implant technology will prove to be even more effective at rehabilitating hearing loss in deaf children.

HOW A COCHLEAR IMPLANT WORKS

There are many types of sensorineural hearing impairment in children. They have been categorized in various ways, from congenital to acquired, and from hereditary to nonhereditary causes. For cases in which a cause can be identified, the cause can be attributed to genetic, infectious, drug-induced, toxin-induced, metabolic, traumatic, or noise-induced causes, among others.[2,14] However, a specific cause of the hearing loss is often not identified.

Despite the wide diversity in categories and causes of hearing loss, there tends to be one common similarity in the mechanism by which nearly all pathologic processes lead to hearing loss. This final common mechanism is damage to the sensory hair cells within the organ of corti of the cochlea.[14] In normal-hearing patients, these small, fragile hair cells serve to translate mechanical movement from sound waves traveling along the basilar membrane into electrical action potentials that are then transmitted via the cochlear nerve ganglia to the brain. In most cases of sensorineural hearing impairment, these sensory hair cells are absent or nonfunctional.[1] A cochlear implant works by bypassing the hair cells with an array of electrodes to directly stimulate the cochlear nerve ganglia, thereby transmitting an electrical signal to the brain that is perceived as sound.[1]

One notable exception to the generalization presented above is auditory neuropathy spectrum disorder (ANSD). Though not yet fully understood, ANSD seems to be a form of SNHL in which at least some of the hair cells within the cochlea (the outer hair cells) do function normally. The problem in ANSD is thought to be secondary to a problem with (1) the inner hair cells, (2) the interface between the inner hair cells and the cochlear nerve, or (3) a problem within the auditory nerve itself, causing dyssynchrony of the action potentials along different nerve axons.[15] Cochlear implants have been found to be helpful in many of these patients as well. For these patients it is presumed that the cochlear implant signal either bypasses the interface between inner hair cells and the cochlear nerve ganglia (a mechanism similar to that described earlier for outer hair cell dysfunction) or that the electrical stimulation from the implant provides a sufficiently strong and organized signal to overcome any lesion that may be causing dyssynchrony in the cochlear nerve.[1]

COMPONENTS OF A COCHLEAR IMPLANT

Modern cochlear implant systems consist of 3 components: (1) the electrode array, (2) the receiver-stimulator, and (3) the external processor (**Figs. 1** and **2**).[16] The electrode array is a small, flexible silicone prosthesis that is the core of the cochlear implant system. It is called an electrode array because it contains 12 to 24 different electrodes arranged serially along its short (15–27 mm) length.[1] The electrode array is placed within the perilymph-filled scala tympani of the cochlea. It is designed to be threaded from the base of the snail-shaped cochlea (at or near the round window) toward the apex of the cochlea. After the electrode array is inserted into the cochlea, each electrode in the array occupies a different location along the length of the cochlea from the base toward the apex. The various spiral ganglia of the cochlear nerve are also arranged inside the cochlea such that the ganglia near the base perceive high-pitched sounds and the ganglia near the apex perceive low-pitched sounds. As a result, stimulation of an electrode near the base of the cochlea results in the perception of a high-pitched sound whereas stimulation of an electrode near the apex results in the perception of a low-pitched sound.[1]

The electrode array is attached by an insulated wire lead to the second component called the receiver-stimulator. The receiver-stimulator is surgically implanted under the skin behind the patient's ear. This portion of the device is about the size of a pacemaker. It communicates via radio signal through the skin with the third component of the cochlear implant system, called the external processor (**Fig. 2**).

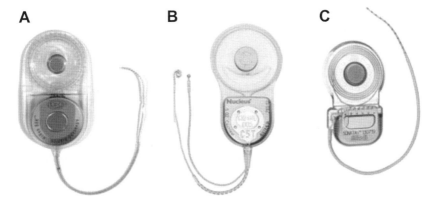

Fig. 1. The most recent cochlear implant models from the 3 major device manufacturers: (*A*) Advanced Bionics Corporation HR90 K; (*B*) Cochlear Corporation Nucleus 5; and (*C*) Med-El GmbH Sonata ti100. ([*A*] *Courtesy of* Advanced Bionics, LLC, Valencia, CA. [*B*] Photo provided *courtesy of* Cochlear™ Americas, © 2011 Cochlear Americas. [*C*] *Courtesy of* Med-EL Inc, Durham, NC; with permission.)

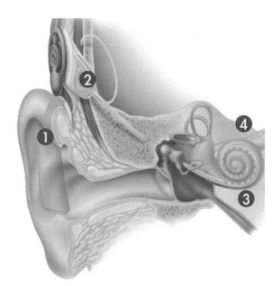

Fig. 2. The cochlear implant: how it works. (1) Sound is received by a microphone located on the external processor, behind the ear. The signal is then processed, coded, and sent via transcutaneous radiofrequency link to the (2) implanted receiver-stimulator. Once received by the receiver-stimulator, the data are decoded and sent to individual electrodes within (3) the intracochlear electrode array. Individual electrodes within the electrode array stimulate spiral ganglion cell populations within their vicinity, causing a signal to be transmitted along (4) the auditory nerve for central processing. (Photo provided *courtesy of* Cochlear™ Americas, © 2011 Cochlear Americas.)

The external processor is worn over the ear, similar to a hearing aid. The external processor contains a microphone for picking up sound and a speech processor that encodes the sound into digital code. The digital code is then transmitted to the receiver-stimulator implanted under the skin. The receiver-stimulator in turn sends the coded signal to the electrode array. The electrode array then stimulates the cochlear nerve at appropriate locations within the cochlea (determined and coded by the processor) to deliver meaningful signals that are perceived as sound by the brain.[1]

SURGERY

In most cases, cochlear implant surgery is straightforward. The procedure is done in the operating room under general anesthesia. Continuous facial nerve monitoring is performed during the procedure because the facial nerve crosses the operative field close to the cochlea. The incision is small and is mostly hidden behind the external ear. A surgical opening (mastoidectomy) is made in the mastoid process of the temporal bone to provide access to the middle ear and cochlea from behind. The facial nerve and the chorda tympani nerve are identified in the mastoid and preserved. The receiver-stimulator is secured in place under the skin behind and slightly above the ear and mastoid. The electrode array and lead connecting it to the receiver-stimulator are threaded through the mastoid and into the middle ear space. The electrode array is then placed into the cochlea either through the round window or through a small surgically created cochleostomy (hole) adjacent to the round window. In normal cases, the procedure takes about 2 to 3 hours and patients go home the same day. A dressing is worn overnight and then removed the following morning. The child is not allowed to wear the external processor for 3 weeks to allow time for the wound to heal. After 3 weeks, the implant is activated and the child begins to wear the external processor and perceive sound for the first time.[17]

WHO IS A CANDIDATE FOR COCHLEAR IMPLANTATION?

Cochlear implantation is considered in patients who cannot be adequately rehabilitated with hearing aids. If a child is expected to have better hearing outcomes with a hearing aid than with a cochlear implant, then cochlear implantation should not be performed.[18,19] Although this concept may seem simple at first, determining the point at which the benefits of cochlear implantation exceed those of hearing amplification is not always straightforward. There are 3 competing factors that complicate this decision in children:

1. Cochlear implantation causes irreversible changes to the inner ear. By definition, cochlear implantation involves a surgical opening of the cochlea for placement of the prosthesis, which often (but not always) results in partial to complete loss of whatever natural hearing was present before cochlear implantation. There is significant interest and research into developing new electrode arrays and atraumatic surgical techniques in an effort to preserve residual natural hearing. However, at present, patients and parents are counseled that cochlear implantation is likely to result in a loss of any residual natural hearing and that they will need to rely on electrical stimulation in the implanted ear.
2. There is clear evidence that children who are implanted at younger ages have significantly better hearing outcomes than children implanted at older ages.[20,21] There is thought to be a window of time in the first few years of life during which implantation is critical to achieve maximum benefit. Beyond that window of time, the child's brain becomes less plastic, or adaptable, and it begins to lose its ability to develop new neural pathways in response to the new auditory input that a cochlear implant provides.[1,2,22,23] At present, although there is no consensus about how narrowly the critical window of time for optimal auditory development is defined, there is a growing body of evidence that supports implantation before 12 months of age.[20,21,24,25] Nevertheless, some of the evidence suggests that the sensitive period may extend to about 3 years of age.[20,22]

    In the United States, the FDA has approved cochlear implantation in children aged 12 months and older.[18,19,26] However, some experienced cochlear implant programs in the United States and cochlear implant programs in countries not bound by FDA criteria are implanting children as young as 6 months.[20,24,25] At present, most cochlear implant programs in the United States try to implant children before the age of 18 to 24 months.
3. The younger children are, the more difficult it is to test their hearing and to determine benefit from wearing a hearing aid.[18,19] One of the most important functions of a hearing aid or cochlear implant is to provide the listener with the ability to recognize and understand oral speech. Although it is easy to test speech discrimination in adults and postlingually deafened children (children deafened after they have learned to speak), such testing is impossible in the congenitally deafened infant or a child who is not mature enough to have developed the ability to understand and produce speech. Preimplant evaluation in such children relies heavily on electrophysiologic testing, such as auditory brainstem-evoked response testing (ABR), which can provide a useful approximation of hearing thresholds in infants and young children.[19] Children are also given a 3-month to 6-month hearing aid trial

to document lack of auditory skills development or minimal auditory skills development with hearing aids. Children older than 2 years can begin to participate in some speech discrimination testing to objectively evaluate how well the hearing aids are working. However, in children younger than 2 years, evidence of auditory improvement (or lack thereof) must be documented by behavioral observations from audiologists, speech pathologists, and parents to determine whether certain auditory milestones are met.[19]

The decision about whether or not to proceed with cochlear implantation early in life can therefore have permanent ramifications on a child's ultimate ability to perceive and understand oral speech. A decision to implant may result in irreversible loss of whatever natural hearing is still present, but delaying that decision beyond the critical window of auditory development results in less than optimal ability to develop speech and language skills. In congenital deafness, that window of time, and therefore the decision about whether or not to implant, occurs within the first 6 months to 3 years of life, precisely at the time when it is most difficult to assess a child's hearing and the helpfulness of hearing aids. However, in many cases the decision to proceed with cochlear implantation is straightforward. Children with profound SNHL, as measured by ABR and lack of progress with hearing aids, are more likely to benefit from a cochlear implant than from hearing aids. In contrast, children with mild to moderate SNHL with evidence of improvement with hearing aids would be better served with hearing aids than with cochlear implantation. Nevertheless, difficult decisions must sometimes be made in cases of children with moderately severe to severe SNHL who are showing only modest evidence of progress on hearing aid trials.[18]

In the United States, FDA guidelines for cochlear implant candidacy specify that children less than 2 years old should have bilateral profound SNHL and that children more than 2 years old should have bilateral severe to profound SNHL to be considered as candidates for cochlear implantation. They further specify that children should undergo a 3-month to 6-month hearing aid trial and show limited benefit from appropriate binaural amplification.[18,19] As with age of implantation, these guidelines are thought to be conservative, and are often exceeded by experienced cochlear implant programs in the United States and by cochlear implant programs in other countries not bound by FDA criteria,[18] because there is growing recognition that some children with greater residual hearing at the time of implantation than specified by FDA criteria may have better outcomes if a prolonged hearing aid trial is avoided.

MEDICAL AND SURGICAL CONSIDERATIONS

In general, patients must be healthy enough to undergo surgery and general anesthesia. Otherwise, the only absolute contraindications to cochlear implantation are (1) absence or agenesis of the cochlea, or (2) absence or aplasia of the cochlear nerve.[19] Patients with incomplete cochlear dysplasias, such as common cavity deformity and various Mondini malformations, can be implanted and often derive significant benefit from cochlear implantation.[19] Noncontrasted imaging studies such as magnetic resonance imaging or computed tomography are obtained before surgery to evaluate for cochlear dysplasia or cochlear nerve anomalies and for preoperative planning.

Ear infections are relative contraindications for cochlear implantation, and in general must be managed before implantation can proceed. Most surgeons recommend removing ventilation tubes before implantation, but cochlear implantation has been performed in patients with patent ventilation tubes and does not seem to lead to complications.[17] For children with recurrent ear infections who already have a cochlear implant in place, management with antibiotics and ventilation tubes should proceed as if they did not have a cochlear implant in place.[17]

Children with hearing loss have a higher risk of developing meningitis than normal children. Cochlear implant recipients have a higher risk of developing meningitis than children with hearing loss who have not been implanted.[17,19] Most cases of meningitis in children with cochlear implants are caused by *Streptococcus pneumoniae* infections. The US Centers for Disease Control and Prevention (CDC) have published recommendations that all cochlear implant recipients receive specific age-appropriate immunization for *S pneumoniae* in addition to the normal immunization for *Haemophilus influenzae* type b (Hib). Children should be up to date with appropriate immunizations at least 2 weeks before implantation.[19]

Children who have hearing loss that was caused by bacterial meningitis are given special attention because it is often necessary to expedite surgery in these cases. Bacterial meningitis can cause permanent, irreversible hearing loss during the active infection, making cochlear implantation necessary. However, after children have recovered from the acute infection, long-term inflammatory changes can continue. This postinfectious inflammatory process is called labyrinthitis ossificans. Within a matter of months following an episode of meningitis it can result in obliteration of the formerly patent cochlea with fibrous or bony tissue that makes surgical placement of the cochlear prosthesis significantly more difficult or even impossible. Although surgical placement can usually be accomplished in these patients by cochlear drill-out, placement of a split electrode array, or other modifications, outcomes may be affected. Therefore, if possible, surgery is expedited in patients with hearing loss from meningitis so that the electrode array can be placed before ossification occurs.[17]

OUTCOMES

A decision to proceed with cochlear implantation involves an educated discussion of the expected outcomes. These outcomes include expected benefits of cochlear implantation and potential risks. As discussed later, the benefits of implantation are far reaching. For the patient, they not only include improved ability to hear but also improved ability to acquire speech and language skills, greater success within the education system, better employment status, and improved quality of life. In addition, cochlear implants provide benefits to society in terms of decreased educational costs and restoration of work productivity potential.

The long-term benefits of cochlear implantation are only beginning to be observed. Multichannel cochlear implants were approved for children in the United States in 1990. Children implanted at that time are now reaching their mid-20s. However, since the 1990s, many improvements have been made within the implant systems that have significantly improved outcomes. In addition, children are receiving implants at younger ages, which has also improved outcomes. Two decades ago, deaf children who received cochlear implants were usually compared with age-matched deaf children who wore high-powered hearing aids as controls; deaf children who receive cochlear implants now have such improved hearing and speech outcomes that they are routinely being compared with age-matched normal-hearing children as controls.

Hearing and Speech Perception Benefits

The primary goal of cochlear implantation is to improve hearing. So how well does a cochlear implant perform in doing that? In a way, what people hear is subjective and difficult for the outsider to observe. Just as beauty is in the eye of the beholder, the hearing that is achieved through cochlear implantation is confined to the experience of the listener. Although that experience is not easily conveyed to others, there are objective measurements of hearing that can be made.

The most practical function of hearing is to provide the ability to perceive and recognize oral speech. Therefore, speech perception testing has become the gold standard for objectively measuring cochlear implant outcomes. Although this kind of testing is easily done in adults and postlingually deafened children, it is not possible in children who are too immature to have developed the ability to speak. Nevertheless, the ability to perceive speech is probably more important to the prelingually deafened child than to anyone else, because that child is in the position of having to use the cochlear implant for the difficult task of learning speech and language.

There are two basic ways to measure speech perception in individuals who have already learned to speak: (1) word recognition tests, and (2) sentence recognition tests.[1] Both are used to evaluate patients receiving cochlear implants. Word recognition tests are more difficult than sentence recognition tests because there are no contextual clues (from the structure of a sentence and surrounding words) in word recognition tests. Various forms of these tests have been devised for different age groups. They can be made easier by providing multiple-choice answers (closed-set testing) or more difficult by requiring an open-ended response (open-set testing).[1]

For children who are too young to speak, observations of the child's hearing-related behavior are made and quantified. For example, one commonly used test, the Infant-Toddler Meaningful Auditory Integration Scale (IT-MAIS), uses a structured parent interview to assess auditory behaviors, such as the child's behavior while using a hearing aid or cochlear implant, the child's response to his or her name, and the child's awareness of environmental sounds.[27] Other behavioral instruments are designed to quantify hierarchical auditory behaviors across broader age ranges. For example, one such instrument, the Categories of Auditory Performance (CAP), grades patients on a hierarchical scale that ranges from 0 points for no sound awareness to 7 points for being able to communicate using a telephone.[28]

So, to determine how well cochlear implant systems perform, it is instructive to first look at adults. In postlingually deafened adults, modern cochlear implant systems consistently show average word recognition scores of 50% to 60% correct and average sentence recognition scores of 80% to 90% correct (using hearing only, without visual clues). However, there is significant variability. Some patients achieve scores of 100% correct, whereas other patients are unable to attain a score of more than 0%. Nevertheless, most patients (ie, three-quarters of them) achieve scores of 80% or higher on sentence recognition testing.[1,29] With scores like these, most deaf patients are able to communicate using the telephone.

Comparing outcomes among children has been more difficult because of the challenges described earlier and because of disparate testing strategies. However, as children implanted in the early to mid-1990s have become older, it has become possible to test them with strategies similar to those used for adults. This testing is beginning to show speech recognition outcomes in children that are similar to the outcomes described above for adults. For example, Davidson and colleagues[30] recently studied 112 teenagers who received cochlear implants in the early to mid-1990s when they were between 2 and 5 years of age. Word recognition and sentence recognition were measured when these children were in elementary school and again when they were in high school. These children with cochlear implants (now in their early 20s) achieved average word recognition scores of 50.6% correct in elementary school and 60.1% correct in high school. They achieved average sentence recognition scores of 63.2% in elementary school and 80.3% correct in high school. Analyzing the individual data, it is clear that most of the high school subjects (about three-quarters of them) achieved sentence recognition scores of at least 80% correct.[30] These results, particularly those achieved in high school, are nearly identical to those achieved by implanted postlingually deafened adults.

It took time (about one decade of cochlear implant use) for children in the study described above to achieve the speech perception scores documented in high school. However, these children were originally implanted with older technology and they were implanted at older ages. The current trend is to implant children at younger ages because outcomes are better. As children have become old enough to participate in speech recognition testing, other investigators have similarly published average word recognition scores ranging from 44% to 72% correct and average sentence recognition scores ranging from 56% to 81% correct.[18,30,31] These data contrast sharply with data from the 1980s showing that no child with profound SNHL who was treated with hearing aids could achieve scores above 30% on word recognition tests.[32] Better outcomes are observed in children implanted at younger ages, children implanted with the latest implants and speech processing strategies, and children who have used their implants for a longer duration of time.[18]

The ability to communicate using the telephone is a good indicator of a patient's speech perception abilities because the telephone removes all visual cues from speech. Before the availability of cochlear implantation, talking on the telephone represented an impossible challenge for severe to profoundly hearing-impaired individuals; however, in 2007, Uziel and colleagues[31] reported that 65 (79%) of 82 profoundly deaf children with at least 10 years of cochlear implant experience could use a telephone with a familiar talker.[33] This rate is on par with rates of telephone use seen in postlingually deafened adults who have cochlear implants and underscores the impact cochlear implants are able to make in the lives of deaf individuals.[34]

Children implanted at younger ages attain better hearing and speech perception outcomes than children implanted at older ages. However, the ideal age for implantation to achieve the optimal outcomes has yet to be defined. Several studies have presented strong evidence that children implanted before 2 years of age have improved hearing and speech perception compared with children implanted at an older age.[24,25] Most of these studies that document improved hearing and speech perception used instruments that are based on observation of the child's auditory behavior. Using this kind of analysis, Govaerts and colleagues[25] reported that children implanted at less than 2 years of age achieved normal speech perception abilities as early as 3 months after implantation (as measured by behavior observation scores). Children implanted after 2 years of age did not do as well.

More recently, there has been growing evidence documenting improved auditory outcomes in children implanted before 12 months of age. In one recent study, Colletti and colleagues[24] implanted 12 children at or before age 6 months. At 4 years after implantation, these implanted children demonstrated speech perception abilities, as demonstrated by behavior observation (CAP) scores, that were equal to similarly measured abilities attained by age-matched normal-hearing peers (**Fig. 3**). Children implanted after age 6 months had less favorable outcomes. However, other studies have not shown clear evidence of improved hearing outcomes in children implanted before age 12 months compared with children implanted a year later.[26] Therefore, the ideal age for implantation to achieve optimal benefit is still in the process of being defined, with some investigators contending that children should be implanted by as young as 6 months and others suggesting that the window for optimal benefit from implantation may extend out to 2 or even 3 years of age.[26]

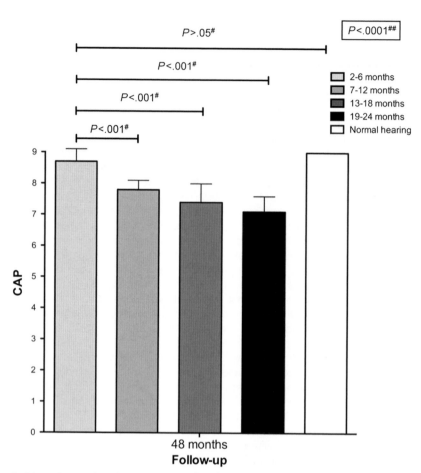

Fig. 3. Mean Categories of Auditory Performance (CAP) II scores at the 48-month follow-up in the 4 groups of children. Note that there is no statistical difference (*P*>.05) between the scores of children implanted at ages 2 to 6 months and normal-hearing children. (*From* Colletti L, Mandalà M, Colletti V. Cochlear implants in children younger than 6 months. Otolaryngol Head Neck Surg 2012;147:142; with permission of SAGE Publications.)

Language Development and Speech Production Benefits

At a deeper level than simply having the ability to recognize speech, parents of deaf children are especially concerned about their child's ability to learn language and to participate or fit in to their communities. This participation begins with their family community, but ultimately extends to the community at large. Ninety percent of deaf children are born to 2 normal-hearing parents and live in normal-hearing families.[35] These families communicate at home using spoken language. When deaf children grow old enough to move out of the home, they have to interact with a world that also uses spoken language for communication. Parents report that the primary reason they seek cochlear implantation for their children is so that they can develop spoken language skills.[6,36] They want their children to hear and speak like children with normal hearing.[37]

One of the more serious consequences of profound deafness is that it results in severe speech and language delay. It has been established by several investigators that profoundly deaf children using hearing aids acquire language at slower rates than normal children.[38–40] In 1997, Robbins and colleagues[38] showed this using the Reynell Developmental Language Scales (RDLS). RDLS is an assessment tool widely used by educators, speech pathologists, and psychologists to identify speech and language delay, often secondary to social deprivation, in young children aged 1 to 8 years. The RDLS is composed of 2 scales. One scale is designed to measure receptive language ability and the other scale is designed to measure expressive language ability. Receptive language ability and expressive language ability are different than speech perception and speech intelligibility.[41–43] Speech perception testing focuses on the degree to which a child recognizes words and sentences, whereas receptive language testing focuses on the degree to which a child is able to comprehend language, or the degree to which the child is able to decode words and sentences into meaningful thoughts. In a similar manner, speech intelligibility testing focuses on the degree to which a child can produce intelligible speech, whereas expressive language testing focuses on the degree to which children are able to encode their thoughts into words and sentences.[41,42] Using the RDLS, Robbins and colleagues[38] showed that the average profoundly deaf child with a hearing aid learns language at about half the rate of normal-hearing peers. However, the same group went on to show that deaf children who receive cochlear implants, on average, begin to learn language at the same rate as normal-hearing peers following implantation (**Fig. 4**).[21,44] Expanding on these findings, Nicholas and Geers[35] showed, through regression analysis of language outcomes of deaf children implanted between 12 and 36 months of age, that the best language development is obtained in children who are implanted before

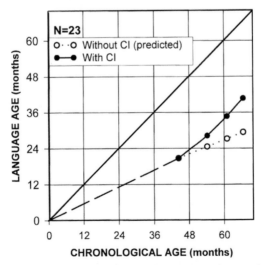

Fig. 4. Average language age as a function of chronologic age for 23 subjects with cochlear implant (CI) before implantation (*dashed line*) and at 3 intervals after implantation (*black circles*). The white circles represent the expressive language growth predicted for these same children had they not received cochlear implants. The solid diagonal line represents the language growth expected of an average normal-hearing child. (*From* Svirsky MA, Robbins AM, Kirk KI. Language development in profoundly deaf children with cochlear implants. Psychol Sci 2000;11:156; with permission of SAGE Publications.)

18 months of age. In addition, their analysis indicates that, for deaf children implanted after age 30 months, the existing speech delay and slower rate of language development may prevent them from ever being able to catch up to their normal-hearing peers. In a separate study, also using the RDLS, Niparko and colleagues[37] confirmed that children who are implanted at less than 18 months of age have the fastest rate of language acquisition, whereas children implanted at ages older than 18 months follow slower language acquisition growth curves.

Cochlear implants also improve expressive vocabulary development as recipients grow older and gain more experience with their devices. The best results are obtained with younger age at implantation and increasing duration of cochlear implant use. Geers and colleagues[13] reported that 58% percent of children implanted before age 5 years and with at least 1 year of cochlear implant experience attained age-appropriate expressive vocabulary scores by kindergarten; higher scores were obtained with decreasing age at implantation. Evaluating a separate group of adolescents implanted between 2 and 5 years of age and who had at least 10 years of implant use, Geers and Sedey[35] showed that the percentage of patients with age-appropriate expressive vocabulary scores increased to 74% by high school.[45]

Cochlear implantation decreases a deaf child's use of sign language and increases the use of oral language; this effect is greater the younger the child is at the time of implantation. Watson and colleagues[46] found that, at 5 years after implantation, 83% of children implanted before age 3 years preferred oral communication with minimal or no signing; this figure decreased to 63.5% in children implanted between the ages of 3 to 5 years, and decreased further to 45.1% in children implanted after age 5 years.

Finally, cochlear implants greatly improve a deaf child's ability to be understood by others. In evaluating the effects of cochlear implantation on speech intelligibility, Tobey and colleagues[47] reported that for deaf adolescents implanted between 2 and 5 years of age and who had at least 10 years of implant use, speech intelligibility scores were 81% to 88%; this is in stark contrast with pre–cochlear implant era data showing speech intelligibility scores of 17% to 21% for deaf children who only had access to hearing aids.

Education Benefits

The success that cochlear implants have in restoring hearing, language, and speech to deaf children produces significant changes in their educational requirements and capacity for achievement. Koch and colleagues[48] developed the education resource matrix in the late 1990s as a model to describe and stratify educational requirements for deaf children. In this matrix, classroom placement ranges from full-time residence in a state school for the deaf (least independence, highest cost) to a self-contained classroom (midlevel independence and cost), to full-time attendance in a mainstream classroom (highest independence, lowest cost). In a more recent study of 35 deaf children who received cochlear implants, the same investigators found that the rate of full-time assignment to a mainstream classroom increased from 12% before implantation to 75% for children with more than 4 years of implant use.[49] In a long-term follow-up of 112 deaf patients with at least 10 years of cochlear implant use, Geers and colleagues[12] showed similar results, with 75% of patients being placed in a full-time mainstream classroom by high school and only 5% requiring full-time special education. This shift toward higher-independence, lower-cost classrooms has substantial implications for cost-benefit analyses of cochlear implantation, as will be discussed below.

In terms of academic achievement, deaf children who receive cochlear implants have substantially better outcomes than their nonimplanted deaf peers. In general, a shorter duration of deafness is associated with improved academic attainment, reading level, academic ability, and classroom participation.[50] Geers and Hayes[51] found that, of 112 high school students who received cochlear implants in childhood for profound SNHL and had at least 10 years experience with their implants, 36% could read at the ninth-grade level. Only 17% read at less than the fourth-grade level, which is the level at which most deaf students scored before the advent of cochlear implantation. Furthermore, on two standardized reading comprehension tests, the Peabody Individual Achievement Test (PIAT) and Test of Reading Comprehension (TORC), 47% and 66% of these students scored at or above the average normal-hearing peer score, respectively. However, the investigators noted that scores on tests of written expression were significantly less than the average scores of normal-hearing peers for more than 50% of the cochlear-implanted students. This finding serves as a reminder that, although deaf children who receive cochlear implants perform better academically than they would without the implants, as a group they have yet to reach performance levels equal to their normal-hearing peers.

Employment Benefits

Employment outcomes for patients who receive cochlear implants in childhood is an area of the literature that is sparse at present, because such data require a minimum of 20 to 30 years of follow-up and it has only been 20 years since widespread cochlear implantation of children began. However, in 2 recent studies that included a small number of adult patients who received cochlear implants in childhood for profound SNHL, the employment levels of these patients were similar to those of their normal-hearing peers.[52,53] There is also evidence from the literature on adult cochlear implantation that cochlear implantation is associated with improved employment outcomes and increases in personal income. In a study of 65 adult cochlear implant recipients, 30.8% were unemployed before cochlear implantation, and this figure decreased to 16.9% following cochlear implantation; these patients also had a statistically significant increase in job satisfaction and confidence at work after implantation.[54] In a study on changes in personal income in adult cochlear implant recipients following cochlear implantation, Monteiro and colleagues[55] reported that median yearly income statistically increased from $30,432 before implantation to $42,672 after implantation.

Quality-of-life Benefits

Cochlear implantation has a profoundly positive impact on a deaf child's quality of life, with benefits seen most clearly in the preteen and teenage years of life. Quality of life (QOL) is defined as an individual's contentment or satisfaction with life.[56] Deaf children have diminished QOL compared with their normal-hearing peers because of feeling less socially accepted, frequently having difficulty making friends, having greater adjustment problems, and being significantly more impulsive.[57] In contrast, Moog and colleagues[58] found that adolescents who undergo cochlear implantation before age 5 years for profound SNHL and have at least 10 years of cochlear implant experience exhibit social skills on par or better than their normal-hearing peers. In addition, 94% participate in sports and other high school activities and 50% hold a part-time job (similar to normal-hearing peers). In a cross-sectional survey of cochlear implant users aged 8 to 16 years and their normal-hearing peers, Loy and colleagues[57] found that overall QOL did not differ between the cochlear implant and normal-hearing groups, further showing that cochlear implantation has the potential to restore normal QOL to deaf children. Similar to other outcome measures of cochlear implantation, Loy and colleagues[57] found that QOL outcomes for cochlear implant users are inversely related to the age at implantation and directly related to the duration of cochlear implant use.

Benefits to Society

Despite the significant benefits that are seen in deaf children with cochlear implants, the cost of undergoing implantation and the necessary rehabilitation that follows remains one of the greatest barriers for a deaf child to undergo timely cochlear implantation.[9] Cheng and colleagues[59] estimated these costs to be approximately $60,000 over the life of the individual (in year 1999 dollars). However, the cost of deafness to society is estimated at more than 1 million dollars (in year 2000 dollars) over the life of one individual, with 67% of this figure caused by lost work productivity and 21% by the costs of special education.[10] Because health care resources are limited, payers require rigorous evidence that a given intervention is worth the resources invested (ie, it is cost-effective).[59]

One simple method of assessing a medical intervention's cost-effectiveness is to compare the intervention's net costs with its net monetary effects; this is termed cost-benefit analysis.[60] As discussed earlier, Francis and colleagues[49] showed that 75% of children who underwent cochlear implantation moved to mainstream classrooms by the time they had 4 or more years of implant experience. Based on this movement to mainstream classrooms and using conservative estimates of the cost of education of profoundly hearing-impaired children, the investigators calculated that cochlear implantation yields net savings of $30,000 to $200,000 per child. However, the total savings to society of cochlear implantation are likely much greater. If lost work productivity in a deaf patient costs society more than 3 times the cost of deaf education, and if cochlear implants are allowing young adults who were implanted as children to attain similar employment levels as their normal-hearing peers, it is reasonable to concluded that the lifetime net savings to society for every deaf child who is implanted is several times the savings seen in education alone.[52,53,59]

Another measure of a medical intervention's cost-effectiveness is cost-utility, which is an intervention's cost per quality-adjusted life-year (QALY) gained.[60] Interventions with a cost-utility less than $20,000 to $25,000 per QALY are considered to be cost-effective.[59] Cheng and colleagues,[59] in a study of 78 profoundly deaf children who received cochlear implants, used 3 different instruments to measure the change in the implanted individuals' QOL from before implantation to after implantation; with these results the investigators then calculated that cochlear implantation has a cost-utility of $5,197 to $9,029 per QALY, indicating that cochlear implantation is very cost-effective. These figures also compare favorably with other medical interventions such as coronary artery bypass grafting ($10,431–$64,033 per QALY), implanted cardiac defibrillator ($29,200 per QALY), and cardiac transplantation ($38,970 per QALY).[61]

RISKS OF COCHLEAR IMPLANTATION

Cochlear implants have made a significant difference in the ability to rehabilitate properly selected hearing-impaired children. However, in addition to evaluating the benefits of cochlear implantation, a decision to proceed with surgery also involves an educated discussion of potential risks so that those risks can be weighed against the expected benefits.

Cochlear implantation is generally well tolerated and has a low rate of complications. The most frequently reported complications occur with a small, but significant and predictable degree of regularity. In descending order of reported incidence, these complications include (1) temporary (or possibly permanent) taste disturbance (19%–45%), (2) need for revision surgery because of device failure (11.2%), (3) wound complications (2.7%–4.8%), and (4) facial nerve stimulation (1%).[62–69]

In addition, there are several other potentially more serious complications that are reported at much less frequent (even remote) rates. When these complications do occur, they are often temporary. These complications include (1) facial nerve injury (0.39%), (2) perilymphatic gusher/cerebrospinal fluid (CSF) fistula (0.25%), (3) postimplantation meningitis (0.115%), and (4) vertigo (0.08%).[65,66]

Taste Disturbance

To obtain adequate access to the middle ear space while protecting the facial nerve, the chorda tympani nerve often must be manipulated, and in some cases it must be divided.[62] Because the chorda tympani nerve provides taste sensation to the anterior two-thirds of the tongue, manipulation or division of this nerve can lead to taste disturbances. In a prospective study of 26 patients who underwent testing of their taste sensation before, 3 days after, and 6 weeks after surgery, 5 (19%) of 26 patients had an immediate postoperative taste disturbance that resolved completely by 6 weeks after surgery.[63] However, one recent study reported this complication at a higher rate. In a retrospective survey by Lloyd and colleagues[62] of 96 adult patients who underwent cochlear implantation, 43 (45%) reported an immediate postoperative taste disturbance; metallic taste and lack of taste were the most commonly reported symptoms. This study reported that a taste disturbance was still present at 51 months after surgery in 18 (19%) of patients. Although these data are not conclusive, it can be inferred that if a taste disturbance occurs following cochlear implantation, it will most likely be transitory. Furthermore, most patients who undergo unilateral division of a chorda tympani nerve retain adequate ability to taste because the contralateral side remains intact. These data may be more significant in cases in which bilateral cochlear implantation is considered.

Revision Cochlear Implantation

Hard or soft failure of a cochlear implant or medical/surgical complications may require a patient to undergo revision cochlear implantation. Cullen and colleagues[64] reported that 107 (11.2%) of 952 children who were implanted over a 15-year period underwent subsequent revision operations during the same time period.[64] Hard failure, defined as complete failure of the cochlear implant, occurred in 49 (46%) of the 107 patients requiring revision. Many of these patients (41%) had a preceding history of head trauma, which may account for the failure of the devices in these patients. Medical and surgical complications accounted for 40 (37%) of the 107 patients undergoing revision. These complications included flap/wound infections or breakdown (50%), electrode extrusion (15%), extracochlear placement of the electrode array (12.5%), and development of cholesteatoma (12.5%). In addition, soft failures, defined as clinical failure of a device while there is still evidence of some auditory input from the device (such as decline in performance), accounted for 16 (15%) of the 107 patients requiring revision. An important finding of this study is that most patients who underwent revision surgery maintained or improved on their best preoperative level of performance after the new implant was in place.[64]

Wound Complications

Complications related to the surgical wound are reported at rates ranging from 2.7% to 4.8%.[65–68] These wound-related complications include infection, flap necrosis, dehiscence of the surgical incision, and extrusion of the receiver-stimulator portion of the implant. These complications are best prevented by administering perioperative antibiotics, avoiding excessive thinning of the skin flaps, not closing the surgical incision under tension, and implanting the receiver-stimulator package at an adequate distance from the surgical incision.[66,69]

Facial Nerve Stimulation

Facial nerve simulation can occur in 1% of children following cochlear implantation because of the close proximity of some of the electrodes to the facial nerve. This problem is usually remedied by reprogramming the patient's implant to not use the offending electrode(s).[65]

Facial Nerve Injury

The facial nerve travels through the operative field and must be navigated carefully during cochlear implantation. This nerve controls the muscles of facial expression and is essential for complete eye closure on the side that is being implanted. Roland[65] reviewed Cochlear Corporation's cumulative data of all complications reported for their devices through July 1998 and found that facial nerve paresis or paralysis occurred in 16 (0.39%) of 4051 children. The number of transient versus permanent injuries was not reported. Roland[65] also reviewed Advanced Bionics' cumulative complication data through July 1998 and found that facial nerve injury occurred in 3 (0.59%) of 510 children; 1 case was caused by a severed facial nerve requiring repair, 1 was a temporary paresis with a full recovery, and 1 was a temporary paresis caused by the electrode array impinging on the facial nerve and resolved completely after repositioning of the electrode array.[65] Facial nerve injury is best avoided by obtaining preoperative imaging and maintaining good surgical technique.[66]

Perilymph Gusher/CSF Leak

Perilymph gusher refers to persistent, often difficult to control leakage of CSF from the perilymphatic space when this space is opened to place the electrode array into the cochlea; this complication is more likely to occur in patients who have congenital malformations of the cochlea.[66] Perilymph gushers must be sealed when encountered to reduce the risk of postoperative meningitis or persistent CSF leak.[66] Overall, this complication is rare, occurring in 10 (0.25%) of 4051 children.[65] The possibility of it occurring can be anticipated by obtaining preoperative imaging of the temporal bones, which identifies malformations of the cochlea.

Postimplantation Meningitis

Meningitis is a severe but rare occurrence following cochlear implantation. A review of Cochlear Corporation's cumulative data from 1982 to 2002 showed that 19 of 16,500 North American patients who received a cochlear implant (children and adults) developed meningitis.[66] This translates into an incidence of meningitis of 18.1 per 100,000/y, which is higher than the incidence of meningitis in the general North American population, which is 2.4 to 10 per 100,000/y.[66] If patients known to be at high risk for meningitis are excluded from the calculation, such as those with cochlear malformations, the incidence of meningitis in the cochlear implant population decreases to 3.9 per 100,000/y.[66] Although there has been debate as to the role of cochlear implantation in causing or predisposing patients to postimplantation meningitis,[5,66] two recent studies by Wei and colleagues[70,71] showed that cochlear-implanted rats were at significantly increased risk of developing bacterial meningitis compared with nonimplanted rats when exposed to S pneumoniae; this risk was significantly reduced by preimplantation vaccination of the rats with the 23-valent pneumococcal polysaccharide vaccine (PPSV23). S pneumoniae is currently responsible for approximately 50% of cases of community-acquired bacterial meningitis; before the development of the H influenzae type b (Hib) vaccine, *H influenzae* was the predominant bacterial pathogen.[66] Therefore, it is important that all children be vaccinated against both of these bacteria before undergoing cochlear implantation. In 2010, the FDA approved the 13-valent pneumococcal conjugate vaccine (PCV13) to replace the 7-valent pneumococcal conjugate vaccine (PCV7).[72] Similar to previous recommendations for the PCV7 vaccine, children less than 2 years old should receive the PCV13 vaccine, children 2 years to 5 years 11 months old should receive both the PCV13 and PPSV23 vaccines, and children 6 years old or older should receive the PPSV23 vaccine.[72] Patients aged 2 years to 5 years 11 months who previously received the full PCV7 vaccine series should receive a single dose of the PCV13 vaccine; furthermore, all patients 6 to 18 years of age who have cochlear implants may receive a single dose of the PCV13 vaccine, regardless of whether or not they have received the PCV7 or PPSV23 vaccines.[72] In addition, all children less than 5 years old should receive the Hib vaccine.[17,66]

Vertigo

Postoperative vertigo is rare in children and is usually transient in nature. Roland[65] found that it was only reported in 7 (0.08%) of 4051 children who underwent cochlear implantation. If vertigo is persistent or severe, a perilymph fistula should be considered.[66]

OTHER MEDICAL/SURGICAL CONSIDERATIONS

Once patients have received a cochlear implant, monopolar cautery can no longer be used in the head and neck region.[17] This is because of the potential for injury to the electrode array or to the cochlea should current travel from the surgical instrument to the electrode array or receiver-stimulator as it passes through the body. Bipolar cautery can be used safely in these patients.[17]

After cochlear implantation, patients must avoid magnetic resonance imaging, although some of the newest implants can be used in low-tesla magnetic fields if left fully in place, and in up to 1.5-telsa fields if the internal magnet is removed surgically before the scan.[73]

Children with cochlear implants are less susceptible to episodes of otitis media in the implanted ear (or both ears for children with bilateral implants); this is thought to be caused by a therapeutic effect from the mastoidectomy that is performed as part of the implantation procedure.[65] Six to 8 weeks after implantation of a structurally normal ear, the risk of otitis media leading to a serious inner ear infection is no higher than that in a normal, nonimplanted ear; however, the risk of serious infection is high if otitis media occurs in the implanted ear within 6 to 8 weeks after surgery.[66] Therefore, otitis media outside of this 6 to 8-week postoperative window can be managed with antibiotics in the same manner as for nonimplanted children (more aggressive therapy is needed for otitis media within the 6 to 8-week window). If episodes of otitis media become frequent, tympanostomy tubes may be placed with the same indications as for nonimplanted children.[74]

RECENT ADVANCES
Bilateral Cochlear Implantation

In the last decade there has been a significant increase in the number of patients who receive bilateral cochlear implants. Initial interest in providing a deaf patient with two implants arose from the recognition that hearing is better if patients have the opportunity to use both ears instead of just one. This observation is true for normal-hearing individuals and it is also true for patients with hearing aids. Therefore, it follows that bilateral cochlear implantation for patients with bilateral deafness should provide better rehabilitation. Numerous studies have been conducted in children in the last decade, and the evidence shows that patients who receive bilateral cochlear implants have superior abilities to localize sound and to understand speech in noisy environments than their unilaterally implanted peers.[4,75–77] Additional benefits for bilateral implantation compared with unilateral implantation include ensuring that the better ear is always implanted and that the patient has a backup should one implant lose power, malfunction, or fail.[75,76] The greatest amount of benefit of bilateral implantation is seen in patients who are implanted at less than 3 years of age and in those who undergo either simultaneous bilateral implantation or sequential bilateral implantation with a duration of less than 12 months between receiving the first and second implants.[77] The disadvantages of bilateral implantation include an increased time of surgery or requirement of 2 separate surgeries, failure to preserve one ear for possible future therapies, and increased expense of implantation.[75] Nevertheless, a growing number of experts in both North America and Europe think that the advantages of bilateral cochlear implantation often outweigh the disadvantages. There has been a recent consensus statement among leaders of European cochlear implant centers that "the infant or child with unambiguous cochlear implant candidacy should receive bilateral cochlear implants simultaneously as soon as possible after definitive diagnosis of deafness to permit optimal auditory development."[4]

Cochlear Implantation for Partial Deafness

Cochlear implantation has traditionally been considered only for patients with bilateral profound deafness. However, in the past decade, cochlear implantation has been shown to be beneficial for patients with some degree of residual hearing as well. In particular, there are some partially deaf patients who have normal or nearly normal low-frequency hearing but who have severe to profound high-frequency hearing loss. These patients often struggle to find a satisfactory solution for rehabilitating their hearing. For these partially deaf patients, hearing aids fail to provide adequate amplification of the higher frequencies necessary for oral communication. In addition, these patients have traditionally not been considered candidates for cochlear implantation because of concern that cochlear implantation may damage the delicate cochlear structures and cause them to lose their residual low-frequency hearing.[78] In the early 2000s, research on adult patients with partial deafness showed that a shortened electrode array could be inserted atraumatically into the cochlea, preserving a patient's low-frequency hearing in most cases, allowing for electrical stimulation in the high frequencies while preserving natural hearing in the lower frequencies.[78,79] This hybrid cochlear implantation technique is based on the way cochlea and spiral ganglion neurons are arranged in the cochlea such that the high frequencies are detected at the base of the cochlea and low frequencies at the apex; thus a shortened electrode implanted at the base of the cochlea reaches the high-frequency spiral ganglion neurons but leaves the apex of the cochlea undisturbed and able to be stimulated in the natural, acoustic manner.[78,80] The patients are then able to use a combination of both a hearing aid or natural hearing for low-frequency hearing and the cochlear implant for high-frequency hearing in the same ear. The high-frequency electrical stimulation provides better speech discrimination, whereas the preserved low-frequency natural hearing provides better environmental awareness and music appreciation than would otherwise be present.[78,79] Inspired by these results, Skarzynski began implanting partially deaf children as young as 4 years of age in Poland in 2004. In 2010, Skarzynski and Lorens[80] reported that, in 84 partially deaf patients (63 adults and 21 children) who received cochlear implants for combined electric and acoustic hearing (EAS), residual hearing was preserved in 97% of patients and, at 12 months after implantation, average single-word recognition increased from 34% to 73% in quiet and from 7% to 54% in noise.[80] For the first group of 9 partially deaf children, the average word recognition scores increased from 30% to 69% in quiet and from 5% to 62% in noise at 12 months after surgery.[80,81] These preliminary results indicate that EAS is likely the best alternative for partially deafened patients of all ages who obtain unsatisfactory hearing results with hearing aids alone.

SUMMARY

Cochlear implants have been widely used for treatment of childhood deafness for more than 20 years. In that time, cochlear implantation has proved to be both safe and highly effective at providing the ability for children with severe to profound deafness to hear and understand speech, and is now considered to be standard of care in the treatment of these patients.

As described earlier, there seems to be a critical window of time in early childhood during which cochlear implantation should be performed to obtain the best outcomes. Although the precise upper limit of that window of time has yet to be established, it seems to be within the first 6 months to 3 years of age, with many investigators arguing that younger is better. It is therefore important that potential candidates be referred for evaluation early. Lester and colleagues[82] found that the primary reasons for delay of cochlear implantation until after 2 years of age included slow referrals for care and parental delays. In addition, lack of newborn hearing screening, failure of the newborn hearing screen to identify hearing loss, and Medicaid insurance alone or in combination with private insurance were risk factors for delayed implantation. These data underscore the importance of every newborn child undergoing hearing screening to identify deaf children at birth and of the need for parent, health care provider, and health care payer education about the indications, important benefits, and reasonable risks of cochlear implantation for deaf children.

REFERENCES

1. Wilson BS, Dorman MF. The design of cochlear implants. In: Niparko JK, editor. Cochlear implants: principles & practice. 2nd edition. Philadelphia: Lippincott Williams & Wilkins; 2009. p. 95–135.
2. Kral A, O'Donoghue GM. Profound deafness in childhood. N Engl J Med 2010; 363:1438–50.
3. Yoon PJ. Pediatric cochlear implantation. Curr Opin Pediatr 2011;23:346–50.
4. Ramsden JD, Gordon K, Aschendorff A, et al. European bilateral pediatric cochlear implant forum consensus statement. Otol Neurotol 2012;33:561–5.
5. Balkany TJ, Brown KD, Gantz BJ. Cochlear implantation: medical and surgical considerations. In: Flint PW, Haughey BH, Lund VJ, et al, editors. Cummings otolaryngology—head and neck surgery. 5th edition. Philadelphia: Mosby Elsevier; 2010. p. 2234–42.
6. Baldassari CM, Schmidt C, Schubert CM, et al. Receptive language outcomes in children after cochlear implantation. Otolaryngol Head Neck Surg 2009;140: 114–9.
7. Harris JP, Anderson JP, Novak R. An outcomes study of cochlear implants in deaf patients: audiologic, economic, and quality-of-life changes. Arch Otolaryngol Head Neck Surg 1995;121:398–404.

8. Blanchfield BB, Feldman JJ, Dunbar JL, et al. The severely to profoundly hearing-impaired population in the United States: prevalence estimates and demographics. J Am Acad Audiol 2001;12:183–9.

9. Parisier SC. Cochlear implants: growing pains. Laryngoscope 2003;113: 1470–2.

10. Mohr PE, Feldman JJ, Dunbar JL, et al. The societal costs of severe to profound hearing loss in the United States. Int J Technol Assess Health Care 2000;16: 1120–35.

11. Clark JH, Wang NY, Riley AW, et al. Timing of cochlear implantation and parents' global ratings of children's health and development. Otol Neurotol 2012;33: 545–52.

12. Geers AE, Brenner CA, Tobey EA. Long-term outcomes of cochlear implantation in early childhood: sample characteristics and data collection methods. Ear Hear 2011;32:2S–12S.

13. Geers AE, Moog JS, Biedenstein J, et al. Spoken language scores of children using cochlear implants compared to hearing age-mates at school entry. J Deaf Stud Deaf Educ 2009;14:371–85.

14. Almond M, Brown DJ. The pathology and etiology of sensorineural hearing loss and implications for cochlear implantation. In: Niparko JK, editor. Cochlear implants: principles & practice. 2nd edition. Philadelphia: Lippincott Williams & Wilkins; 2009. p. 43–81.

15. Berlin CI, Morlet T, Hood LJ. Auditory neuropathy/dyssynchrony: its diagnosis and management. Pediatr Clin North Am 2003;50:331–40.

16. Carlson ML, Driscoll CL, Gifford RH, et al. Cochlear implantation: current and future device options. Otolaryngol Clin North Am 2012;45:221–48.

17. Tucci DL, Pilkington TM. Medical and surgical aspects of cochlear implantation. In: Niparko JK, editor. Cochlear implants: principles & practice. 2nd edition. Philadelphia: Lippincott Williams & Wilkins; 2009. p. 161–86.

18. Leigh J, Dettman S, Dowell R, et al. Evidence-based approach for making cochlear implant recommendations for infants with residual hearing. Ear Hear 2011;32:313–22.

19. Heman-Ackah SE, Roland JT, Haynes DS, et al. Pediatric cochlear implantation: candidacy evaluation, medical and surgical considerations, and expanding criteria. Otolaryngol Clin North Am 2012;45:41–67.

20. Cosetti MK, Waltzman SB. Outcomes in cochlear implantation: variables affecting performance in adults and children. Otolaryngol Clin North Am 2012; 45:155–71.

21. Ganek H, Robbins AM, Niparko JK. Language outcomes after cochlear implantation. Otolaryngol Clin North Am 2012;45:173–85.

22. Sharma A, Dorman MF, Spahr AJ. Rapid development of cortical auditory evoked potentials after early cochlear implantation. Neuroreport 2002;13: 1365–8.

23. Flexer C. Cochlear implants and neuroplasticity: linking auditory exposure and practice. Cochlear Implants Int 2011;12(Suppl 1):S19–21.

24. Colletti L, Mandalà M, Colletti V. Cochlear implants in children younger than 6 months. Otolaryngol Head Neck Surg 2012;147:139–46.

25. Govaerts PJ, De Beukelaer C, Daemers K, et al. Outcome of cochlear implantation at different ages from 0 to 6 years. Otol Neurotol 2002;23:885–90.

26. Tajudeen BA, Waltzman SB, Jethanamest D, et al. Speech perception in congenitally deaf children receiving cochlear implants in the first year of life. Otol Neurotol 2010;31:1254–60.

27. Robins AM, Rensaw JJ, Berry SW. Evaluating meaningful auditory integration in profoundly hearing-impaired children. Am J Otol 1991;12(Suppl):144–50.
28. Archbold S, Lutman M, Marshall D. Categories of auditory performance. Ann Otol Rhinol Laryngol 1995;104(Suppl 166):312–4.
29. Helms J, Muller J, Schon F, et al. Evaluation of performance with the COMBI40 cochlear implant in adults: a multicentric clinical study. ORL J Otorhinolaryngol Relat Spec 1997;59:23–35.
30. Davidson LS, Geers AE, Blamey PJ, et al. Factors contributing to speech perception scores in long-term pediatric cochlear implant users. Ear Hear 2011;32:19S–26S.
31. Uziel AS, Sillon M, Vieu A, et al. Ten-year follow-up of a consecutive series of children with multichannel cochlear implants. Otol Neurotol 2007;28:615–28.
32. Worthington DW, Stelmachowicz P, Larson L, et al. Language and learning skills of hearing-impaired students: audiological evaluation. ASHA Monogr 1986;23: 12–20.
33. Clinkard D, Shipp D, Friesen LM, et al. Telephone use and the factors influencing it among cochlear implant patients. Cochlear Implants Int 2011;12:140–6.
34. Cray JW, Allen RL, Stuart A, et al. An investigation of telephone use among cochlear implant recipients. Am J Audiol 2004;13:200–12.
35. Nicholas JG, Geers AE. Will they catch up? The role of age at cochlear implantation in the spoken language development of children with severe to profound hearing loss. J Speech Lang Hear Res 2007;50:1048–62.
36. Kluwin TN, Stewart DA. Cochlear implants for younger children: a preliminary description of the parental decision process and outcomes. Am Ann Deaf 2000;145:26–32.
37. Niparko JK, Tobey EA, Thal DJ, et al. Spoken language development in children following cochlear implantation. JAMA 2010;303:1498–506.
38. Robbins AM, Svirsky M, Kirk KI. Children with implants can speak, but can they communicate? Otolaryngol Head Neck Surg 1997;117:155–60.
39. Osberger MJ. Language and learning skills of hearing-impaired students: summary and implications for research and educational management. ASHA Monogr 1986;23:92–8.
40. Levitt H, McGarr N, Geffner D. Development of language and communication skills in hearing-impaired children: concluding commentary. ASHA Monogr 1987;26:140–5.
41. Reynell JK, Huntley M. Reynell developmental language scales. 2nd edition. Windsor (United Kingdom): NFER Publishing; 1985.
42. Reynell J, Huntley RM. New scales for the assessment of language development in young children. J Learn Disabil 1971;4:549–57.
43. Reynell JK. Reynell developmental language scales. Manual (Exper. Ed.). Windsor (United Kingdom): NFER Publishing; 1969.
44. Svirsky MA, Robbins AM, Kirk KI. Language development in profoundly deaf children with cochlear implants. Psychol Sci 2000;11:153–8.
45. Geers AE, Sedey AL. Language and verbal reasoning skills in adolescents with 10 or more years of cochlear implant experience. Ear Hear 2011;32:39S–48S.
46. Watson LM, Archbold SM, Nikolopoulos TP. Children's communication mode five years after cochlear implantation: changes over time according to age at implant. Cochlear Implants Int 2006;7:77–91.
47. Tobey EA, Geers AE, Sundarrajan M, et al. Factors influencing speech production in elementary and high school-aged cochlear implant users. Ear Hear 2011; 32:27S–38S.

48. Koch ME, Wyatt JR, Francis HW, et al. A model of educational resource use by children with cochlear implants. Otolaryngol Head Neck Surg 1997;117:174–9.

49. Francis HW, Koch ME, Wyatt JR, et al. Trends in educational placement and cost-benefit considerations in children with cochlear implants. Arch Otolaryngol Head Neck Surg 1999;125:499–505.

50. Bond M, Mealing S, Anderson R, et al. The effectiveness and cost-effectiveness of cochlear implants for severe to profound deafness in children and adults: a systematic review and economic model. Health Technol Assess 2009;13:1–330.

51. Geers AE, Hayes H. Reading, writing, and phonological processing skills of adolescents with 10 or more years of cochlear implant experience. Ear Hear 2011; 32:49S–59S.

52. Beadle EA, McKinley DJ, Nikolopoulos TP, et al. Long-term functional outcomes and academic-occupational status in implanted children after 10 to 14 years of cochlear implant use. Otol Neurotol 2005;26:1152–60.

53. Venail F, Vieu A, Artieres F, et al. Educational and employment achievements in prelingually deaf children who receive cochlear implants. Arch Otolaryngol Head Neck Surg 2010;136:366–72.

54. Fazel MZ, Gray RF. Patient employment status and satisfaction following cochlear implantation. Cochlear Implants Int 2007;8:87–91.

55. Monteiro E, Shipp D, Chen J. Cochlear implantation: a personal and societal economic perspective examining the effects of cochlear implantation on personal income. J Otolaryngol Head Neck Surg 2012;41:S43–8.

56. Lin FR, Niparko JK. Measuring health-related quality of life after pediatric cochlear implantation: a systematic review. Int J Pediatr Otorhinolaryngol 2006;70:1695–706.

57. Loy B, Warner AD, Tong L, et al. The children speak: an examination of the quality of life of pediatric cochlear implant users. Otolaryngol Head Neck Surg 2010; 142:247–53.

58. Moog JS, Geers AE, Gustus CH. Psychosocial adjustment in adolescents who have used cochlear implants since preschool. Ear Hear 2011;32:75S–83S.

59. Cheng AK, Rubin HR, Powe NR, et al. Cost-utility analysis of the cochlear implant in children. JAMA 2000;284:850–6.

60. Lin FR, Niparko JK, Francis HW. Outcomes in cochlear implantation: assessment of quality-of-life impact and economic evaluation of the benefits of the cochlear implant in relation to costs. In: Niparko JK, editor. Cochlear implants: principles & practice. 2nd edition. Philadelphia: Lippincott Williams & Wilkins; 2009. p. 229–44.

61. Wyatt JR, Niparko JK, Rothman ML, et al. Cost effectiveness of the multichannel cochlear implant. Am J Otol 1995;16:52–62.

62. Lloyd S, Meerton L, Di Cuffa R, et al. Taste change following cochlear implantation. Cochlear Implants Int 2007;8:203–10.

63. Alzhrani F, Lenarz T, Teschner M. Taste sensation following cochlear implantation surgery. Cochlear Implants Int 2012. [Epub ahead of print].

64. Cullen RD, Fayad JN, Luxford WM, et al. Revision cochlear implant surgery in children. Otol Neurotol 2008;29:214–20.

65. Roland JT. Complications of cochlear implant surgery. In: Waltzman S, Cohen N, editors. Cochlear implants. New York: Thieme; 2000. p. 171–5.

66. Clark G. Surgery. In: Cochlear implants: fundamentals and applications. New York: Springer-Verlag; 2003. p. 595–653.

67. Johnston JC, Smith AD, Fitzpatrick E, et al. Estimation of risks associated with paediatric cochlear implantation. Cochlear Implants Int 2010;11:146–69.

68. Francis HW, Buchman CA, Visaya JM, et al. Surgical factors in pediatric cochlear implantation and their early effects of electrode activation and functional outcomes. Otol Neurotol 2008;29:502–8.
69. Luxford WL, Cullen RD. Surgery for cochlear implantation. In: Brackmann DE, Shelton C, Arriaga MA, editors. Otologic surgery. 3rd edition. Philadelphia: Saunders Elsevier; 2010. p. 373–81.
70. Wei BP, Shepherd RK, Robins-Browne RM, et al. Threshold shift: effects of cochlear implantation on the risk of pneumococcal meningitis. Otolaryngol Head Neck Surg 2007;136:589–96.
71. Wei BP, Shepherd RK, Robins-Browne RM, et al. Assessment of the protective effect of the pneumococcal vaccination in preventing meningitis after cochlear implantation. Arch Otolaryngol Head Neck Surg 2007;133:987–94.
72. Centers for Disease Control and Prevention. Licensure of a 13-valent pneumococcal conjugate vaccine (PCV13) and recommendations for use among children – Advisory Committee on Immunization Practices (ACIP), 2010. MMWR Morb Mortal Wkly Rep 2010;59:258–61.
73. Fritsch MH, Mosier KM. MRI compatibility issues in otology. Curr Opin Otolaryngol Head Neck Surg 2007;15:335–40.
74. Preciado D, Choi S. Management of acute otitis media in cochlear implant recipients: to tube or not to tube? Laryngoscope 2012;122:709–10.
75. Basura GJ, Eapen R, Buchman CA. Bilateral cochlear implantation: current concepts, indications, and results. Laryngoscope 2009;119:2395–401.
76. Lovett RE, Kitterick PT, Hewitt CE, et al. Bilateral or unilateral cochlear implantation for deaf children: an observational study. Arch Dis Child 2010;95:107–12.
77. Gordon KA, Papsin BC. Benefits of short interimplant delays in children receiving bilateral cochlear implants. Otol Neurotol 2009;30:319–31.
78. Wilson BS. Partial deafness cochlear implantation (PDCI) and electric-acoustic stimulation (EAS). Cochlear Implants Int 2010;11(Suppl 1):56–66.
79. Lorens A, Polak M, Piotrowska A, et al. Outcomes of treatment of partial deafness with cochlear implantation: a DUET study. Laryngoscope 2008;118:288–94.
80. Skarzynski H, Lorens A. Partial deafness treatment. Cochlear Implants Int 2010;11(Suppl 1):29–41.
81. Skarzynski H, Lorens A, Piotrowska A, et al. Partial deafness cochlear implantation in children. Int J Pediatr Otorhinolaryngol 2007;71:1407–13.
82. Lester EB, Dawson JD, Gantz BJ. Barriers to the ear cochlear implantation of deaf children. Otol Neurotol 2011;32:406–12.

Laryngopharyngeal Reflux Disease in Children

Naren N. Venkatesan, MD, Harold S. Pine, MD,
Michael Underbrink, MD*

KEYWORDS

- Laryngopharyngeal reflux disease • Extraesophageal reflux disease • Diagnosis

KEY POINTS

- Extraesophageal symptoms of gastroesophageal reflux disease (GERD) have long been recognized and referred to as laryngopharyngeal reflux disease (LPRD).
- Despite its similarities with GERD, LPRD has been more difficult to diagnose accurately and consistently.
- This variability has made creating comprehensive treatment guidelines difficult.
- Currently, the treatment of LPRD seems to provide symptomatic benefits as well as improvements in these concomitant diseases.
- LPRD should be considered as a chronic disease with a variety of presentations.

INTRODUCTION

Gastroesophageal reflux disease (GERD) is a complex problem in the pediatric population and has received significant attention in the literature. Extraesophageal reflux disease, commonly called laryngopharyngeal reflux disease (LPRD), continues to be an entity with more questions than answers. Although the role of LPRD has been implicated in various pediatric diseases, it has been inadequately studied in others. LPRD is believed to contribute to failure to thrive, laryngomalacia, recurrent respiratory papillomatosis (RRP), chronic cough, hoarseness, esophagitis, and aspiration among other pathologies.

Although the exact prevalence is unknown, it is estimated that nearly 1 in 5 children likely suffers from reflux disease.[1] Currently, given that childhood obesity is on the increase, and with the association between obesity and reflux, it is likely that the incidence is increasing. As our understanding of various diseases of the aerodigestive tract increases, the role of reflux as a contributing factor continues to gain attention. Although the definitions have not changed dramatically, knowledge regarding the

Department of Otolaryngology—Head and Neck Surgery, University of Texas Medical Branch, 301 University Boulevard, Route 0521, Galveston, TX 77555, USA
* Corresponding author.
E-mail address: mpunderb@utmb.edu

Pediatr Clin N Am 60 (2013) 865–878
http://dx.doi.org/10.1016/j.pcl.2013.04.011   **pediatric.theclinics.com**

benefits of treating LPRD as a contributing factor in many afflictions of the upper aero-digestive tract has certainly increased.

LPRD is defined by the reflux of either gastric acid or refluxate (containing pepsin) into the larynx, oropharynx, and/or nasopharynx.[2] Although once believed to be an extension of gastroesophageal reflux disease, the differences in symptoms, findings, and treatments has led to the evolution of LPRD as a unique and distinct disease process.[3] It is a disease classically diagnosed by symptomatology in the patient. Although confirmation of the disease requires objective findings on various tests, including endoscopy, pH probes, and radiographic studies, a high index of suspicion must be maintained to diagnose the child.

Although LPRD is present in both infants and younger children, it usually presents with a different set of symptoms depending on age (**Box 1**). Infants typically present with regurgitation, vomiting, dysphagia, anorexia, failure to thrive, apnea, recurrent croup, laryngomalacia, subglottic stenosis, or chronic respiratory issues. School-age children tend to demonstrate chronic cough, dyspnea, dysphonia, persistent sore throat, halitosis, and globus sensation. Older children may also complain of regurgitation, heartburn, vomiting, nausea, or have chronic respiratory issues. The symptoms in these children tend to bridge the gap between those seen in infants and those in teenagers/adults.[2] Certain complaints, including dysphagia, vomiting,

---

Box 1
Various extraesophageal manifestations of GERD

Infants

Failure to thrive

Wheezing

Stridor

Persistent cough

Apnea

Feeding difficulties

Aspiration

Regurgitation

Recurrent croup

Children

Cough

Hoarseness

Stridor

Sore throat

Asthma

Vomiting

Globus sensation

Wheezing

Aspiration

Recurrent pneumonia

regurgitation, dyspnea, and globus sensation, are more broad. The role and manifestations of LPRD in specific disease processes requires further attention (**Box 2**).

IMPAIRED SWALLOWING AND ASPIRATION

In infants, swallowing is a highly coordinated function requiring the infant to perform and coordinate the actions of suck-swallow-breathe, in that order, to avoid aspiration.[4] Performing this sequence requires an intact laryngeal sensation, which explains why children with neurologic deficits tend to have greater feeding difficulties and increased episodes of microaspirations.

Understanding the effects of reflux on the larynx is the key to better treatment of the neonate and infant. The supraglottic mucosa must be able to sense the upcoming food bolus. This sensation leads to appropriate vocal fold closure, while also stimulating the opening of the hypopharynx and upper esophageal sphincter. This highly sensitive mechanism is important at all ages, but more so in newborns as they begin to learn cognitive functioning. Edema from chronic irritation by gastric aspirate causes decreased sensation in these tissues, and thereby increases the risk of aspiration in these patients.[5-7]

Testing of the laryngeal adductor reflex can be checked by endoscopy combined with a pulse of air to the aryepiglottic folds to simulate a food bolus. This testing begins with a pressure of 2.5 mm Hg and gradually increases in increments of 0.5 mm Hg to 10 mm Hg. The goal is to identify at what pressure the reflex is triggered, with a positive response being a cough or break in respiration. The need for greater than 4.5 mm Hg of pressure to obtain a positive response is suggestive of microaspiration and poor laryngeal adductor reflex in children.

Suskind and colleagues[4] showed significant improvement in videofluoroscopic swallow evaluations and pharyngeal impairment scores when infants with swallowing issues were treated for GERD. Aviv and colleagues[5] demonstrated that just 3 months of GERD treatment was sufficient time to demonstrate normalization of laryngopharyngeal sensation. This improvement in turn led to improved swallowing function and decreased posterior laryngeal edema. In addition to antireflux medication, thickening of feeds has always been a traditional method of preventing microaspiration. Thickening helps by improving overall laryngopharyngeal sensing of the bolus and thus improves the coordination of swallowing.[8,9]

Box 2
Diseases affected by reflux

Subglottic stenosis

Laryngomalacia

Asthma

Recurrent otitis media

Vocal cord nodules

Vocal cord granuloma

Eosinophilic esophagitis

Allergic rhinitis

Recurrent respiratory papillomatosis

Although swallowing is a highly coordinated activity, laryngopharyngeal reflux likely plays a role in dysfunction of the swallow reflex and therefore requires treatment. Currently, there are no universally accepted methods for evaluating the role of LPRD in these patients, although fiber-optic endoscopy can provide visual clues of changes in the larynx. Empirical trials of a proton pump inhibitor and thickening of feeds can delineate the role of LPRD and therefore benefit the child in most cases.

LARYNGOMALACIA

In the pediatric population, laryngomalacia is one of the most common causes of airway distress.[10] It typically presents as inspiratory stridor, coughing, choking, or regurgitation. The lack of inherent strength in the larynx leads to collapse of tissues and subsequent upper airway obstruction. A recent meta-analysis[11] showed that 65% of patients with severe laryngomalacia had reflux. Further analysis revealed that those children with moderate to severe laryngomalacia were nearly 10 times more likely to suffer from reflux than those with only mild laryngomalacia. The proposed mechanism is that aerophagia during feedings causes gastric distention leading to vagal reflexes followed by postprandial vomiting and regurgitation.

The increased association between laryngomalacia and reflux has led to the question of whether reflux causes laryngomalacia or is simply present concurrently. Although supraglottic biopsies did show mild intraepithelial infiltrate, pathognomonic for reflux, the gross morphologic changes did not seem to correspond to laryngomalacia.[12,13] These findings only seem to confuse the issue regarding the role of reflux in laryngomalacia. On the other hand, 2 studies using 24-hour dual-probe pH manometry showed 100% correlation between laryngomalacia and reflux, where reflux is defined as at least 1 episode of pH less than 4 for at least 4 seconds.[14,15] Unfortunately, there is still some uncertainty regarding the role of pharyngeal pH monitoring in these patients. Little and colleagues[16] demonstrated that nearly half of patients with extraesophageal reflux were only accurately diagnosed after pharyngeal monitoring and a negative esophageal study. Rabinowitz and colleagues[17] stated that

> Beyond its value in clinical practice, upper esophageal reflux testing should be employed in research studies that evaluate the impact of GER [gastroesophageal reflux] therapy on ENT [ear, nose, and throat] symptoms.

Although several retrospective studies have reported an improvement in laryngomalacia symptoms (cough, stridor, choking) with antireflux treatment, a prospective trial done by Thompson[15] indicates a strong correlation between reflux treatment and decreased laryngomalacia symptoms. Three levels of laryngomalacia severity were categorized, ranging from mild (inconsequential stridor during feeding) to moderate (inspiratory stridor, no failure to thrive, and inconsequential dyspnea, cyanosis, or brief apneas) to severe (inspiratory stridor and life-threatening complications). Nearly 89% of patients in the moderate and severe groups showed improvement in coughing and choking after 7.3 months of GERD therapy. Improvements in regurgitation were reported in nearly 70% of patients.

These findings seem to encourage the treatment of laryngomalacia with LPRD. However, resolution of symptoms may simply be attributed to the natural course of the disease. Thompson[18] commented on the natural history of laryngomalacia in infants, noting, "Symptoms worsen at 4–8 months, improve between 8 and 12 months, and usually resolve by 12–18 months of age." The mean age at diagnosis for patients in the 2007 study was older than 3 months (102.8 days). Therefore, it seems possible that many of the symptom improvements reported in this study reflect the natural history of the disease. No studies have compared the outcome of patients with laryngomalacia treated for LPRD with those who receive no treatment. In summary, although further studies are needed, treatment of laryngomalacia with antireflux therapy may be beneficial. Each patient should be evaluated independently by an otolaryngologist to determine disease severity and decide on therapy.

SUBGLOTTIC STENOSIS

Subglottic stenosis typically presents in the neonate/infant with recurrent crouplike episodes and chronic cough. Often, these patients may not demonstrate any difficulty breathing at rest; however, episodes of dyspnea and stridor can quickly develop, caused by the limited airway circumference in young children, which cannot handle even minimal inflammatory insults. Three major causes of subglottic stenosis are trauma, infection, and LPRD.[19]

The role of LPRD in causing subglottic stenosis has been studied in canine models, giving it significant credence; however, the effect of acid and pepsin on the human subglottic mucosa has not been as thoroughly studied. The formation of vocal cord granulomas has long been known as a sequela of reflux, and these same histologic changes were noted in early subglottic stenosis lesions.[20] Although irritation and mucosal damage begin the stenosis process, the role of reflux in preventing reepithelialization should not be understated.[21] Further studies have demonstrated the effect of reflux at the cellular level, including downregulation of epidermal growth factor receptor, which reduces mucosal turnover, increased transforming growth factor $\beta1$, which causes fibroblast differentiation, and excessive connective tissue deposition.[22,23]

Although the correlation between reflux and subglottic mucosal changes has been evaluated, no prospective data are available to better correlate the clinical relationship. Reports of children whose stridor and degree of stenosis decreases with reflux management advocate for LPRD treatment in this patient population.[24] Reviews show that nearly two-thirds of children with subglottic stenosis have reflux disease to some extent.[24-31] Furthermore, subglottic stenosis correlates with reflux disease with a relative risk of 2.5.[26-28,32] In 1 study, nearly one-third of patients with subglottic stenosis who were treated for reflux were able to avoid surgical intervention.[24] With these findings and correlations in mind, early evaluation for and treatment of LPRD may lead to prevention of disease progression and should be encouraged in patients with subglottic stenosis.

RRP

RRP is a complex, often prolonged, infection of the upper airway by the human papilloma virus. The complexity of this disease is beyond the scope of this article; however, LPRD treatment provides benefit to these patients. There has been increased anecdotal evidence in the literature of cases where children with mild to moderate LPRD have shown improvement or even resolution of disease with antireflux therapy.[33,34] The ciliated respiratory epithelium of the larynx has increased sensitivity when chronically exposed to pepsin and gastric refluxate. This increased sensitivity may contribute to more advanced presentations of the disease or a more frequent need for surgical debridement. Some of the concerning findings in disease progression of RRP, such as laryngeal webs, may be diminished or even prevented if these children receive antireflux therapy.[35] Although treatment of RRP with LPRD therapy alone is not recommended, ensuring that these patients are placed on adjuvant antireflux therapy may help to minimize the consequences or progression of their disease and in some cases may even lead to resolution.

ASTHMA

Because of concerns about the airway often noted in children with LPRD, asthma and the role of treatment of LPRD to improve asthma has been postulated. It has been estimated that gastroesophageal reflux may be present in 40% to 80% of children with asthma.[36] There is a growing belief that rhinitis and asthma are often present together, and that rhinitis can cause laryngeal changes that may mimic LPRD changes. Therefore, when evaluating asthmatics for LPRD with laryngoscopy, strict criteria should be used, such as limiting positive findings to vocal cord nodules and granulomas.[37] Among asthmatic adults and children, LPRD changes in the larynx have been identified on laryngoscopy in nearly 70% of cases.[37,38] Thus, any patient with suspected LPRD in addition to asthma and/or allergic rhinitis should undergo pH probe testing to confirm the diagnosis.

The use of β-agonists has also been studied as a possible trigger for reflux by reducing the tone of the lower esophageal sphincter.[39] However, a recent study seems to prove that no such correlation exists.[37] Another belief was that uncontrolled asthma may worsen LPRD, but it seems that children with asthma, whether controlled or uncontrolled, have similar rates of LPRD.[16] From the literature to date, the main concept to note is that these 2 conditions, LPRD and asthma, are often present together, and they both require treatment. The effect of treatment of one on the status of the other unfortunately requires further research.

HOARSENESS

Although laryngopharyngeal reflux is often described as a significant contributor to adult hoarseness, its role in children has not been as well established. Vocal cord nodules are widely considered to be the most common cause of pediatric hoarseness.[40] Various studies have begun to question whether LPRD should be given greater consideration as a cause of this problem. Gumpert and colleagues[41] counted interarytenoid edema or chronic inflammation as a sign of LPRD and found these findings in 90% of children with hoarseness. Although this was a retrospective study, it does consider the prevalence of at least some LPRD changes in children with hoarseness.

A possible explanation as to why LPRD can often be underdiagnosed is that findings on endoscopy may mimic vocal cord nodules. There is a subtle difference between nodules seen at the junction between the anterior one-third and posterior two-thirds of the vocal folds and the pseudonodules of LPRD noted as edema in the anterior one-third of the vocal folds.[42] Although direct laryngoscopy under general anesthesia may easily highlight these differences, it is significantly more challenging to note these subtle changes on flexible fiber-optic laryngoscopy in an awake child. This difficulty may be a key reason why the prevalence of LPRD in children may be underappreciated.

Early recognition of the role of LPRD and appropriate treatment are key to the most effective management of the hoarse patient. In adults, the finding of vocal cord nodules[43] is managed with a combination of speech therapy and antireflux medication, typically a proton pump inhibitor. Block and Brodsky[42] found similar such benefits in children. Children with only LPRD findings showed some improvement with pharmacotherapy and speech therapy compared with pharmacotherapy alone. Perhaps more remarkable was the improvement seen in children with nodules who were treated with a combination of pharmacotherapy and speech therapy compared with those treated with only 1 modality.

These findings, in addition to the treatment of LPRD and nodules in the adult population, seem to imply that appropriate treatment of a child with hoarseness would be to combine pharmacotherapy with speech therapy.[44] Unfortunately, there has been limited objective evidence in children with hoarseness, specifically with respect to pH probe findings and pepsin immunoassays. Although further studies are necessary, it seems prudent that the treatment of children with hoarseness attributed to LPRD and/or nodules should include pharmacotherapy as well as speech therapy.

COUGH

Cough is a typical complaint in children seen by a pediatrician; it is seen in the clinic in nearly 35% of preschool children.[45] The cough mechanism itself is a complex process generated in the cerebral cortex. It can be generated spontaneously or occur involuntarily as a protective mechanism. Rapidly adapting receptors as well as nocireceptors are the primary sensory receptors involved in chronic cough.[46] Rapidly adapting receptors are typically involved in response to physical stimuli such as smoke, ingested solutions, and pulmonary congestion.[47] On the other hand, nocireceptors respond to chemical stimuli (histamines, bradykinins, prostaglandins, and substance P).[48]

Although nocireceptors tend to maintain their sensitivity, rapidly adapting receptors respond and transform based on frequency of involvement. Children with chronic allergies, postnasal drainage, asthma, or GERD may demonstrate changes in the severity and frequency of their cough over time. Thus, some of these diseases may silently worsen despite no overt symptoms. Recognizing the role of reflux as a cause of a cough is imperative and should be high in the differential diagnosis once infection has been ruled out. Specifically, in the setting of a chronic cough (cough for more than 4 weeks), LPRD, allergy, and asthma should be strongly suspected.[49]

As described in other sections, irritation of the larynx by reflux is best categorized by the frequency and severity of reflux events. Although it may seem that these acute events should trigger a spell of coughing, this relationship is not so direct. A recent study[50] evaluating 20 children with reflux evaluated their coughing spells while being monitored with a pH probe. Findings showed that most coughs, nearly 90%, did not correspond with a reflux event. The chronic irritation of laryngeal tissues from reflux is the predominant culprit, rather than acute events, thereby stressing the importance of long-term treatment to reverse the process.

In the evaluation of chronic cough, it is always possible for 2 pathologies to be present simultaneously. In 1 study,[25] children with chronic cough underwent esophageal biopsies for evaluation of GERD. Of those children with positive biopsies, 75% also had a history of asthma. In a unique study[51] involving multiple disciplines, several specialists evaluated 40 children with cough for longer than 8 weeks. They found that reflux and asthma were present in nearly half the patients and another quarter of the patients had multiple causes.

Thus, the evaluation of chronic cough should be extensive with the idea that multiple factors may be playing a role. LPRD can often be considered as a possible primary cause. Furthermore, the possibility of a second contributory cause such as LPRD, allergies, or asthma should always be evaluated in patients who are unresponsive to therapy (**Fig. 1**).

DIAGNOSIS

Because of its subtlety, LPRD may be difficult to recognize in patients with the chronic effects of this disease. To the otolaryngologist, many physical examination findings may suggest LPRD; however, most of these findings can only be seen when viewing the larynx (**Box 3**).[52] Without the ability to view the larynx, the index of suspicion must be even higher for the pediatrician. A child with any of the conditions discussed as well

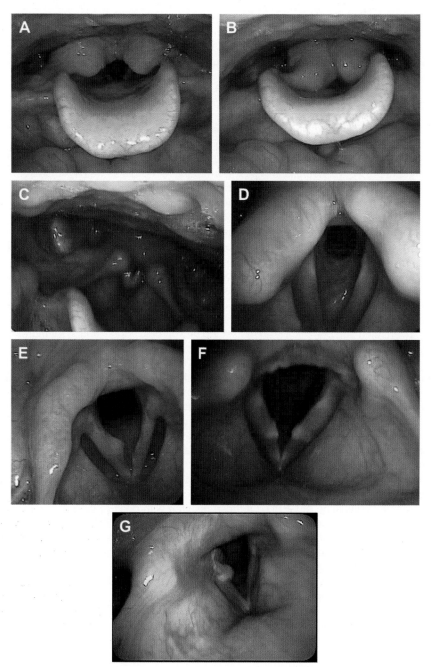

Fig. 1. (*A*) Laryngomalacia with vocal cords open. (*B*) Laryngomalacia with collapse and obstruction of airway in same patient. (*C*) Posterior pharyngeal wall cobblestoning. (*D*) Subglottic stenosis. (*E*) Right true vocal fold cyst. (*F*) Bilateral true vocal fold nodules. (*G*) Early formation of right true vocal fold granuloma (Noted posteriorly).

Box 3
Reflux findings seen on laryngoscopy

Lingual tonsil swelling

Postglottic edema

Postglottic erythema

Arytenoid edema

Arytenoid erythema

Laryngeal ventricle obliteration

True vocal fold edema

Laryngomalacia

Tracheomalacia

Vocal fold nodules

Subglottic stenosis

Hypopharyngeal cobblestoning

Narrowed trachea

Increased secretions

---

as unresponsive or unexplained difficulty with feeding or the airway should suggest the possibility of reflux as a contributing factor and prompt a referral to a specialist.

Diagnosis of reflux begins with a thorough history paying special attention to feeding and airway symptoms. With regard to feeding, it is crucial to know if a child has regurgitation or emesis and the timing of these events (ie, how long after meals?). Deciding if the child has adequate weight gain that correlates with oral intake is also important. Previous airway issues should be identified as well, because diseases such as subglottic stenosis, laryngomalacia, and RRP may have already been diagnosed. Knowledge of choking incidents, chronic cough, and recurrent crouplike episodes may suggest an underlying anatomic airway issue or even microaspiration. If there is a sufficient index of suspicion, the practitioner should enlist the help of specialists and obtain objective data for the evaluation of LPRD.

Reflux disease has been evaluated and diagnosed using a variety of objective tests, including histopathology from esophageal biopsies, barium esophograms, and double and/or single pH probes. The 24-hour pH probe study is considered the current gold standard for the diagnosis of LPRD and can be helpful in evaluating the severity of disease.

TREATMENT

Although diagnostic measures can be used to determine if a child has LPRD, the decision to proceed with work-up and treatment is key. Empirical therapy with either proton pump inhibitors or histamine (H2) blockers is often the preferred initial approach in children with presumed GERD. The primary care practitioner must decide when to initiate diagnostic work-up of LPRD/GERD.

With regard to extraesophageal symptoms and laryngopharyngeal involvement of reflux, there are certain diseases that can be readily diagnosed by simple endoscopy, such as subglottic stenosis, laryngomalacia, laryngeal edema, RRP, vocal cord granulomas, or vocal cord nodules. The diagnosis of 1 of these conditions should prompt a course of medical therapy and a period of observation for symptomatic improvement. In the case of more complex issues (swallowing difficulty, aspiration, cough) additional diagnostic testing before medical therapy is often warranted. Treatment options for LPRD include lifestyle modifications, medical therapy, and/or surgical therapy.[1,53]

Lifestyle modification for reflux typically centers on 3 actions: altering food composition, adjusting the diet to eliminate known triggers of reflux, and adjusting postural positioning. As children grow older, they can begin to follow similar guidelines as for adults. As stated earlier, thickening of feeds improves laryngeal sensation and overall swallowing function. Frequent but smaller meals can also help to reduce reflux. Sleep positioning may provide further benefit to infants by encouraging sleep in the lateral position as well as elevating the head of the bed if possible.[3] Avoidance of known triggers of LPRD is often a key dietary modification that improves symptoms in older children. Much like GERD, avoidance of certain foods (ie, juices and spicy foods, chocolates, and mints) and not eating meals just before sleep can help to decrease reflux.[2] These changes alone (elevating the head of the bed, milk thickening, and fasting before bedtime) may even lead to complete resolution of LPRD.[54,55]

If lifestyle changes are insufficient in resolving symptoms of LPRD, medical therapy is the next avenue to explore. As with adults, the recommended first-line therapy is proton pump inhibitors (PPIs). They bind irreversibly to active proton pumps and provide greatest efficacy when taken just before a meal.[55] In adults, a 30-minute gap between consumption of medication and commencing a meal is typically recommended. Among the various PPIs, esomeprazole has been shown to provide the greatest benefit.[56] In children, similar studies have not been performed; however, in neonates and infants, lansoprazole and omeprazole are the only PPIs approved by the US Food and Drug Administration.

Histamine-2 receptor antagonists (H2RAs), once a mainstay in treatment, have now become second-line therapy. They have typically been used to either help wean patients off PPIs or to supplement PPI therapy. Unlike PPIs, they are typically taken at night to provide nocturnal suppression of acid as they reduce meal-stimulated gastric acid production by nearly 70%.[57] In children, the use of a H2RA is most helpful for weaning off PPIs. Ranitidine is available as a syrup, which may help to increase patient compliance. Although the use of PPIs and H2RAs have been studied in adults, there is no consensus on their role in the treatment of reflux.[58] Although further studies are needed, the use of a PPI or H2RA in short courses of therapy can often yield beneficial results. The failure to respond to either a PPI or H2RA in cases of suspected reflux indicates a lack of significant reflux, insufficient dosage, or the need to consider surgical intervention.

Surgical therapy for reflux should be reserved for those children whose symptoms are life threatening or drastically affecting their quality of life despite maximum medical therapy. Although surgery may seem appealing by promising the possibility of eliminating the need for medication, it carries with it the risk of high failure rates, significant morbidity, and even death.[59] As some of these situations (coughing, choking, aspiration, or recurrent pneumonias) compromise a patient's respiratory status, the risks of surgery may greatly outweigh the projected benefits. If all factors have been considered, fundoplication can be entertained as a possibility. Nissen fundoplication is the gold standard procedure performed for the surgical treatment of GERD. This procedure attempts to restore the integrity of the lower esophageal sphincter. When performed on appropriate patients, it has a 90% symptom control rate.[60,61] Furthermore, when performed on patients without respiratory issues, the success rate increases even further.[62]

SUMMARY

Extraesophageal symptoms of GERD have long been recognized and referred to as LPRD. Despite its similarities with GERD, LPRD has been more difficult to diagnose accurately and consistently. This variability has made creating comprehensive treatment guidelines difficult. Much of the current information regarding the role of LPRD has been learned by noting its presence in conjunction with another well-understood disease (laryngomalacia, subglottic stenosis, vocal cord nodules, and so forth). Currently, the treatment of LPRD seems to demonstrate symptomatic benefits as well as improvements in these concomitant diseases. Thus, LPRD should be considered as a chronic disease with a variety of presentations. High clinical suspicion along with consultation with an otolaryngologist, who can evaluate for laryngeal findings, is necessary to accurately diagnose LPRD. Future studies will work to illuminate the role of gastric acid and refluxate on the upper aerodigestive tract. However, until excluded, the role of LPRD should never be underestimated and should always be treated in symptomatic patients.

REFERENCES

1. Vandenplas Y, Sacre-Smith L. Continuous 24-hour esophageal pH monitoring in 285 asymptomatic infants 0 to 15 months old. J Pediatr Gastroenterol Nutr 1987; 6:220–4.
2. Stavroulaki P. Diagnostic and management problems of laryngopharyngeal reflux disease in children. Int J Pediatr Otorhinolaryngol 2006;70:579–90.
3. McGuirt WF Jr. Gastroesophageal reflux and the upper airway. Pediatr Clin North Am 2003;50:487–502.
4. Suskind DL, Thompson DM, Gulati M, et al. Improved infant swallowing after gastroesophageal reflux disease treatment: a function of improved laryngeal sensation? Laryngoscope 2006;116:1397–403.
5. Aviv JE, Liu H, Parides M, et al. Laryngopharyngeal sensory deficits in patients with laryngopharyngeal reflux and dysphagia. Ann Otol Rhinol Laryngol 2000; 109:1000–6.
6. Link DT, Willging JP, Miller CK, et al. Pediatric laryngopharyngeal sensory testing during flexible endoscopic evaluation of swallowing: feasible and correlative. Ann Otol Rhinol Laryngol 2000;109:899–905.
7. Thompson DM. Laryngopharyngeal sensory testing and assessment of airway protection in pediatric patients. Am J Med 2003;115(Suppl 3A):166S–8S.
8. Orenstein SR, Magill HL, Brooks P. Thickening of infant feedings for therapy of gastroesophageal reflux. J Pediatr 1987;110:181–6.
9. Henry SM. Discerning differences: gastroesophageal reflux and gastroesophageal reflux disease in infants. Adv Neonatal Care 2004;4:235–47.
10. Holinger LD. Etiology of stridor in the neonate, infant, and child. Ann Otol Rhinol Laryngol 1980;89:397–400.
11. Hartl TT, Chadha NK. A systematic review of laryngomalacia and acid reflux. Otolaryngol Head Neck Surg 2012;147(4):619–26.
12. Chandra RK, Gerber ME, Holinger LD. Histological insight into the pathogenesis of severe laryngomalacia. Int J Pediatr Otorhinolaryngol 2001;61: 31–8.
13. Iyer VK, Pearman K, Raafat F. Laryngeal mucosal histology in laryngomalacia: the evidence for gastro-oesophageal reflux laryngitis. Int J Pediatr Otorhinolaryngol 1999;49:225–30.

14. Matthews BL, Little JP, Mcguirt WF Jr, et al. Reflux in infants with laryngomalacia: results of 24-hour double-probe pH monitoring. Otolaryngol Head Neck Surg 1999;120:860–4.

15. Thompson DM. Abnormal sensorimotor integrative function of the larynx in congenital laryngomalacia: a new theory of etiology. Laryngoscope 2007; 117(6 Pt 2 Suppl 114):1–33.

16. Little JP, Matthews BL, Glock MS, et al. Extraesophageal pediatric reflux: 24-hour double-probe pH monitoring of 222 children. Ann Otol Rhinol Laryngol Suppl 1997;169:7.

17. Rabinowitz SS, Piecuch S, Jibaly R, et al. Optimizing the diagnosis of gastro-esophageal reflux in children with otolaryngologic symptoms. Int J Pediatr Oto-rhinolaryngol 2003;67:625.

18. Thompson DM. Laryngomalacia: factors that influence disease severity and out-comes of management. Curr Opin Otolaryngol Head Neck Surg 2010;18:564–70.

19. Karkos PD, Leong SC, Apostolidou MT, et al. Laryngeal manifestations and pediatric laryngopharyngeal reflux. Am J Otol 2006;27(3):200–3.

20. Delahunty JE, Cherry J. Experimentally produced vocal cord granulomas. Laryngoscope 1968;78(11):1941–7.

21. Little FB, Koufman JA, Kohut RI, et al. Effect of gastric acid on the pathogenesis of subglottic stenosis. Ann Otol Rhinol Laryngol 1985;94(5):516–9.

22. Yellon RF, Parameswarran M, Brandom BW. Decreasing morbidity following laryngotracheal reconstruction in children. Int J Pediatr Otorhinolaryngol 1997; 41(2):145–54.

23. Jarmuz T, Roser S, Rivera H, et al. Transforming growth factor-beta 1, myofibro-blasts, and tissue remodelling in the pathogenesis of tracheal injury: potential role of gastroesophageal reflux. Ann Otol Rhinol Laryngol 2004;113(6):488–97.

24. Halstead LA. Gastroesophageal reflux: a critical factor in pediatric subglottic stenosis. Otolaryngol Head Neck Surg 1999;120:683–8.

25. Yellon RF, Coticchia J, Dixit S. Esophageal biopsy for the diagnosis of gastro-esophageal reflux-associated otolaryngologic problems in children. Am J Med 2000;108(Suppl 4a):131S–8S.

26. Mitzner R, Brodsky L. Multilevel esophageal biopsy in children with airway man-ifestations of extraesophageal reflux disease. Ann Otol Rhinol Laryngol 2007; 116:571–5.

27. Halstead LA. Role of gastroesophageal reflux in pediatric upper airway disor-ders. Otolaryngol Head Neck Surg 1999;120:208–14.

28. Carr MM, Nagy ML, Pizzuto MP, et al. Correlation of findings at direct laryngos-copy and bronchoscopy with gastroesophageal reflux disease in children: a prospective study. Arch Otolaryngol Head Neck Surg 2001;127:369–74.

29. Carr MM, Abu-Shamma U, Brodsky LS. Predictive value of laryngeal pseudosul-cus for gastroesophageal reflux in pediatric patients. Int J Pediatr Otorhinolar-yngol 2005;69:1109–12.

30. Giannoni C, Sulek M, Friedman EM, et al. Gastroesophageal reflux association with laryngomalacia: a prospective study. Int J Pediatr Otorhinolaryngol 1998; 43:11–20.

31. Can MM, Nguyen A, Poje C, et al. Correlation of findings on direct laryngoscopy and bronchoscopy with presence of extraesophageal reflux disease. Laryngo-scope 2000;110:1560–2.

32. Stroh BC, Faust RA, Rimell FL. Results of esophageal biopsies performed during triple endoscopy in the pediatric patient. Arch Otolaryngol Head Neck Surg 1998;124:545–9.

33. McKenna M, Brodsky L. Extraesophageal acid reflux and recurrent respiratory papillomatosis in children. Int J Pediatr Otorhinolaryngol 2005;69: 597–605.
34. Borkowski G, Sommer P, Stark T, et al. Recurrent respiratory papillomatosis associated with gastroesophageal reflux disease in children. Eur Arch Otorhinolaryngol 1999;256(7):370–2.
35. Holland BW, Koufman JA, Postma GN, et al. Laryngopharyngeal reflux and laryngeal web formation in patients with pediatric recurrent respiratory papillomas. Laryngoscope 2002;112(11):1926–9.
36. Thakkar K, Boatright RO, Gilger MA, et al. Gastroesophageal reflux and asthma in children: a systematic review. Pediatrics 2010;125:925–30.
37. Kilic M, Ozturk F, Kirmemis O, et al. Impact of laryngopharyngeal and gastroesophageal reflux on asthma control in children. Int J Pediatr Otorhinolaryngol 2013;77(3):341–5.
38. Eryuksel E, Dogan M, Golabi P, et al. Treatment of laryngo-pharyngeal reflux improves asthma symptoms in asthmatics. J Asthma 2006;43:539–42.
39. Parsons JP, Mastronarde JG. Gastroesophageal reflux disease and asthma. Curr Opin Pulm Med 2010;16:60–3.
40. Wohl DL. Nonsurgical management of pediatric vocal fold nodules. Arch Otolaryngol Head Neck Surg 2005;131(1):68–70.
41. Gumpert L, Kalach N, Dupont C, et al. Hoarseness and gastroesophageal reflux in children. J Laryngol Otol 1998;112(1):49–54.
42. Block BB, Brodsky L. Hoarseness in children: the role of laryngopharyngeal reflux. Int J Pediatr Otorhinolaryngol 2007;71:1361–9.
43. Kuhn J, Toohill RJ, Ulualp SO, et al. Pharyngeal acid reflux events in patients with vocal cord nodules. Laryngoscope 1998;108:1146–9.
44. Karkos PD, Wilson JA. Empiric treatment of laryngopharyngeal reflux with proton pump inhibitors; a systematic review. Laryngoscope 2006;116:144–8.
45. Kogan MD, Pappas G, Yu SM, et al. Over-the-counter medication use among preschool-age children. JAMA 1994;272:1025–30.
46. Mazzone SB. Sensory regulation of the cough reflex. Pulm Pharmacol Ther 2004;17:361–8.
47. Palmer R, Anon JB, Gallagher P. Pediatric cough: what the otolaryngologist needs to know. Curr Opin Otolaryngol Head Neck Surg 2011;19:204–9.
48. Millqvist E, Bende M. Role of the upper airways in patients with chronic cough. Curr Opin Allergy Clin Immunol 2006;6:7–11.
49. Chang AB, Landau LI, van Asperen PP, et al. Cough in children: definitions and clinical evaluation. Med J Aust 2006;184:398–403.
50. Chang AB, Connor FL, Petsky HL, et al. An objective study of acid reflux and cough in children using an ambulatory pHmetry-cough logger. Arch Dis Child 2011;96(5):468–72.
51. Khoshoo V, Edell D, Mohnot S, et al. Associated factors in children with chronic cough. Chest 2009;136:811–5.
52. May JG, Shah P, Lemonnier L, et al. Systematic review of endoscopic airway findings in children with gastroesophageal reflux disease. Ann Otol Rhinol Laryngol 2011;120(2):116–22.
53. Cezard JP. Managing gastro-oesophageal reflux disease in children. Digestion 2004;69(Suppl):3–8.
54. Bach KK, McGuirt WF Jr, Postma GN. Pediatric laryngopharyngeal reflux. Ear Nose Throat J 2002;81(9 Suppl 2):27–31.

55. Meyer TK, Olsen E, Merati A. Contemporary diagnostic and management techniques for extraoesophageal reflux disease. Curr Opin Otolaryngol Head Neck Surg 2004;12(6):519–24.

56. Miner P Jr, Katz PO, Chen Y, et al. Gastric acid control with esomeprazole, lansoprazole, omeprazole, pantoprazole, and rabeprazole: a five-way crossover study. Am J Gastroenterol 2003;98:2616–20.

57. Katz PO. Optimizing medical therapy for gastroesophageal reflux disease: state of the art. Rev Gastroenterol Disord 2003;3:59–69.

58. Chang A, Lasserson T, Gaffney J, et al. Gastro-oesophageal reflux treatment for prolonged non-specific cough in children and adults. Cochrane Database Syst Rev 2005;(2):CD004823.

59. Hassall E. Wrap session: is the Nissen slipping? Can medical treatment replace surgery for severe gastroesophageal reflux disease in children? Am J Gastroenterol 1995;90(8):1212–20.

60. Fung KP, Seagram G, Pasieka J, et al. Investigation and outcome of 121 infants and children requiring Nissen fundoplication for management of gastroesophageal reflux. Clin Invest Med 1990;13:237–46.

61. Little AG, Ferguson MK, Skinner DB. Reoperation for failed antireflux operations. J Thorac Cardiovasc Surg 1986;91:511–7.

62. Pennell RC, Lewis JE, Cradock TV, et al. Management of severe gastroesophageal reflux in children. Arch Surg 1984;119:553–7.

Voice Disorders in Children

Victoria Possamai, MBChB, FRCS (ORL-HNS)*,
Benjamin Hartley, MBBS, BSc, FRCS (ORL-HNS)

KEYWORDS

- Pediatric • Child • Voice • Dysphonia

KEY POINTS

- Understanding the distinct anatomy of the pediatric larynx and changes that occur through to adolescence is key to effectively managing voice disorders in children.
- Multidisciplinary pediatric voice clinics are increasing, and provide an excellent setting for detailed assessment in an office environment.
- Awake laryngoscopic examination in the office is possible in most children and provides superior dynamic information compared with a rigid laryngoscopy under anesthetic.
- It is important to distinguish those conditions that may recover spontaneously, those that respond to speech and language therapy, and those that require surgical intervention to allow appropriate patient and parent counseling.

INTRODUCTION

There have been great advances in knowledge regarding voice disorders and strategies for managing them in recent years. This initially occurred in adult practice, with the development of the subspecialty of phoniatrics, which has evolved rapidly. It is now common for ear, nose, and throat (ENT) departments to have a clinician with a specialist interest in phoniatrics and a multidisciplinary voice clinic. This experience has more recently been applied in the pediatric setting to guide assessment and management of voice disorders in children.

THE PEDIATRIC LARYNX IS DIFFERENT

To effectively manage childhood voice disorders, it is important to consider the differences between the child and adult larynx and indeed the transition between the 2 during adolescence. In a child, the larynx is relatively smaller, and sits in a higher position, with the cricoid at the level of the fourth cervical vertebra compared with the sixth in an adult, which can have an impact on endoscopic access. The epiglottis

No financial interests to declare.
Department of ENT Surgery, Great Ormond Street Hospital for Children, Great Ormond Street, London NW1N 3JH, UK
* Corresponding author.
E-mail address: victoriapossamai@mac.com

Pediatr Clin N Am 60 (2013) 879–892
http://dx.doi.org/10.1016/j.pcl.2013.04.012
0031-3955/13/$ – see front matter © 2013 Elsevier Inc. All rights reserved.

has a more tightly curled shape. The vocal folds are shorter with a reduced membranous–to–cartilaginous fold ratio. The structure of the vocal fold is immature, lacking the 5 layers seen in the adult vocal fold. The mucosa of the subglottis is more reactive and therefore prone to edema, hence the predisposition to croup and laryngeal obstruction in children. The suggestion that the subglottis is the narrowest level of the pediatric airway has been challenged, with the finding that in children the narrowest part is also at the glottic level, with no evidence of the classically described funnel-shaped larynx; however, this observation has been made in anesthetized paralyzed children (**Table 1**).[1]

EPIDEMIOLOGY

Epidemiologic data suggest that the prevalence of voice disorders in children is high, with figures in the 1960s to 1980s reported between 6% and 23% in 5-year-olds to 18-year-olds.[2–4] In most of these cases, the voice problem is not perceived to be a concern by the parents or children, and they therefore do not seek medical attention. They have often become accustomed to a slightly abnormal pitch or tone, and the suggestion that this may represent an abnormality often comes from an external individual (eg, a teacher when a child starts school), which may trigger a medical review. The range of voice problems that do present varies widely, from those child performers with normal conversational voice but concern about loss in the upper range of their singing voice, to those with severe laryngeal pathology and no voice at all. After a thorough assessment, the appropriate voice therapy, and, on occasion, surgical treatment, most voice disorders in children can be improved.

There is evidence in the literature to demonstrate the impact of voice disorders in children, both in terms of the child's perception of themselves and how they are perceived by others. A study carried out in the United States in 2008 used the pediatric voice-related quality-of-life instrument in 95 children with vocal nodules, vocal fold paralysis, and paradoxic vocal fold dysfunction. The study found reduced total scores, and reduced scores in social-emotional and physical-functional domains compared with children without voice dysfunction.[5] A separate study assessed the attitudes of adults in response to listening to children with dysphonia, finding significant negative perceptions of the children as "dirty, weak, sick, ugly" compared with their peers without dysphonia.[6]

DEVELOPMENT OF THE LARYNX

It is beyond the scope of this review to discuss the embryology of the larynx, which is well described elsewhere, although it is important to bear in mind that some causes of voice disorders may be congenital and relate to the embryologic development of the larynx. An example is a glottic web, resulting from incomplete recanalization of the

Table 1 Differences between the pediatric and adult larynx		
Features	**Pediatric**	**Adult**
Position	Higher (cricoid T4)	Lower (cricoid T6)
Shape	Curled epiglottis	More open epiglottis
Vocal fold structure	Immature	Mature: 5 layers
Vocal cords	Membranous:Cartilage ratio 1.0:1.5	Membranous:Cartilage ratio 1.0:5.0
Mucosa	Reactive, prone to edema	Less reactive

embryonic larynx at approximately 10 weeks' gestation. The postnatal changes that occur during the growth and development of the larynx are also pertinent to development and management of voice disorders and therefore a description of those is included. The work of Hirano and colleagues during the 1980s informs much of this knowledge.[7,8]

Vocal Fold Growth

The length of the vocal folds is equal in both genders (6–8 mm) until the age of 10 years. Following this, there is significant growth in both boys and girls; however, more marked in boys, with the membranous vocal fold increasing to 14.8 to 18.0 mm, compared with 8.5 to 12.0 mm in girls. The cartilaginous part of the vocal cord also lengthens with age, but relatively less, so that the ratio of membranous-to-cartilaginous fold is 1.5:1.0 in the newborn, 4.0:1.0 in the adult female, and 5.5:1.0 in the adult male. Hirano and colleagues[8] also derived the concept that the posterior wider glottis acts as the respiratory glottis, with the phonatory glottis anteriorly. This is an important consideration when planning phonosurgery, such as arytenoidectomy in bilateral cord palsy. Increasing the airway size exclusively posteriorly should have a limited impact on the voice outcome.

Vocal Fold Structure

The understanding of the layered vocal fold structure is key to phonosurgery in adults. The 5 layers are the epithelium; the superficial, intermediate, and deep layers of the lamina propria; and the muscle layer. The 2 most superficial layers are known as "the cover," moving freely over the deeper layers. These form the vocal ligament and body of the vocal fold, and care should be taken to maintain these intact to preserve voice. Hirano and colleagues[8] and others have observed that this structure is not present at birth, but rather starts to develop during the first months of life, reaching recognizable adult structure by puberty. This provides a challenge in phonosurgery in young children, as the lack of a clear plane of dissection in the superficial lamina propria makes raising microflaps more difficult.

The pitch of the voice in children is a characteristic difference from the adult voice. Pitch lowers gradually throughout infancy and childhood in both genders, with a more marked change at puberty, most significant in boys. This pitch change relates to the anterior growth of the thyroid cartilage, driven by testosterone, and corresponds to the external development of the thyroid prominence or Adam's apple.

ASSESSMENT

Children with voice disorders may be seen in a general or specialist voice clinic. The history and basic ENT examination are the same in both settings; however, the specialist clinic provides the added benefit of the combined expertise of an otolaryngologist and speech and language therapist. There should also be the availability of videostroboscopic equipment and expertise to use it for a more detailed assessment. The availability of this clinic is likely to vary and, therefore, whether all children are seen in such a clinic or whether screened initially in a general clinic will differ between departments. The general trend is toward children with dysphonia being seen in specialist pediatric voice clinics.

HISTORY

A key step early on when taking the history is to distinguish whether the child has a voice disorder rather than a problem with speech, articulation, or language. The presenting symptom in voice disorders is, classically, hoarseness, whereas mispronunciation suggests a problem with speech and articulation, and inability to find the correct words relates to a disorder of language (**Table 2**).

Where possible, information should be sought from both the parents and the child. The chronology of the symptom is helpful. If the problem has been present since birth, a congenital pathology is likely, although a history of intubation in the perinatal period may be more suggestive of an acquired pathology, such as subglottic stenosis, formation of cysts, or cricoarytenoid fibrosis. It is common for later-onset symptoms to be related to an upper respiratory tract infection with associated laryngitis, with persistence of the hoarseness exacerbated by voice misuse. The severity of the problem ranges from a complete loss of voice to loss of singing voice in certain situations. The perceived importance of the disorder is also variable, with very mild dysphonia a serious concern to children who perform, or aspire to. The time course of the dysphonia is also important, an intermittent dysphonia is less likely to indicate a discrete vocal cord lesion, although the symptom may fluctuate and fatigue throughout the day.

The presence of associated laryngeal symptoms is an indicator of possible serious underlying pathology and must not be missed. Stridor and reduced exercise tolerance suggest an obstructive pathology, such as laryngeal stenosis or papillomas. Swallowing problems or choking may suggest vocal fold paralysis.

Other pathologies may influence the health of the larynx. It is helpful to inquire about symptoms suggestive of laryngopharyngeal reflux, which may cause local irritation and dysphonia. Throat clearing related to postnasal drip in allergic rhinitis will do the same. Respiratory disease may also cause dysphonia via several mechanisms. Persistent cough can lead to hoarseness, restrictive pathology reduces infraglottic pressure affecting the strength of the voice, and corticosteroid inhalers used to treat asthma can also cause dysphonia,[9] which may be amenable to modification of the regimen or inhaler technique.

Less direct symptoms may also have an impact; for example, hearing loss may encourage the child to shout, leading to voice misuse–related dysphonia. It is helpful to ask about voice use in general and in the home environment. It has been noted that children with larger sibling groups have a higher prevalence of dysphonia associated with voice misuse.[10] This can be related to development of vocal nodules. Asking about smoking and alcohol use may also be relevant.

EXAMINATION

A general otolaryngologic examination should be performed, including examination of the ears and hearing. Assessment of the voice should be thorough and may use a combination of subjective and objective voice analysis measures, including perceptual evaluation of voice, videostroboscopic imaging of vocal cord movement, and acoustic analysis. Self-assessment tools are also valuable. In the authors' practice, children and their parents attending voice clinic are asked to complete the voice

Table 2 Presenting symptoms in voice, speech, and language disorders	
Symptom	**Classification of Problem**
Hoarseness	Disorder of voice
Mispronunciation	Disorder of speech/articulation
Problems with word finding	Disorder of language

handicap index and a vocal tract discomfort scale, which was modified from a study in adults with muscle tension dysphonia by Mathieson and colleagues in 2009.[11] These are repeated following voice therapy or surgical intervention to aid assessment of the outcome of these interventions.

The aims of examining the larynx can be considered as twofold. First, to assess for any evidence of a structural abnormality, such as a cyst, nodule, or papillomata. Second, to assess the dynamic view of laryngeal function during phonation to identify problems, such as vocal cord paralysis or muscular hyperfunction. There are several methods of laryngoscopic examination, each of which has advantages and disadvantages (**Table 3**).

Laryngoscopy Under General Anesthetic

Traditionally, the pediatric larynx has been examined under general anesthetic. This allows excellent visualization of structural abnormalities, but very limited information regarding function. Vocal cord movement can be crudely assessed while the child is waking. This form of assessment is used in younger or poorly compliant children, but all efforts should be made to attempt awake laryngeal and voice examination, and this is achievable in most children.

Awake Fiberoptic Laryngoscopy

Awake fiberoptic laryngoscopy is capable of excluding most focal laryngeal lesions and can provide images of adequate quality to allow stroboscopy to examine the mucosal wave. It is usually achievable transnasally with the choice of a 2.2-mm or 4.0-mm fiberoptic endoscope. The optics are superior in the larger endoscope, so it is preferred if possible. It can be performed on a child of almost any age. Younger children aged 1 to 5 years may be less tolerant of the procedure; however, with the assistance of the parents and appropriate encouragement, it is frequently achievable.

Awake Rigid Laryngoscopy

Awake rigid laryngoscopy requires a higher level of cooperation from the child, so is used as the technique of choice in those older than 6 years. It involves asking the child to stick out his or her tongue, grasping the tongue with a gauze swab and introducing a 70° rigid Hopkins rod endoscope into the oropharynx to gain a view of the larynx. The images obtained are of excellent quality, giving unparalleled information regarding the structure and movement of the vocal folds. The images also provide a very useful tool to educate the child and parents regarding the voice disorder. Vocal cord paralysis is usually obvious with any form of laryngoscopy; however, this technique can highlight

Table 3		
Advantages and disadvantages of different modalities of examining the larynx		
Modality	**Advantages**	**Disadvantages**
Microlaryngoscopy (general anaesthetic [GA])	Full cooperation Ability to biopsy/excise	Invasive Limited dynamic view
Flexible nasendoscopy	Well tolerated Awake Good view	Limited time Limited stroboscopy
Awake rigid endoscopy	Awake Best dynamic view Teaching aid	Less well tolerated

more subtle motility disorders, such as supraglottic constriction and reduced posterior glottic closure.

Additional Tests

Laryngeal electromyography (EMG) is performed using electrodes placed in the thyro-arytenoid and posterior cricoarytenoid muscles. In children, this requires general anesthesia. It has a role in the assessment of children with vocal fold paralysis, in particular, to help to predict return of function. There is evidence that this recovery may be apparent on EMG studies months before becoming visible on laryngoscopy, and may, therefore, have a role in predicting outcome in vocal fold paralysis, aiding decisions regarding management.[12] A further study has proposed a grading system to denote severity, and found that this correlated well with the need for tracheostomy.[13]

Further tests to assess for evidence of reflux can also be considered, although are not always conclusive. These include standard pH monitoring and multichannel impedance testing to assess for nonacid reflux. Esophageal biopsy and brochoalveolar lavage have also been described, but correlate poorly with each other and endoscopic findings.[14] Many specialists therefore advocate a trial of antireflux treatment in suspected cases in preference to invasive investigations.

COMMON DISORDERS
Vocal Nodules and Functional Voice Disorders

Vocal nodules are the commonest cause of hoarseness in children and are regarded as the organic manifestation of laryngeal hyperfunction.[15] They are commoner in boys, with a study of 617 school children in Turkey suggesting a prevalence of 21% in boys and 11% in girls.[16] The severity of the voice disorder has also been shown to correlate with nodule size.[17] These respond well to voice therapy and surgical treatment is rarely indicated, although, interestingly, the evidence is lacking, with no trials eligible for inclusion in a recent Cochrane review of surgical versus nonsurgical interventions for vocal nodules.[18] In adolescents, the therapy is similar to that used with adults; however, younger children require strategies to be adapted. A key objective is to reduce voice strain, which is achieved by various strategies to eliminate shouting, whispering, throat clearing, and cough. Allowing voice rest and recovery after a "noisy activity," such as playing football, with periods of quiet play are advised. Traditional teaching, based on clinical experience, suggests that most vocal nodules improve during puberty, and this theory fits with the significant changes that occur in the membranous vocal fold during this period. A study carried out by Mori,[19] however, found that a proportion of nodules (12%) did not improve at puberty. This study also suggested that vocal hygiene alone did not improve nodules, but voice therapy did have a positive impact, with increasing benefit with the greater the number of sessions attended. Tezcaner and colleagues[20] describe using a combination of subjective (GRBAS: Grade, Roughness, Breathiness, Asthenia, Strain) and objective (multidimensional voice program) measures to assess outcome after speech therapy, with good voice improvements reported.

Surgery has a limited role, predominantly because of the real concerns about scarring resulting in poor voice outcomes. In those children who fail to respond to a long course of voice therapy, it can be useful to perform microlaryngoscopy, which may help to exclude other pathology that may be amenable to microsurgical excision. Bouchayer and Cornut[21] found microlaryngoscopy evidence of cysts, sulci, and polyps in children with a prior diagnosis of nodules. Occasionally, a cyst can be present on one vocal cord, with a nodule on the contralateral cord, which may explain a poor response to voice therapy. There have also been reports of microwebs found at microlaryngoscopy in both children and adults with vocal nodules.[22] With increasing expertise and use of videostroboscopy, these conditions should be possible to identify in the clinic.

A range of functional voice disorders can also be demonstrated in children without the presence of vocal nodules. When these behaviors become entrenched, the way the voice is produced becomes persistently abnormal with signs of muscle tension, such as supraglottic constriction, on laryngoscopy. Children may present with dysphonia or aphonia related to underlying psychological factors, and this is particularly suggested by a significant dysphonia with normal laryngoscopic examination. The presence of a normal cough or laugh would further support this. These children may require voice therapy and a careful psychological assessment. Puberphonia, when the prepubertal voice persists through adolescence into adulthood, is also associated with psychological problems. The combination of specialist voice therapy and psychological therapy may be needed to achieve an adult voice.

A complex relationship exists between vocal disorders and behavior. Children with vocal cord nodules showed significantly increased scores in domains of acting out, distractibility, disturbed peer relations, and immature behaviors compared with peers without nodules.[23] The question of cause and effect needs to be considered.

Laryngeal Papillomatosis

Laryngeal papillomatosis is an important condition to identify, as the often initial symptom of voice disturbance may progress to symptoms of airway obstruction (**Fig. 1**). Papillomata are caused by human papilloma viruses (HPVs) 6 and 11. Transmission is materno-fetal and thought to be related to the passage through the birth canal, although birth by cesarean section is not completely protective, suggesting a more complex route of transmission in utero.[24] With respect to surgical therapy, the aim is to remove bulky disease to improve voice and airway, while avoiding damage and scarring to the underlying laryngeal structures, which would jeopardize long-term voice outcomes. Particular care is therefore required at the anterior commissure to prevent glottic webbing. Scarring and webbing are known complications from laser removal of papillomata and the use of cold steel or microdebrider techniques may therefore be favorable. As early as 2004, a survey of members of the American Society

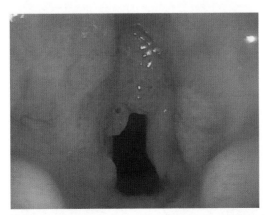

Fig. 1. Laryngoscopic image showing recurrent respiratory papillomatosis involving the glottis and supraglottis.

of Pediatric Otolaryngology worldwide found that 53% were favoring the microdebrider, and 42% were using laser.[25] Adjunctive medical treatments have been trialed with some success. These include interferon; virostatics, such as acyclovir, valaciclovir, and cidofavir; indole-3-carbinol; mumps vaccination; and photodynamic therapy. There are several case series reported in Europe showing very good treatment responses with intralesional cidofavir injection,[26,27] one of which carried out in Germany reported a "clear voice improvement" in most patients.[28] However, the only prospective double-blind trial has not shown significant benefit when compared with placebo,[29] and there have been recent concerns raised regarding possible carcinogenic effects observed in in vitro studies.[30] There is also recent interest in the use of the quadravalent HPV vaccination, Gardasil, with a case report of its successful administration in a child with recurrent respiratory papillomatosis.[31] These adjunctive treatments are reserved for those requiring surgical removal of papillomata at frequent intervals to aim to limit the number of surgical procedures needed and thereby potentially improve voice outcomes.

Postintubation Voice Disorders

The risk of developing acquired subglottic stenosis following a prolonged period of intubation, usually in premature infants, is well documented (**Fig. 2**). There has been an evolution of surgical techniques to address and correct the stenosis and achieve decannulation in those who have required tracheostomy. It is common for the voice following this type of surgery to be impaired. Less serious types of postintubation injury do occur, which predominantly affect the voice, rather than airway, and they may be overlooked. During the process of intubation, the vocal fold or underlying lamina propria may be damaged, resulting in dysphonia (**Fig. 3**). The mobility of the vocal folds can also be affected by posterior scarring or cricoarytenoid joint fixation secondary to intubation. It is important to distinguish these causes from vocal cord paralysis.

In some cases, these children can gain some improvement from voice therapy. Surgery in this group of children is a challenge and needs to be tailored to each individual case. Vocal fold medialization techniques may provide benefit, but this is limited when there is loss of the mucosal wave from damage to the vocal fold. Its application is also limited by the need to maintain an adequate airway.

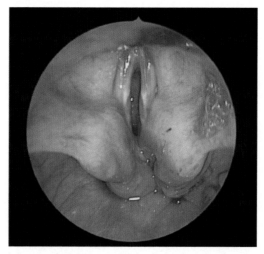

Fig. 2. Laryngoscopic image showing acquired subglottic stenosis.

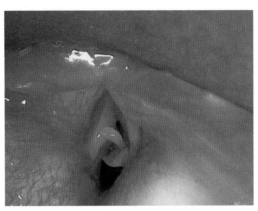

Fig. 3. Laryngoscopic image showing vocal cord granulomas following intubation.

Vocal Fold Paralysis

In bilateral vocal fold paralysis, the voice does not usually severely affect the child maintaining a strong voice or cry; it is the airway that causes symptoms and the need for treatment. Approximately 50% of children require tracheostomy.[32] In congenital cases, spontaneous recovery may occur, although if there is no evidence of this after waiting for at least 2 years, it is unlikely that it will happen beyond this time. Surgical treatment involves widening the glottis using a lateralization procedure. Several have been described, including laser arytenoidectomy and suture lateralization of the vocal fold. The principle is to increase the space posteriorly to improve the airway while preserving maximal anterior glottic closure to maintain voice.

Unilateral vocal fold paralysis, in contrast, causes symptoms of weak voice or cry and aspiration. It is unusual for the airway to be greatly compromised. Improvement in symptoms over time is the norm and may be attributable to spontaneous recovery of function or compensation by the contralateral vocal fold. In the minority who have persistent dysphonia, medialization techniques can be used. Medialization thyroplasty is an option, although in the prepubertal age group, there is concern about whether the placement of a silastic implant may interfere with the expected physiologic growth spurt and may be in the wrong position following this. Its utility is also reduced in children, as the procedure is best done under local anesthetic. A less invasive option is vocal fold injection, which is Dr Hartley's preference in prepubertal children. The author has experience with the use of autologous fat, which can pose difficulties both in the harvest, in very lean children, and in its insertion into and administration via a spinal needle. More recently, injectable calcium hydroxylapatite has been used with greater ease, and preliminary results are encouraging (**Figs. 4–6**); however, published data on the efficacy of radiesse in children are not yet available.

Reinnervation techniques are an attractive concept. The techniques are able to restore laryngeal tone, but a limitation is that they are less successful in achieving voluntary movement. The pediatric population is most likely to benefit, as nerve-grafting techniques are more successful in general (see later section on future directions).

A key point is to not assume an immobile vocal cord is paralyzed. The same appearances can be caused by posterior glottic scarring or cricoarytenoid joint fixation, which need to be carefully assessed. The appropriate treatment is very different, with a wait and watch policy for paralysis with a tendency for spontaneous resolution.

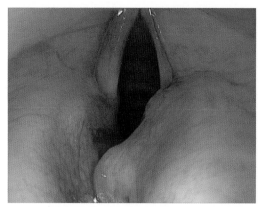

Fig. 4. Laryngoscopic image showing atrophic right vocal card due to right vocal fold paralysis.

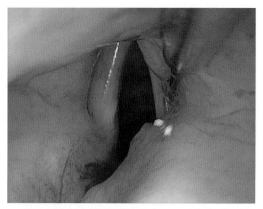

Fig. 5. Laryngoscopic image showing right vocal fold injection for vocal cord palsy.

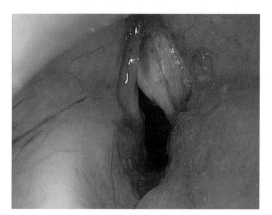

Fig. 6. Laryngoscopic image of immediate postinjection appearance. Note well-preserved posterior glottic airway.

Scarring and fixation will not improve without treatment by lateralization procedure, and there is nothing to gain from the child waiting several years with a tracheostomy in these cases.

Tracheostomy and Voice

Voice impairment is common in children with tracheostomies. The main cause of this is frequently the underlying laryngeal pathology, which requires management with a tracheostomy. The tracheostomy tube then diverts air from the glottis, causing further compromise; however, those children with a tracheostomy and a healthy larynx can achieve good voice by occluding the tube during expiration, projecting the air up through the glottis and upper airway. This depends on there being adequate space around the tube, which may require downsizing, and can usually be achieved while maintaining an adequate airway. Speech valves can be a very useful adjunct to facilitate this, with the additional benefit of a positive impact on secretion management and swallowing.

FUTURE DIRECTIONS
Laryngeal Transplantation for Voice

Occasionally one encounters a child with such severe laryngeal stenosis that it is not amenable to surgical treatment. The etiology is normally severe burns or caustic ingestion. The child is dependent on a tracheostomy and has no voice; therefore, communicating using signing or nonoral devices. Replacement of the larynx with transplantation would provide the best prospect of a positive outcome, but has so far been performed in only 2 adult patients. The first took place in 1998 and was successful, but there have remained barriers to further developments in this area, in particular concerns regarding reinnervation, immunosuppression, patient selection, and cost-benefit analysis.[33]

Reinnervation of Paralyzed Larynx

The dysphonia associated with vocal fold paralysis can be successfully treated with phonosurgery to medialize the vocal cord; however, these techniques do not reliably improve aspiration and this can therefore be the most troublesome symptom to manage. Laryngeal reinnervation may provide a solution, but is not widely practiced currently in children. In adults, a systematic review in 2010 found that the most commonly performed and successful reinnervation technique is ansa cervicalis to recurrent laryngeal nerve anastomosis.[34] It has been performed with success in adults, with a large series of 237 patients with unilateral vocal fold paralysis after thyroid surgery finding significantly improved vocal parameters and confirmation of successful reinnervation on EMG.[35] In adult patients, laryngeal reinnervation has been directly compared with vocal fold medialization in the treatment of unilateral vocal cord palsy in a prospective randomized trial.[36] Both groups showed significant improvements; however, interestingly, the group aged older than 50 did better with medialization, whereas the group younger than 50 did better with reinnervation, implying that nerve-grafting techniques have better outcomes in younger patients, making the pediatric group particularly suitable. The technique has been used in the pediatric age group with some success, although current reports are mainly of small case series with short-term follow-up.[37,38]

Repair of Damaged Vocal Cords with Synthetic Superficial Lamina Propria

Medialization of cords with damage to the superficial lamina propria (SLP) and loss of the normal mucosal wave has limited benefit in voice improvement. An alternative approach is to develop a synthetic substitute for this important gel layer to be injected into the Reinke space. A US study in 2011 describes the injection of a polyethylene glycol polymer in canines with promising effects on phonatory mucosa.[39] A different approach harvested fibroblast from patients' buccal mucosa, and injected them into the SLP following cell culture, with improved outcomes sustained for 12 months measured by voice handicap index (VHI), voice quality questionnaire, and mucosal wave grade.[40]

SUMMARY

Management of voice disorders is an exciting area of pediatric otolaryngology that is evolving rapidly. With careful assessment and directed management, using voice therapy alone or in conjunction with surgery, most children will gain improvement in their voice.

REFERENCES

1. Dalal PG, Marray D, Messner AH, et al. Pediatric laryngeal dimensions: an age-based analysis. Anesth Analg 2009;108:1475–9.
2. Aram D, Ekelman B, Nation J. Preschoolers with language disorders—10 years later. J Speech Hear Res 1984;27:232–44.
3. Senturia BH, Wilson FB. Otolaryngorhinic findings in children with voice deviations. Preliminary report. Ann Otol Rhinol Laryngol 1968;77:1027–41.
4. Silverman EM, Zimmer CH. Incidence of chronic hoarseness among school age children. J Speech Hear Disord 1975;40:211–5.
5. Merati AL, Keppel K, Braun NM, et al. Pediatric voice-related quality of life: findings in healthy children and in common laryngeal disorders. Ann Otol Rhinol Laryngol 2008;117(4):259–62.
6. Ruscello DM, Lass NJ, Podbesek J. Listeners' perceptions of normal and voice-disordered children. Folia Phoniatr 1988;40(6):290–6.
7. Hirano M, Kurita S, Nakashima T. Growth, development and aging of the human vocal folds. In: Bless DM, Abbs JH, editors. Vocal fold physiology:contemporary research and clinical issues. San Diego (CA): College Hill Press; 1983. p. 22–43.
8. Hirano M, Kurita S, Kiyokawa K. Posterior glottis. Morphological study in excised human larynges. Ann Otol Rhinol Laryngol 1986;95:576–81.
9. Roland NJ, Bhalla RK, Earis J. The local side effects of corticosteroids. Chest 2004;126(1):213–9.
10. Angelillo N, Di Costanzo B, Angelillo M. Epidemiological study on vocal disorders in paediatric age. J Prev Med Hyg 2008;49(1):1–5.
11. Mathieson L, Hiani S, Epstein R, et al. Laryngeal manual therapy: a preliminary study to examine its treatment effects in the management of muscle tension dysphonia. J Voice 2009;23(3):353–66.
12. Maturo SC, Braun N, Brown DJ, et al. Intraoperative laryngeal electromyography in children with vocal fold immobility: results of a multicenter longitudinal study. Arch Otolaryngol Head Neck Surg 2011;137(12):1251–7.
13. AlQudehy Z, Norton J, El-Hakim H. Electromyography in children's laryngeal mobility disorders: a proposed grading system. Arch Otolaryngol Head Neck Surg 2012;138(10):936–41.
14. Mandell DL, Kay D, Dohar JE, et al. Lack of association between esophageal biopsy, bronchoalveolar lavage, and endoscopy findings in hoarse children. Arch Otolaryngol Head Neck Surg 2004;130(11):1293–7.

15. Koufman JA, Blalock PD. Functional voice disorders. Otolaryngol Clin North Am 1991;24:1059–73.
16. Akif Kilic M, Okur E, Yildirim I, et al. The prevalence of vocal fold nodules in school age children. Int J Pediatr Otorhinolaryngol 2004;68(4):409–12.
17. Shah RK, Woodnorth GH, Glynn A, et al. Pediatric vocal nodules: correlation with perceptual voice analysis. Int J Pediatr Otorhinolaryngol 2005;60(7):903–9.
18. Pedersen M, McGlashan J. Surgical versus non-surgical interventions for vocal fold nodules. Cochrane Database Syst Rev 2012;(6):CD001934.
19. Mori K. Vocal fold nodules in children: preferable therapy. Int J Pediatr Otorhinolaryngol 1999;49(Suppl 1):S303–6.
20. Tezcaner CZ, Karatayli Ozgursoy S, Sati I, et al. Changes after voice therapy in objective and subjective measurements of pediatric patients with vocal nodules. Eur Arch Otorhinolaryngol 2009;266(12):1923–7.
21. Bouchayer M, Cornut G. Microsurgical treatment for benign vocal fold lesions: indications, technique, results. Folia Phoniatr 1992;44(3–4):155–84.
22. Ford CN, Bless DM, Campos G, et al. Anterior commissure microwebs associated with vocal nodules: detection, prevalence and significance. Laryngoscope 1994;104(11 Pt 1):1369–75.
23. Green G. Psycho-behavioural characteristics of children with vocal nodules: WPBIC ratings. J Speech Hear Disord 1989;54(3):306–12.
24. Kosko JR, Derkay CS. Role of cesarean section in prevention of recurrent respiratory papillomatosis—is there one? Int J Pediatr Otorhinolaryngol 1996;35(1):31–8.
25. Schraff S, Derkay CS, Burke B, et al. American Society of Paediatric Otolaryngology members' experience with recurrent respiratory papillomatosis and the use of adjuvant therapy. Arch Otolaryngol Head Neck Surg 2004;130(9):1039–42.
26. Wierzbicka M, Jackowska J, Bartochowska A, et al. Effectiveness of cidofovir intralesional treatment in recurrent respiratory papillomatosis. Eur Arch Otorhinolaryngol 2011;268(9):1305–11.
27. Pontes P, Weckx LL, Pignatari SS, et al. Local application of cidofavir as adjuvant therapy in recurrent laryngeal papillomatosis in children. Rev Assoc Med Bras 2009;55(5):581–6.
28. Pudszuhn A, Welzel C, Bloching M, et al. Intralesional cidofavir application in recurrent laryngeal papillomatosis. Eur Arch Otorhinolaryngol 2007;264(1):63–70.
29. McMurray JS, Connor N, Ford CN. Cidofovir efficacy in recurrent respiratory papillomatosis: a randomized, double-blind, placebo-controlled study. Ann Otol Rhinol Laryngol 2008;117:477–83.
30. Donne AJ, Hampson L, He XT, et al. Potential risk factors associated with the use of cidofovir to treat benign human papillomavirus-related disease. Antivir Ther 2009;14(7):939–52.
31. Forster G, Boltze C, Seidel J, et al. Juvenile laryngeal papillomatosis—immunisation with the polyvalent vaccine Gardasil. Laryngol Rhinol Otol 2008;87(11):796–9.
32. Daya H, Hosni A, Bejar-Solar I, et al. Pediatric vocal fold paralysis: a long-term retrospective study. Arch Otolaryngol Head Neck Surg 2000;126(1):21–5.
33. Birchall M, Macchiarini P. Airway transplantation: a debate worth having? Transplantation 2008;85(8):1075–80.
34. Aynehchi BB, McCoul ED, Sundaram K. Systematic review of laryngeal reinnervation techniques. Otolaryngol Head Neck Surg 2010;143(6):749–59.

35. Wang W, Chen D, Chen S, et al. Laryngeal reinnervation using ansa cervicalis for thyroid surgery-related unilateral vocal fold paralysis: a long-term outcome analysis of 237 cases. PLoS One 2011;6(4):e19128.

36. Paniello RC, Edgar JD, Kallogjeri D. Medialization versus reinnervation for unilateral vocal fold paralysis: a multicentre randomized clinical trial. Laryngoscope 2011;121(10):2172–9.

37. Marcum KK, Wright SC, Kemp ES, et al. A novel modification of the ansa to recurrent laryngeal nerve reinnervation procedure for young children. Int J Pediatr Otorhinolaryngol 2010;74(11):1335–7.

38. Smith ME. Pediatric ansa cervicalis to recurrent laryngeal nerve anastomosis. Adv Otorhinolaryngol 2012;73:80–5.

39. Karajanagi SS, Lopez-Guerra G, Park H, et al. Assessment of canine vocal fold function after injection of a new biomaterial designed to treat phonatory mucosal scarring. Ann Otol Rhinol Laryngol 2011;120(3):175–84.

40. Chetri DK, Berke GS. Injection of cultured autologous fibroblasts for human vocal fold scars. Laryngoscope 2011;121(4):785–92.

Laryngomalacia

Allison M. Dobbie, MD*, David R. White, MD

KEYWORDS

- Stridor • Laryngomalacia • Upper airway obstruction • Supraglottoplasty
- Aryepiglottoplasty

KEY POINTS

- Laryngomalacia is the most common congenital laryngeal anomaly, accounting for up to 70% of patients who present with stridor. Most cases are mild and self-resolve, but severe symptoms require investigation and treatment.
- Laryngomalacia presents as a spectrum of disease, from mild intermittent stridor to life-threatening airway compromise.
- There is a strong association of laryngomalacia with gastroesophageal reflux disease (GERD), which warrants medical treatment of GERD in many cases.
- In children with severe laryngomalacia, supraglottoplasty is the preferred surgical option, which can achieve improvement in both airway and feeding symptoms.
- Laryngomalacia can play a role in sleep-disordered breathing and obstructive sleep apnea.

 Videos of flexible fiberoptic laryngoscopy and supraglottoplasty accompany this article at http://www.pediatric.theclinics.com/

INTRODUCTION: NATURE OF THE PROBLEM

Laryngomalacia is the most common congenital laryngeal anomaly and accounts for 60% to 70% of cases of stridor in neonates and infants.[1] The physical finding of stridor is a manifestation of upper airway obstruction caused by collapse of the supraglottic tissue because of excess mucosa, and abnormal and/or reduced laryngeal tone. Symptoms generally become apparent after the first 2 weeks of life, and, in most cases, resolve between 12 and 18 months of age. Most cases resolve with minimal or no treatment; approximately 10% of cases require surgical intervention.

The term laryngomalacia, or soft larynx in Latin, replaced the more antiquated term congenital laryngeal stridor, which had previously been used to describe the

Division of Pediatric Otolaryngology, Department of Otolaryngology-Head and Neck Surgery, Medical University of South Carolina, 135 Rutledge Avenue, MSC 550, Charleston, SC 29425, USA
* Corresponding author.
E-mail address: allison.dobbie@gmail.com

Pediatr Clin N Am 60 (2013) 893–902
http://dx.doi.org/10.1016/j.pcl.2013.04.013
0031-3955/13/$ – see front matter © 2013 Elsevier Inc. All rights reserved.

condition. First coined by Jackson and Jackson[2] in 1942, the term differentiated the condition from other causes of stridor and more clearly depicted the flaccidity of the larynx.[3]

THE INFANT LARYNX: ANATOMIC CONSIDERATIONS

A review of laryngeal anatomy aids in the understanding of pathophysiology in laryngomalacia. The structure of the larynx is divided into 3 areas: the supraglottis, glottis, and subglottis. Laryngomalacia affects the supraglottic structures, which include the portions of the larynx above the level of the vocal cords. Important supraglottic structures that can be involved in laryngomalacia include the epiglottis, arytenoid cartilages, and aryepiglottic folds (which connect the epiglottis to the arytenoids).

Neonatal and infantile larynges have several important differences from those of older children and adults. At birth, the position of the larynx is higher than in older children and adults.[4] The growth of the larynx is accelerated during the first 3 years of postnatal life and gradually achieves its final shape. Postnatal descent of the hyoid and larynx is unique to humans. The high position of the larynx at the time of birth facilitates transition to spontaneous breathing and prevention of aspiration, and this also accounts for obligate nasal breathing in neonates. The descent of the larynx is crucial for appropriate development of speech. Major postnatal changes to the larynx occur in the first year of life.

The infantile epiglottis is longer than the laryngeal length in older children, which may predispose it to posterior displacement. The cartilage of the infantile larynx is also more pliable than that of the larynx later in life, a property that has been proposed to play a role in the collapsibility of the laryngeal airway.

CLINICAL PRESENTATION

Inspiratory stridor is the primary feature of laryngomalacia. Characterized by a harsh, high-pitched sound, stridor as it presents in laryngomalacia often worsens while the infant is supine, feeding, or crying. Feeding difficulties also often accompany the presence of stridor in patients with laryngomalacia, because the delicate balance between the suck-swallow sequence and respiration is often disrupted.[5] Coughing, choking, regurgitation with feedings, and slow oral intake are all common symptoms. There is thought to be a close relationship between laryngomalacia and gastroesophageal/laryngopharyngeal reflux, although the exact mechanism has yet to be fully elucidated.

Other causes of stridor must also be considered when evaluating a patient with these symptoms (Table 1). One of the most useful ways to differentiate between causes of noisy breathing is to identify in which phase of the respiratory cycle the sound is heard. Different causes of airway obstruction can lead to stridor during different phases of respiration: inspiration, expiration, or both (biphasic).

Stridor present during inspiration is usually caused by partial obstruction at the level of the supraglottic tissues. Variable extrathoracic obstruction results in primarily inspiratory stridor. During inspiration, atmospheric pressure is greater than extrathoracic intraluminal airway pressure, leading to collapse of supraglottic structures. During the expiratory phase, the exhalatory breath increases extrathoracic airway pressure such that it overcomes the collapse. Stridor primarily present during expiration is usually caused by obstruction in the lower tracheal airway. Negative intrathoracic pressure during inspiration allows air movement into the lungs, but the increase in intrathoracic pressure during expiration causes affected portions of the tracheal airway to collapse, leading to expiratory stridor.

Table 1
Causes of infantile stridor

Inspiratory Phase	Expiratory Phase	Biphasic
Laryngomalacia	Tracheomalacia	Subglottic stenosis
Vallecular cyst	Complete tracheal rings	Subglottic cyst
Epiglottitis	Vascular anomalies • Pulmonary artery sling • Double aortic arch • Aberrant innominate artery	Subglottic hemangioma
—	—	Vocal cord paralysis
—	—	Laryngeal web
—	—	Respiratory papillomatosis

WORK-UP: PATIENT HISTORY

A complete patient history should be obtained when evaluating a patient with stridor. History should include a focus on antenatal and perinatal events, as well as current symptoms (**Table 2**).

WORK-UP: PHYSICAL EXAMINATION

A complete physical examination should be performed, taking special note of the following:

- Vital signs
- Weight
- General appearance
- Presence of upper airway sounds and their timing within the respiratory cycle
- Work of breathing, such as the presence of suprasternal retractions or abdominal muscle usage
- Auscultation of lung fields
- Chest wall structural abnormalities (eg, pectus excavatum)

WORK-UP: DIAGNOSTIC TESTING

When laryngomalacia is suspected, diagnosis is confirmed with flexible fiberoptic laryngoscopy (Video 1). Flexible laryngoscopy can, in most cases, be performed easily

Table 2
Key components in patient history

Antenatal/Perinatal Events	Respiratory Symptoms	Other Symptoms
Prenatal complications	Stridor	Weight gain
Gestational age and weight at birth	Ameliorating or aggravating factors (positioning, sleep, crying)	Feeding problems (coughing, choking, gagging)
History of endotracheal intubation	Cyanosis	Prolonged feeding time
Other congenital anomalies	Apneas	Reflux
—	—	History of pneumonias (suspected aspiration)

in the otolaryngologist's office or at the bedside without sedation. A small, flexible fiberoptic endoscope is passed from the child's nostril through the nasal cavity and is positioned just above the larynx, allowing observation of the dynamic states of the larynx. Topical anesthetic such as lidocaine has been shown to exaggerate laryngomalacia[6] and should not be used during flexible laryngoscopy in patients suspected to have the disease. Flexible fiberoptic laryngoscopy has been found to have good reliability (88%) for diagnosis of laryngomalacia, regardless of physician experience.[7]

The key findings on flexible laryngoscopy, which may be present in any combination, are:

- A tightly curled, omega-shaped epiglottis
- Retroflexion (posterior displacement) of epiglottis
- Short aryepiglottic folds
- Redundant, prolapsing arytenoid mucosa and cartilage

Formal direct laryngoscopy and bronchoscopy under general anesthesia is not necessary in every patient with findings of laryngomalacia on flexible endoscopy. Most patients only require confirmation of diagnosis by flexible endoscopy alone. Rigid direct laryngoscopy should be performed in the following situations:

- Absence of any abnormality in a patient with clinical stridor
- When the symptom severity does not correlate with laryngoscopic examination, raising suspicion for another cause or secondary lesion
- Clinical signs and symptoms of severe disease, in patients for whom surgical intervention is considered
- Significant aspiration symptoms that cause concern for a posterior laryngeal cleft or tracheoesophageal fistula

Other diagnostic tests may be considered, including modified barium swallow or functional endoscopic evaluation of swallowing, particularly if concern for aspiration exists. In addition, esophageal pH probe studies should be considered if moderate to severe laryngomalacia symptoms persist despite antireflux treatment. Some investigators propose formal pH studies on all patients with laryngomalacia.[8]

CLASSIFICATION

Many classification schemes have been proposed for laryngomalacia, but no single system has been universally adopted. All schemes center on defining the site at which the supraglottic collapse is present.[9–13] There are 4 main categories:

- Posterior collapse: primarily caused by redundant arytenoid mucosa and/or excess cuneiform cartilage that prolapses into the airway
- Lateral collapse: from foreshortened aryepiglottic folds
- Anterior collapse: obstruction from retroflexed epiglottis
- Combined: 2 or more of the patterns coexistent

If surgical intervention becomes necessary, classification of anatomic site of collapse can help direct surgical approach.[12]

ETIOLOGIC THEORIES

The exact pathophysiology of laryngomalacia has yet to be fully elucidated and is the subject of much ongoing research. Since the original description of this disease process, several theories have been proposed to explain its pathogenesis, which include anatomic, cartilaginous, and neurologic theories. The anatomic theory purports that the cause of laryngomalacia is abnormal shape and structure of the larynx. In a prospective study by Manning and colleagues,[14] laryngeal dimensions were compared between patients with laryngomalacia and controls. The mean ratio of aryepiglottic fold/glottic length of patients with severe laryngomalacia was significantly lower than that of controls without laryngomalacia. Within the group of patients with severe laryngomalacia, the ratio for those without associated neurologic conditions did not differ from that of the other patients.

The cartilaginous theory attributes the cause to an intrinsic structural difference in the laryngeal cartilages of infants with laryngomalacia, but this has been refuted by recent studies that showed histologically normal fibroelastic arytenoid cartilage from patients with laryngomalacia.[15]

At present, the neurologic theory has the most support in recent studies. The neurologic theory proposes that neurosensory dysfunction leads to lack of neuromuscular coordination of the supraglottic airway. Increased laryngopharyngeal sensory thresholds were observed in patients with laryngomalacia,[16] indicating that peripheral afferent function of laryngeal sensation is altered. This is a plausible clinical explanation for the weak laryngeal tone seen in infants with laryngomalacia, because studies have shown that alteration of laryngeal afferents is associated with changes in laryngeal motor function.

A recent histopathologic study lends support to this theory. Munson and colleagues[17] showed that nerve perimeter and surface area of the superior laryngeal nerve branches of the vagal nerve within supra-arytenoid tissue obtained from patients with severe laryngomalacia are significantly greater compared with age-matched autopsy tissue, thereby providing histologic confirmation of altered vagal nerve function in this patient population.

Gastroesophageal reflux disease (GERD) has also been implicated as a causative factor because of the high prevalence of reflux seen in patients with laryngomalacia.[18,19] GERD is observed in about 70% of patients with laryngomalacia.[20] Despite this strong association, systematic review of the literature has not found support for a direct causal relationship.[21] Nevertheless, laryngomalacia and extraesophageal reflux disease seem to have a propagating relationship. First, the negative intrathoracic pressure generated by breathing against an airway obstruction likely encourages contents of the stomach to be drawn into the esophagus, larynx, and pharynx. This mechanism has been proved in an animal model.[22] Second, supporters of the neuromuscular theory of laryngomalacia[16] point out that the same efferent vagal signals responsible for laryngeal muscular tone, which are thought to be underdeveloped in patients with laryngomalacia, control the tone of the lower esophageal sphincter.[23]

There is some evidence to support that the presence of extraesophageal reflux may in turn worsen symptoms of laryngomalacia by causing edema and inflammation of laryngeal tissues. In a study of specimens taken from patients with laryngomalacia of tissue excised during supraglottoplasty, histologic analysis revealed marked submucosal edema and dilated lymphatic channels.[15] In addition, laryngopharyngeal reflux may lead to impaired laryngopharyngeal sensation with resultant swallowing dysfunction and microaspiration in children.[24]

NONPHARMACOLOGIC TREATMENT

In patients in whom disease presentation is mild, with only intermittent stridor and absence of feeding difficulty, no intervention other than periodic monitoring is warranted (**Fig. 1**). Even mild cases can be treated with alterations in feeding techniques.

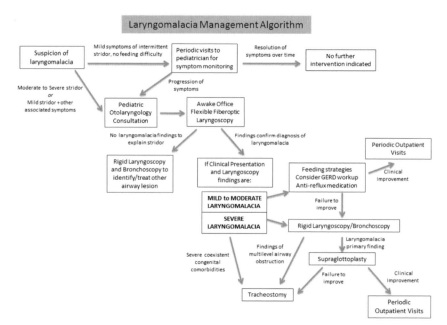

Fig. 1. Algorithm for management of laryngomalacia.

Feeding modifications include pacing, texture change by thickening the formula, and upright positioning during feeding.

PHARMACOLOGIC TREATMENT

The association between laryngomalacia and GERD is well established; however, the role of antireflux medications remains controversial.[25] There is a paucity of good evidence evaluating efficacy of antireflux medical treatment, because nearly all of the studies are limited by patient selection bias as well as the lack of randomization and control groups.[8,20]

However, acid suppression therapy should be implemented in patients with laryngomalacia who have a confirmed diagnosis of GERD. In patients with laryngomalacia with feeding difficulties and GERD-related symptoms, infants with laryngomalacia have improved feeding symptoms with high-dose H2-blocker therapy (ranitidine 3 mg/kg, 3 times a day).[16] Proton pump inhibitors (PPI) should be considered for refractory or breakthrough symptoms. They should also be implemented in patients who undergo surgical therapy, in the immediate perioperative and postoperative period until complete healing has occurred. Those with refractory symptoms may benefit from combined daytime PPI therapy and nighttime H2-blocker therapy.

SURGICAL MANAGEMENT

The decision to proceed with surgical management of laryngomalacia is determined by the severity of the patient's symptoms rather than by the severity of the endoscopic appearance of the airway (**Table 3**). Before the development of supraglottoplasty, tracheostomy was the standard treatment of severe laryngomalacia. Although tracheostomy is effective in bypassing the laryngeal obstruction, there are numerous risks, complications, and challenges associated with pediatric tracheostomy.

Table 3	
Indications for surgical intervention	
Absolute Indications	**Relative Indications**
Cor pulmonale and/or pulmonary hypertension	Weight loss with feeding difficulty
Pectus excavatum	Aspiration
Hypoxia/hypercapnea	Obstructive sleep apnea/sleep-disordered breathing
Respiratory compromise	—
Failure to thrive	—

Supraglottoplasty, also termed aryepiglottoplasty, is an endoscopic procedure designed to modify the anatomy of the supraglottic larynx to reduce collapse and prolapse into the airway. It has become the preferred primary surgical intervention for laryngomalacia. Supraglottoplasty typically involves division of the aryepiglottic folds and excision of arytenoid mucosa and/or cartilage (Video 2). A wide variety of techniques have been used. The first reported procedure of this type was in 1984 by Lane and colleagues[26] using cold steel instruments, followed by Seid and colleagues[27] using carbon dioxide laser.

Subjective improvement of stridor is seen in almost all patients after supraglottoplasty. Success rates of the procedure are around 90%. Polysomnography has recently been used as an objective test to evaluate success of the procedure, with postsurgical improvement in most measures.[28]

Supraglottoplasty has also been shown to reduce gastroesophageal reflux. In one study, all patients with laryngomalacia and coexistent GERD had significant reduction in reflux indices (defined as the percentage of time the pH is below 4 during pH probe study; $P = .02$).[23] Growth curves after supraglottoplasty have been studied as well. A study by Meier and colleagues[29] noted that within 3 months after surgery, significant improvement on the growth curve was seen in patients treated with supraglottoplasty ($P = .009$) compared with those either observed or treated with acid suppression therapy. After 12 months, all 3 groups approached the mean on the growth curve.

Risk factors for supraglottoplasty failures have been studied. Most often, lower success rates are seen in patients with other medical comorbidities.[30,31] In one recent study,[32] prematurity was an independent risk factor for a poor outcome after supraglottoplasty, even after correction for age and weight.

Complications of supraglottoplasty are rare, but include laryngeal edema, granuloma formation, and supraglottic stenosis.[30] Aspiration after supraglottoplasty has also been studied as a potential complication of the procedure.[33,34] However, postsupraglottoplasty aspiration recently has been found to be a continuation of aspiration that was present preoperatively rather than as a consequence of the operation.[5]

Contraindications for supraglottoplasty are few, but include presence of multilevel airway obstruction and severe neurodevelopmental comorbidities. Moreover, supraglottoplasty should be postponed if possible when upper or lower respiratory tract infections are present.

STATE-DEPENDENT AND LATE-ONSET LARYNGOMALACIA

Laryngomalacia has also been reported in children presenting with sleep-induced stridor, upper airway obstruction, and apnea.[35,36] In these patients, diagnosis is often much later, because in many cases there are no symptoms of laryngomalacia while the patient is awake. Many undergo adenotonsillectomy on diagnosis with obstructive sleep apnea as the standard first-line surgical treatment. On failure of improvement after adenotonsillectomy, sedated flexible bronchoscopy or sleep endoscopy can reveal the presence of laryngomalacia. Supraglottoplasty can be implemented to treat obstructive sleep apnea in patients with laryngomalacia observed during sleep endoscopy.

Another subtype of laryngomalacia is the exercise-induced variant.[37,38] This has been observed most often in older children and teenagers. Endoscopic findings in older children with laryngomalacia usually show collapse of supra-arytenoid tissue with normal-appearing epiglottis and aryepiglottic folds, in contrast with what is often observed in congenital laryngomalacia.[39]

SUMMARY

Laryngomalacia is a common disease of infancy and childhood and is certain to be encountered by the pediatrician. Most patients have a benign disease course; however, some present with more severe symptoms and develop life-threatening airway obstruction and failure to thrive. Proper identification of those patients who require medical and surgical intervention is key to treatment proceeding in timely fashion with successful outcomes. Additional consideration of the role of laryngomalacia in feeding disorders and sleep-disordered breathing aids in comprehensive care of patients with this disease.

SUPPLEMENTARY DATA

Supplementary data related to this article can be found online at http://dx.doi.org/10.1016/j.pcl.2013.04.013

REFERENCES

1. Daniel SJ. The upper airway: congenital malformations. Paediatr Respir Rev 2006;7(Suppl 1):S260–3.
2. Jackson C, Jackson CL. Diseases and injuries of the larynx. New York: The Macmillan company; 1942. p. xi, 1 l.
3. Richter GT, Thompson DM. The surgical management of laryngomalacia. Otolaryngol Clin North Am 2008;41(5):837–64, vii.
4. Lieberman DE, McCarthy RC, Hiiemae KM, et al. Ontogeny of postnatal hyoid and larynx descent in humans. Arch Oral Biol 2001;46(2):117–28.
5. Richter GT, Wootten CT, Rutter MJ, et al. Impact of supraglottoplasty on aspiration in severe laryngomalacia. Ann Otol Rhinol Laryngol 2009;118(4):259–66.
6. Nielson DW, Ku PL, Egger M. Topical lidocaine exaggerates laryngomalacia during flexible bronchoscopy. Am J Respir Crit Care Med 2000;161(1):147–51.
7. Lima TM, Goncalves DU, Goncalves LV, et al. Flexible nasolaryngoscopy accuracy in laryngomalacia diagnosis. Braz J Otorhinolaryngol 2008;74(1):29–32.
8. Bouchard S, Lallier M, Yazbeck S, et al. The otolaryngologic manifestations of gastroesophageal reflux: when is a pH study indicated? J Pediatr Surg 1999;34(7):1053–6.
9. Shah UK, Wetmore RF. Laryngomalacia: a proposed classification form. Int J Pediatr Otorhinolaryngol 1998;46(1–2):21–6.
10. Holinger LD, Konior RJ. Surgical management of severe laryngomalacia. Laryngoscope 1989;99(2):136–42.

11. Roger G, Denoyelle F, Triglia JM, et al. Severe laryngomalacia: surgical indications and results in 115 patients. Laryngoscope 1995;105(10):1111–7.
12. Olney DR, Greinwald JH Jr, Smith RJ, et al. Laryngomalacia and its treatment. Laryngoscope 1999;109(11):1770–5.
13. Lee KS, Chen BN, Yang CC, et al. CO_2 laser supraglottoplasty for severe laryngomalacia: a study of symptomatic improvement. Int J Pediatr Otorhinolaryngol 2007;71(6):889–95.
14. Manning SC, Inglis AF, Mouzakes J, et al. Laryngeal anatomic differences in pediatric patients with severe laryngomalacia. Arch Otolaryngol Head Neck Surg 2005;131(4):340–3.
15. Chandra RK, Gerber ME, Holinger LD. Histological insight into the pathogenesis of severe laryngomalacia. Int J Pediatr Otorhinolaryngol 2001;61(1):31–8.
16. Thompson DM. Abnormal sensorimotor integrative function of the larynx in congenital laryngomalacia: a new theory of etiology. Laryngoscope 2007; 117(6 Pt 2 Suppl 114):1–33.
17. Munson PD, Saad AG, El-Jamal SM, et al. Submucosal nerve hypertrophy in congenital laryngomalacia. Laryngoscope 2011;121(3):627–9.
18. Giannoni C, Sulek M, Friedman EM, et al. Gastroesophageal reflux association with laryngomalacia: a prospective study. Int J Pediatr Otorhinolaryngol 1998; 43(1):11–20.
19. Matthews BL, Little JP, McGuirt WF Jr, et al. Reflux in infants with laryngomalacia: results of 24-hour double-probe pH monitoring. Otolaryngol Head Neck Surg 1999;120(6):860–4.
20. Bibi H, Khvolis E, Shoseyov D, et al. The prevalence of gastroesophageal reflux in children with tracheomalacia and laryngomalacia. Chest 2001;119(2):409–13.
21. Hartl TT, Chadha NK. A systematic review of laryngomalacia and acid reflux. Otolaryngol Head Neck Surg 2012;147(4):619–26.
22. Wang W, Tovar JA, Eizaguirre I, et al. Airway obstruction and gastroesophageal reflux: an experimental study on the pathogenesis of this association. J Pediatr Surg 1993;28(8):995–8.
23. Hadfield PJ, Albert DM, Bailey CM, et al. The effect of aryepiglottoplasty for laryngomalacia on gastro-oesophageal reflux. Int J Pediatr Otorhinolaryngol 2003; 67(1):11–4.
24. Suskind DL, Thompson DM, Gulati M, et al. Improved infant swallowing after gastroesophageal reflux disease treatment: a function of improved laryngeal sensation? Laryngoscope 2006;116(8):1397–403.
25. Apps JR, Flint JD, Wacogne I. Towards evidence based medicine for paediatricians. Question 1. Does anti-reflux therapy improve symptoms in infants with laryngomalacia? Arch Dis Child 2012;97(4):385–7 [discussion: 387].
26. Lane RW, Weider DJ, Steinem C, et al. Laryngomalacia. A review and case report of surgical treatment with resolution of pectus excavatum. Arch Otolaryngol 1984; 110(8):546–51.
27. Seid AB, Park SM, Kearns MJ, et al. Laser division of the aryepiglottic folds for severe laryngomalacia. Int J Pediatr Otorhinolaryngol 1985;10(2):153–8.
28. Powitzky R, Stoner J, Fisher T, et al. Changes in sleep apnea after supraglottoplasty in infants with laryngomalacia. Int J Pediatr Otorhinolaryngol 2011;75(10):1234–9.
29. Meier JD, Nguyen SA, White DR. Improved growth curve measurements after supraglottoplasty. Laryngoscope 2011;121(7):1574–7.
30. Denoyelle F, Mondain M, Gresillon N, et al. Failures and complications of supraglottoplasty in children. Arch Otolaryngol Head Neck Surg 2003;129(10):1077–80 [discussion: 1080].

31. Senders CW, Navarrete EG. Laser supraglottoplasty for laryngomalacia: are specific anatomical defects more influential than associated anomalies on outcome? Int J Pediatr Otorhinolaryngol 2001;57(3):235–44.

32. Day KE, Discolo CM, Meier JD, et al. Risk factors for supraglottoplasty failure. Otolaryngol Head Neck Surg 2012;146(2):298–301.

33. Schroeder JW Jr, Bhandarkar ND, Holinger LD. Synchronous airway lesions and outcomes in infants with severe laryngomalacia requiring supraglottoplasty. Arch Otolaryngol Head Neck Surg 2009;135(7):647–51.

34. Eustaquio M, Lee EN, Digoy GP. Feeding outcomes in infants after supraglottoplasty. Otolaryngol Head Neck Surg 2011;145(5):818–22.

35. Amin MR, Isaacson G. State-dependent laryngomalacia. Ann Otol Rhinol Laryngol 1997;106(11):887–90.

36. Smith JL 2nd, Sweeney DM, Smallman B, et al. State-dependent laryngomalacia in sleeping children. Ann Otol Rhinol Laryngol 2005;114(2):111–4.

37. Bent JP 3rd, Miller DA, Kim JW, et al. Pediatric exercise-induced laryngomalacia. Ann Otol Rhinol Laryngol 1996;105(3):169–75.

38. Smith RJ, Bauman NM, Bent JP, et al. Exercise-induced laryngomalacia. Ann Otol Rhinol Laryngol 1995;104(7):537–41.

39. Richter GT, Rutter MJ, deAlarcon A, et al. Late-onset laryngomalacia: a variant of disease. Arch Otolaryngol Head Neck Surg 2008;134(1):75–80.

Nasal Obstruction in Newborns

Sharon H. Gnagi, MD[a], Scott A. Schraff, MD[b],*

KEYWORDS

- Nasal obstruction • Choanal atresia • Pyriform aperture stenosis
- Nasolacrimal duct cyst • Rhinitis • Nasal dermoid • Glioma • Encephalocele

KEY POINTS

- Nasal obstruction in newborns can range in severity from a mild irritant to a life-threatening situation with potentially devastating consequences including respiratory distress and failure to thrive.
- The differential diagnosis for nasal obstruction of the newborn is vast, requiring a thorough history, physical examination, nasal endoscopy, and imaging for accurate diagnosis and treatment.
- The most common etiology of nasal obstruction is simple inflammation of the nasal mucosa, which may be managed conservatively.
- Several etiologies of nasal obstruction may warrant further evaluation and genetic workup to diagnose associated conditions.

INTRODUCTION

Newborn infants are obligate nasal breathers for the first several months of life, with more than 50% of infants desaturating if nasally obstructed.[1] Anatomically, their entire tongue length is in contact with the hard and soft palate, and the epiglottis is superior to the soft palate, causing difficulty with oral breathing.[2] This allows for concomitant respiration with oral intake while the infant is learning to mouth breathe in the first 4 to 6 weeks after birth. Therefore, nasal obstruction may lead to serious consequences in the neonate, including respiratory distress or failure to thrive. Thus, nasal obstruction is an important clinical entity to recognize, effectively diagnose, and treat.

EVALUATION
History

Appropriate evaluation of nasal obstruction in newborns requires a thorough neonatal history. Signs and symptoms consistent with nasal obstruction may be described by

The authors have nothing to disclose.
[a] Department of Otolaryngology, Mayo Clinic Arizona, 5777 East Mayo Boulevard, Phoenix, AZ 85054, USA; [b] Department of Otolaryngology, Phoenix Children's Hospital, 1919 East Thomas Road, Phoenix, AZ 85006, USA
* Corresponding author.
E-mail address: schraffs@hotmail.com

the parents, family, or care providers (**Box 1**). Maternal history is equally important, as maternal medical conditions, drug ingestion, and sexually transmitted diseases can be etiologies of nasal obstruction in the newborn. Familial genetic disorders, and/or prenatally diagnosed conditions should also be noted. Birth history including prematurity, length of labor, presentation, and trauma during delivery (eg, use of forceps) can implicate a potential iatrogenic cause of nasal obstruction.

Additionally, timing and onset of symptoms can provide clues as to the etiology of nasal obstruction. While bilateral nasal obstruction often presents in the neonatal period, unilateral nasal obstruction may not present until much later in life, with chronic nasal drainage, skin irritation, and congestion. Intermittent respiratory distress at birth may be associated with a ball-valving obstruction or intermittent nasal congestion associated with the physiologic nasal cycle.[3] Thus, Apgar scores and need for resuscitation and/or intubation at birth may help delineate the severity and anatomic extent of the obstruction.

Physical Examination

The first task when assessing the newborn with nasal obstruction is to determine the degree of respiratory difficulty and establish a safe airway. Tachypnea, nasal flaring, substernal and costal retractions, and irritability suggest respiratory distress. Lethargy and cyanosis are more concerning and suggest respiratory fatigue, impending failure, and need for an immediate intervention.

If an adequate airway exists, the physical examination begins with external inspection for a gross deformity, asymmetry, or pit. Then, nasal patency should then be assessed. Anterior rhinoscopy with an otoscope may also help visualize anterior stenosis, masses, or obstructive mucus. Application of a decongestant may enhance the

Box 1
Signs and symptoms of nasal obstruction
Stuffy nose
Rhinorrhea
Mucus
Stertor
Snoring/snorting
External deformity
Nasal flaring
Chest Retractions
Cyanosis ($\pm$ cyclical nature)
Feeding difficulties
Hyponasal cry
Failure to thrive
Dyspnea/apnea
Aerophagia with abdominal distention
Difficulty sleeping
Epiphora

examination and enable the provider to compare the congested and decongested extent of obstruction to distinguish between anatomic obstruction and mucosal edema.[4] Alternative methods of assessing patency include placing a mirror or spoon under the nare and visualizing condensation, administering nasal saline and observing bubbles, or closing 1 nare and the mouth and auscultating for air movement.[5] Another option includes gently passing a small (5 or 6 French) catheter through the nose into the nasopharynx to confirm an open communication. Obstruction at the anterior inlet may suggest pyriform aperture stenosis, while obstruction posteriorly (approximately 32 mm) may suggest choanal atresia.[6] Visualizing or palpating the tube through the mouth confirms that the tube is not coiled in the nose to prevent misdiagnosis. In infants with craniofacial abnormalities or visible nasal masses, care must be taken when attempting to pass a nasal catheter, as these may be associated with skull base defects and risk intracranial passage of the catheter.[7] Additional studies to assess nasal patency include the use of a tympanometer placed at the nare to confirm or exclude a closed cavity.[8]

Nasal Endoscopy

Nasal endoscopy is typically the next step to determine the location or causality of the obstruction. A flexible endoscopic nasal examination is a simple and minimally invasive diagnostic procedure that can be performed in the office or at bedside with no sedation by trained specialists. The examination poses essentially no risk and causes minimal distress to the patient and family. In the rare instance that an adequate endoscopic nasal examination cannot be completed at the bedside, further evaluation in the operating room may be warranted. If a nasal mass is identified on endoscopy, it should be assumed to have intracranial extent until proven otherwise. Therefore, no biopsy of a mass should be performed until appropriate imaging has been undertaken.[9]

Imaging

There are multiple imaging modalities available for assessing nasal obstruction and the upper airway of newborns. Historically, plain radiographs with radiopaque contrast in the nasal cavity have been used to assess for obstruction. With the advent of more sophisticated imaging technology, plain films are rarely employed because of poor sensitivity and specificity. Computed tomography CT scans allow the best bony definition, and are typically the test of choice to assess choanal atresia and pyriform aperture stenosis. Suctioning of the nose before CT scanning is helpful to clear secretions that may be confused with a soft tissue or membranous obstruction.[10] Magnetic resonance imaging (MRI) is a better choice to evaluate nasal masses to delineate intracranial involvement and extent. MRI also avoids radiation exposure in infants and may be preferentially selected over CT for this reason.

DIFFERENTIAL DIAGNOSIS

The differential diagnosis for nasal obstruction in newborns is vast (**Box 2**). A thorough evaluation includes careful consideration of each potential etiology, and acknowledgment that more than 1 etiology may coexist.

Congenital Etiologies

There are countless congenital malformations secondary to aberrant embryogenesis of both the internal and external nose potentially causing nasal obstruction. These include but are not limited to: midfacial hypoplasia, craniosynostosis, arhinia

Box 2
Differential diagnosis of neonatal nasal obstruction

Congenital
- Choanal atresia
- Congenital nasal pyriform aperture stenosis
- Midfacial hypoplasia
- Nasolacrimal duct cysts
- Midline nasal masses
  - Nasal dermoid
  - Glioma
  - Encephalocele/meningocele
  - Thornwaldt cyst

Neoplasms
- Teratoma
- Hamartoma
- Hemangioma
- Lymphangioma
- Lipoma
- Neurofibroma
- Rhabdomyosarcoma
- Lymphoma

Infectious
- Upper respiratory infection
- Respiratory syncytial virus
- STDs
  - Chlamydia
  - Gonorrhea
  - Syphilis

Foreign body
Traumatic/iatrogenic
- Septal dislocation
- Septal hematoma
- Nasal tip depression
- Rhinitis medicamentosa
- Instrumentation: suction trauma, nasogastric tube, CPAP, nasal prongs

Inflammatory
- Allergic rhinitis (cow's milk, soy)
- Gastroesophageal reflux
- Recurrent emesis
- Idiopathic

Metabolic
- Hypothyroidism

Maternal
- Estrogenic stimuli
- Drug ingestion (methimazole, methyldopa, opiates, tricyclic antidepressants, propranolol)

Associated syndromes
- Cystic fibrosis
- Kartagener
- CHARGE
- Apert
- Crouzon
- Treacher-Collins
- Fetal alcohol syndrome
- Down

(complete absence of the nose), nasal hypoplasia (congenitally absent nasal bones), complete or partial nasal duplication, single centrally placed nostril, supernumerary teeth in the nose, Thornwaldt cyst, nasopharyngeal stenosis (incomplete separation of the soft palate and posterior pharyngeal wall), and others. Of these numerous congenital causalities, the most common and clinically significant will be discussed.

Choanal atresia
Normally, the nasal cavity is connected to the remainder of the airway via the nasopharynx. Choanal atresia is the failure of the nasal cavity to connect to the naso- and oropharynx. Theoretically, this results from alterations in embryogenesis with persistence of the buccopharyngeal membrane or failure of the oronasal membrane

to rupture, although no theory has been proven.[2] It occurs in approximately 1 of 5000 to 8000 live births and is twice as common in girls.[11] Unilateral choanal atresia is more common than bilateral involvement, accounting for 65% to 75% of cases. Comparatively, bilateral choanal atresia has more serious clinical implications and is associated with other congenital abnormalities in 50% of patients.[6] Although most readily associated with CHARGE syndrome (**Box 3**), it is also seen with polydactyly, Crouzon syndrome, craniosynostosis, microencephaly, meningocele, facial asymmetry, cleft palate, hypertelorism, and nasal and auricular deformities.[2]

Nasal endoscopy demonstrates a blind sac with a lack of communication from the nasal cavity to the nasopharynx (**Fig. 1**). CT is the radiographic imaging method of choice and reveals narrowing of the posterior nasal cavity, medialization of the lateral nasal wall, and thickening of the vomer; it may be classified as bony, membranous, or mixed (**Fig. 2**).[12] Because of its association with multiple other anomalies, a genetic evaluation and thorough workup of possible associated conditions should be completed.

Treatment for choanal atresia requires surgical intervention. The timing of intervention is largely dependent on bilateral verses unilateral involvement. Newborns with bilateral choanal atresia typically present with respiratory distress at birth and may require intubation to establish an airway. In bilateral cases, surgical correction is typically performed in the first week of life and has been described via transnasal puncture, transpalatal and endoscopic transnasal approaches plus or minus postoperative stenting, mitomycin C application, and laser use.[7] In unilateral cases, treatment is typically delayed until just before school attendance to allow growth and development of the midface, while stopping embarrassing nasal drainage and resultant skin irritation, and relieving nasal obstruction before interaction with peers.[2]

Congenital nasal pyriform aperture stenosis

Congenital nasal pyriform aperture stenosis (CNPAS) is an uncommon etiology of nasal obstruction resulting from bony overgrowth of the nasal process of the maxilla.[13] The pyriform aperture is a pear-shaped bony inlet comprising the most anterior and narrowest bony portion of the nasal airway; therefore, any overgrowth causes a decrease in cross-sectional area with resultant exponential increase in airway resistance and associated obstruction.[14] Anterior rhinoscopy reveals a narrowed anterior nasal passage with bony thickening medially, typically affecting bilateral nares (**Fig. 3**). Nasal endoscopy may not be able to be performed secondary to the small anterior passage. CT is typically the imaging method of choice and confirms the diagnosis if the pyriform aperture measures less than 11 mm at the level of the inferior meatus (**Fig. 4**).[15]

Box 3
CHARGE association
C: Colobomas
H: Heart abnormalities
A: Choanal atresia
R: Growth or mental retardation
G: Genitourinary anomalies
E: Ear abnormalities

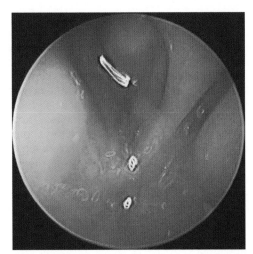

Fig. 1. Nasal endoscopy revealing membranous occlusion of the posterior nasal cavity consistent with choanal atresia.

CNPAS may occur as an isolated anomaly or in association with absence of the anterior pituitary, diabetes insipidus, submucous cleft palate, and hypoplastic maxillary sinuses. Oral examination may reveal an absent upper labial frenulum and a prominent central mega incisor (**Fig. 5**). It may manifest as part of the holoprosencephaly

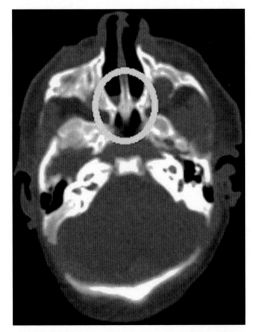

Fig. 2. Axial CT showing atretic choanae. Circle encompasses atresia at posterior nasal vault. Note the champagne flute appearance of the nasal caults characteristic for choanal atresia. (*From* Shah UK, Daniero JJ, Clary MS, et al. Low birth weight choanal atresia repair using image guidance. Int J Pediatr Otorhinolaryngol 2011;75:1339; with permission.)

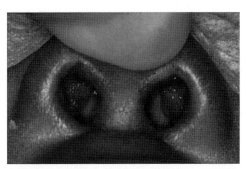

Fig. 3. Congenital nasal pyriform aperture stenosis, as seen on anterior rhinoscopy. (*From* Elluru RG, Wootten CT. Congenital malformations of the nose. In: Flint PW, Haughey BH, Lund VJ, et al, editors. Cummings otolaryngology: head & neck surgery. 5th edition. Philadelphia: Mosby; 2010. p. 2693; with permission.)

sequence (HPE), characterized by failure of the prosencephalon (forebrain) to divide into bilateral cerebral hemispheres.[14,16,17] Suspicion of HPE warrants chromosomal analysis, genetic consultation, and possibly an endocrinology workup and electrolyte evaluation. Further imaging of the brain may be required with MRI.

Management is dependent on the severity of symptomatology, but may require surgical intervention to drill and widen the pyriform aperture (**Fig. 6**). This is typically performed via a sublabial approach and may require nasal stents left up to a month postoperatively to prevent restenosis.

Nasolacrimal duct cysts

Nasolacrimal duct obstruction is a common congenital abnormality and occurs in approximately 30% of neonates.[18] In most cases, the obstruction is asymptomatic

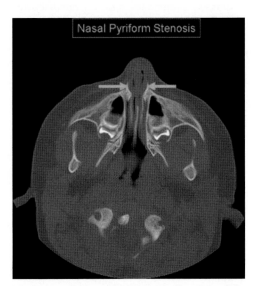

Fig. 4. CT scan of a child who has CNPAS. Note the inward bowing of the nasal processes of the maxillary bone with the pyriform aperture measuring 7 mm (*arrows*). (*From* Tate JR, Sykes J. Congenital nasal pyriform aperture stenosis. Otolaryngol Clin North Am 2009;42:523; with permission.)

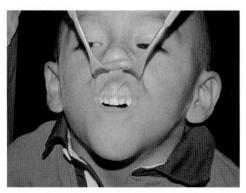

Fig. 5. Child who has CPAS and evidence of a single central megaincisor. (*From* Tate JR, Sykes J. Congenital nasal pyriform aperture stenosis. Otolaryngol Clin North Am 2009;42:523; with permission.)

and resolves spontaneously within the first year of life.[19] However, if there are both a proximal obstruction and a distal obstruction within the duct, a cyst known as a dacryocystocele forms, which may herniate into the nasal cavity and cause obstruction. Distal obstruction typically occurs at the valve of Hasner, which normally ruptures with neonatal respirations at birth.[20] Bilateral obstruction occurs in approximately 14% of congenital dacryocystoceles, and a fraction of these protrude into the nasal cavity causing resultant respiratory distress.[21]

Associated findings include epiphora and facial swelling with blue-to-red discoloration inferior to the medial canthus of the eye. Nasal endoscopy reveals a mass protruding below the inferior turbinate (**Fig. 7**). Nasolacrimal duct cysts can be differentiated from midline nasal masses by the ability to bypass them medially on endoscopy.[20] Imaging reveals cystic masses projecting into the nasal cavity with superomedial displacement of the inferior turbinate, and may demonstrate dilation of the lacrimal duct and sac (**Fig. 8**). Conservative management including warm compresses and gentle massage may be effective for simple dacryocystoceles without intranasal extension. However, for those with intranasal extension, management normally consists of probing of the duct and/or surgical marsupialization of the intranasal cyst.[3]

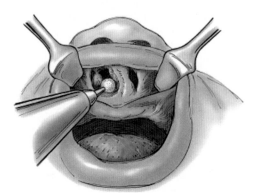

Fig. 6. Sublabial approach to the pyriform aperture. A drill is used to increase the cross-sectional area of the pyriform aperture. (*From* Tate JR, Sykes J. Congenital nasal pyriform aperture stenosis. Otolaryngol Clin North Am 2009;42:522; with permission.)

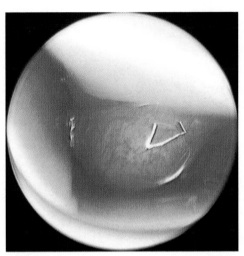

Fig. 7. Endoscopic view of a nasolacrimal duct cyst lateral and inferior to the inferior turbinate resulting in superomedial displacement of the turbinate.

Congenital frontonasal masses

Congenital midline nasal masses may cause nasal obstruction in the newborn and present a diagnostic challenge for the clinician, as they may represent several different underlying pathologies. Although the most common etiologies are nasal dermoid, encephalocele, and glioma, the differential consists of other neoplasms will be discussed (**Fig. 9**). Frontonasal masses are rare and occur in only 1 of every 20,000 to 40,000 births.[22] All result from aberrant embryogenesis of the anterior neuropore, typically producing a skull base defect with risk of intracranial connection. Because of this, children presenting with midline nasal masses may be at increased risk of developing meningitis, and a biopsy should not be performed before imaging.

Midline nasal masses may present with an external deformity or may be solely intranasal with no external sign on physical examination. Nasal endoscopy can help delineate the extent of intranasal involvement. MRI is the imaging modality of choice for assessing all masses of the frontonasal region (**Fig. 10**). Advantages include multiplanar imaging, distinguishing cartilage, bone, brain, and fluid interfaces; diffusion imaging to detect epidermoid tumors; and the capacity to evaluate the brain for associated cerebral anomalies.[23] Management often requires surgical correction, classically via a combined approach with multiple surgical subspecialties such as otolaryngology, plastic surgery, and neurosurgery.

Nasal dermoid

Nasal dermoids total 1% to 3% of all dermoid cysts and approximately 4% to 12% of head and neck dermoids.[24] They result from faulty involution of a neuroectodermal tract through the anterior neuropore, pulling outlying skin internally. This creates a pit, sinus tract, or cyst containing mesodermal and ectodermal components. There is a slight male predominance, and although most cases are sporadic, a familial predisposition has been reported.[25] Associated abnormalities such as craniosynostosis, hemifacial microsomia, lacrimal duct cysts, cleft lip/palate, pinna deformity, hydrocephalus, and hypertelorism have been described.[26] Intracranial extension has a variable incidence, with 5% to 45% reported in the literature, and resulting intracranial infection is rare.[27]

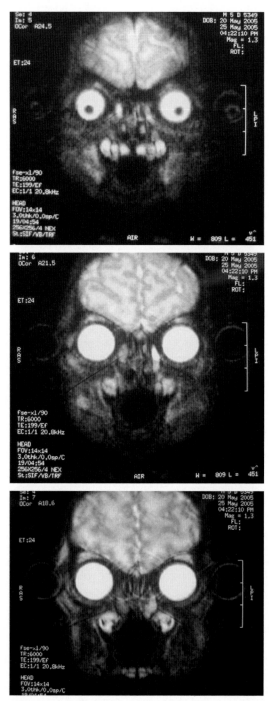

Fig. 8. Sequential MRI images demonstrating dilated lacrimal ducts bilaterally terminating in dilated intranasal mucoceles or dacryocystocoeles. (*From* Leonard DS, O'Keefe M, Rowley H, et al. Neonatal respiratory distress secondary to bilateral intranasal dacryocystocoeles. Int J Pediatr Otorhinolaryngol 2008;72:1875; with permission.)

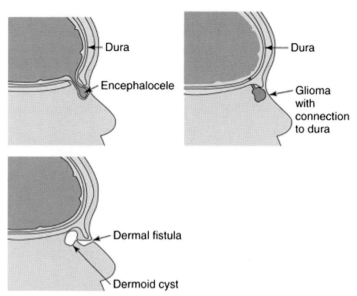

Fig. 9. Schematic view of the common midline nasal masses. (*From* Elluru RG, Wootten CT. Congenital malformations of the nose. In: Flint PW, Haughey BH, Lund VJ, et al, editors. Cummings otolaryngology: head & neck surgery. 5th edition. Mosby; 2010. p. 2687; with permission.)

These present as a midline mass ranging in location from the base of the columella, along the nasal dorsum, to the nasoglabellar region.[28] A sinus opening along this route, with a protruding hair is pathognomonic, and may have discharge or local infection associated with it (**Fig. 11**).[26] Similar to gliomas, they are noncompressible, nonexpansile, and do not transilluminate.

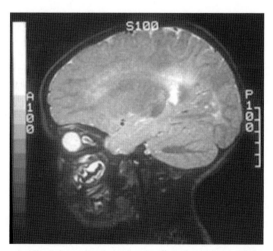

Fig. 10. Sagittal magnetic resonance image of a basal meningocele protruding into the nasopharynx. (*From* Elluru RG, Wootten CT. Congenital malformations of the nose. In: Flint PW, Haughey BH, Lund VJ, et al, editors. Cummings otolaryngology: head & neck surgery. 5th edition. Mosby; 2010. p. 2688; with permission.)

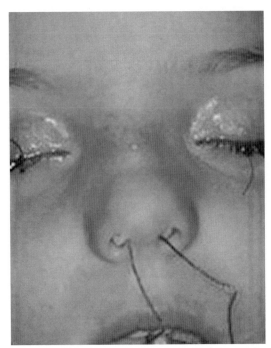

Fig. 11. Nasal dermoid manifesting as a firm midline nasal swelling associated with a sinus opening. (*From* Elluru RG, Wootten CT. Congenital malformations of the nose. In: Flint PW, Haughey BH, Lund VJ, et al, editors. Cummings otolaryngology: head & neck surgery. 5th edition. Mosby; 2010. p. 2689; with permission.)

Nasal glioma

Nasal glioma, or more precisely nasal glial heterotopia, consists of isolated extracranial glial tissue which may or may not be connected to the brain by a fibrous stalk. They are rare, with a male-to-female ratio of 3:2, and no familial predisposition.[28] Presentation has a 6:3:1 ratio of extranasal:intranasal:combined lesions.[9] Presentation varies from an overt external mass to subtle findings including telecanthus and a widened nasal bridge. Intranasal lesions are typically seen as pale masses arising from the lateral nasal wall or middle turbinate, but they can arise from the septum. In rare instances, gliomas may extend into the orbit, frontal sinus, oral cavity, or nasopharynx.[28]

Encephalocele

Encephaloceles are extracranial protrusions of meninges, cerebrospinal fluid, and neural tissue. Meningoceles may present similarly without herniation of brain tissue. They are rare with no gender predilection.[29] There are several different subclassifications of encephaloceles depending on the location of dehiscence in the skull base, and they may present either as external or internal nasal masses (**Fig. 12**). They are pale, compressible, pulsatile, and transilluminate with light. Compression of the jugular vein with resultant expansion, known as Furstenberg's test, is present. They may also expand with crying or straining. Associated abnormalities are present in 30% to 40% of cases.[29]

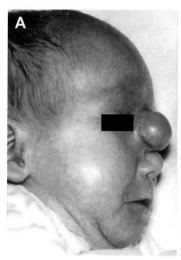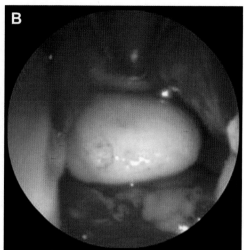

Fig. 12. (*A*) Sincipital encephalocele. A soft, bluish compressible mass protruding from the glabellar region. (*B*) Basal encephalocele seen in nasopharynx with a 120° angled telescope. (*From* Elluru RG, Wootten CT. Congenital malformations of the nose. In: Flint PW, Haughey BH, Lund VJ, et al, editors. Cummings otolaryngology: head & neck surgery. 5th edition. Mosby; 2010. p. 2687–8; with permission.)

Neoplastic Etiologies

In addition to congenital midline nasal masses, congenital neoplasms should be considered, including both benign and malignant forms. Reported prevalence for all congenital tumors is in the range of 1.7 to 13.5 cases per 100,000 live births.[30] These may present similarly to the previously mentioned nasal masses both within the nasal cavity and externally. Differential diagnosis of congenital nasal neoplasms includes teratomas, harmartomas, rhabdomyosarcoma, hemangiomas, neurofibromas, epidermoid cysts, lipoma/lipoblastomas, and lymphatic malformations among other rare neoplasms. Radiographic imaging with CT or MRI is recommended to evaluate for extent of the lesion (**Fig. 13**). Any prenatal ultrasound imaging concerning for a nasal or head and neck mass should alert the clinician to the risk of respiratory distress and elicit appropriate perinatal planning (**Fig. 14**). The first step in treatment is securing an airway, followed by treatment specific to etiology. This may include consideration of an ex utero intrapartum treatment (EXIT) procedure, in which the fetus is delivered via cesarean section while maintaining the placenta and umbilical cord, allowing an airway to be established by means of intubation or tracheostomy.[30]

Infectious Etiologies

Viral and bacterial infections may lead to partial nasal obstruction in newborns either independently or coexisting with other causes of nasal obstruction. Infections of the nasolacrimal duct, termed dacryocystitis, may also lead to nasal obstruction with a presentation similar to nasolacrimal duct cysts. Sexually transmitted diseases (STDs) in the mother, such as chlamydia, gonorrhea, and syphilis, are important bacterial pathogens to recognize as possible etiologies of nasal congestion and obstruction requiring prompt treatment with antibiotics. Clinical suspicion based on maternal sexual history, substance abuse, prior STD diagnosis, poor prenatal care, and perinatal STD testing should guide further investigation.

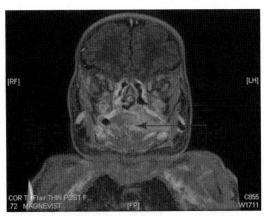

Fig. 13. Nasopharyngeal teratoma on a coronal magnetic resonance image with characteristic heterogeneous signal intensity (*arrow*). (*From* Elluru RG, Wootten CT. Congenital malformations of the nose. In: Flint PW, Haughey BH, Lund VJ, et al, editors. Cummings otolaryngology: head & neck surgery. 5th edition. Mosby; 2010. p. 2696; with permission.)

Although chlamydial and gonorrheal infection in infants most commonly present as conjunctivitis, both may also present with nasopharyngitis and rhinitis responsive to oral antibiotics.[31,32] Conjunctivitis associated with *Chlamydia trachomatis* typically develops 5 to 12 days after birth and can be associated with an afebrile, subacute pneumonia at 1 to 3 months of age.[33] In contrast, conjunctivitis associated with gonorrhea

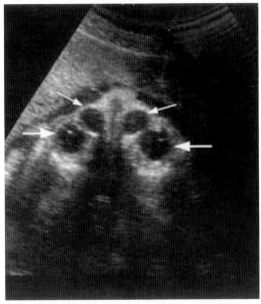

Fig. 14. Anterior coronal view of fetal face demonstrating bilateral dacrocystoceles (*small arrows*) anterior-medial to the orbits (*large arrows*). (*From* Goldberg H, Sebire NJ, Holwell D, et al. Prenatal diagnosis of bilateral dacrocystoceles. Ultrasound Obstet Gynecol 2000;87:448, with permission.)

typically manifests 2 to 5 days after birth and may be associated with sepsis, arthritis, meningitis, vaginitis, urethritis, and infection at fetal monitoring sites such as abscesses from scalp electrodes.[33]

Congenital syphilis commonly presents with nasal discharge, often referred to as syphilitic snuffles. Initially it is seen as watery discharge, but it becomes progressively thick and purulent, causing nasal obstruction. Differentiating features of syphilis include nonimmune hydrops, jaundice, hepatosplenomegaly, skin rash, and pseudo-paralysis of an extremity.[33] It is responsive to standard antibiotic therapy.[34]

Iatrogenic Etiologies

Trauma during delivery or postnatal care can cause or exacerbate nasal obstruction. Birth trauma affecting the head and neck occurs in 0.82% of births and is associated with vaginal delivery, primiparity, forceps delivery, infants large for gestational age, and male gender.[35]

Dislocation of the cartilaginous nasal septum from the vomerine groove occurs in 0.6% to 0.93% of newborns and may result in nasal obstruction because of the deviated septum.[35,36] The exact etiology is debatable; however, it is most commonly attributed to birth trauma, although abnormal intrauterine pressures or other prenatal causes may play a role.[37] Physical examination reveals a deviated nasal tip with an angulated columella and flattened, asymmetric nasal ala. The nasal tip flattens easily with light pressure on palpation, and inspection with an otoscope or speculum reveals dislocation of the cartilage toward the narrowed nostril.[37] In comparison, a flattened nose is a frequent normal finding in newborns that may also cause transient nasal obstruction, typically resolving within 48 hours. It can be distinguished from septal dislocation by pressing lightly on the nasal tip and meeting resistance. Septal dislocation treatment is controversial and may consist of either observation or bedside manual manipulation of the septum back into the septal groove and columella.

Another iatrogenic etiology of nasal obstruction is nasal vestibular stenosis, resulting from soft tissue damage to the external nare.[38] In addition to this, trauma from nasal prongs, continuous positive airway pressure (CPAP), nasogastric feedings tubes, and suction trauma from overvigorous suctioning of secretions can cause clinically significant nasal obstruction and possible synechia formation (**Fig. 15**).[39,40] Septal hematomas may occur during birth or from the previously mentioned causes and require incision and drainage to avoid cartilage necrosis and subsequent saddle nose deformity.

Inflammatory, Systemic, and Other Etiologies

Neonatal rhinitis, or inflammation of the nasal mucosa, is the most common cause of nasal congestion and partial obstruction.[39] Infants present with typical symptoms of nasal obstruction, and physical examination reveals mucosal edema and secretions. This can occur alone, as a manifestation of another condition, or in tandem with other etiologies of nasal obstruction, thereby exacerbating the underlying cause.

Mucus production varies from 0.1 to 0.3 mg/kg/d; therefore, mucus itself may cause significant nasal occlusion independently. Deficiencies of mucociliary clearance such as Kartagener syndrome or cystic fibrosis are especially prone to mucoid obstruction. While rhinitis with obstruction has been reported with cow's milk allergy/intolerance[41] or hypothyroidism,[42] more common associations would be gastroesophageal reflux disease (GERD), inferior turbinate hypertrophy, or adenoid enlargement. Maternal etiologies include estrogenic stimuli (similar to rhinitis of pregnancy)[43] or maternal drug ingestion, such as methyldopa,[44] methimazole,[45] tricyclic antidepressants, narcotics,

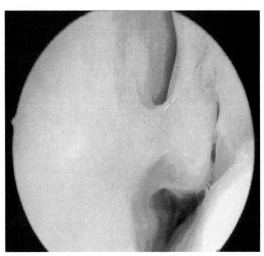

Fig. 15. Naso-endoscopy revealing synechia on the right side from CPAP catheters. (*Adapted from* DeRoew A, Landsberg R, Fishman G, et al. Neonatal iatrogenic nasal obstruction. Int J Pediatr Otorhinolaryngol 2004;68:615; with permission.)

or antihypertensive medications such as propranalol.[39] Most neonatal rhinitis cases are idiopathic in nature.

Treatment for neonatal rhinitis includes humidification, gentle suction of secretions, and topical steroids or nasal decongestants. Limitation of vasoconstrictive agents to 3 days in infants is crucial to avoid rhinitis medicamentosa, which could be life threatening secondary to rebound congestion and obstruction in the neonate.[46] Rhinitis associated with a specific ingestion is diagnosed via history and treated by maternal avoidance or change of formula. No response to conservative management would warrant further evaluation.

Gastroesophageal reflux

Gastric content reflux into the nasal cavity may cause chronic inflammation and subsequent nasal obstruction. The resulting inflammation has been associated with adenoid enlargement[47] and alteration of mucosal conditions increasing susceptibility to bacterial and/or viral infections, which may further exacerbate nasal obstruction.[48] Other symptoms in affected infants include episodes of spitting up, irritability, and possibly arching or torticollis. The current gold standards for diagnosing otolaryngologic manifestations of GERD are the dual-channel 24-hour pH or impedence probe.[49,50]

Airway obstruction has been demonstrated as a contributing factor in the pathogenesis of GERD in animal models, whereby by the mechanical force required to overcome upper airway obstruction during expiration resulted in gastric reflux.[48,51] In addition to this, aspirated reflux contents with resultant coughing further promotes GERD secondary to increased intra-abdominal pressure. As a result, children with other etiologies of nasal obstruction may subsequently be affected by GERD, which can aggravate the underlying obstruction via mucosal edema and inflammation resulting in a vicious cycle. Therefore, antireflux medications in infants with nasal obstruction are a valid consideration, especially if other symptoms of reflux are present. GERD has also been shown as a complicating factor in choanal atresia repair, further supporting the use of antireflux medications in these patients.[52] Currently, proton pump inhibitor use in the newborn is controversial, and some studies have shown no benefit. This may be explained by the fact that even nonacidic reflux has been shown to induce inflammation. In addition to a reflux medication trial, modifications such as propping infants up after feedings and thickening formula may be helpful.[39]

SYNDROMIC ASSOCIATIONS

Several etiologies of nasal obstruction may present with concurrent abnormalities that may require further assessment, including genetic evaluation. Nasal obstruction has been described in association with Crouzon, CHARGE, Pfeiffer, Apert, Treacher-Collins, Down, and fetal alcohol syndromes, among others.[39,53–56] Infants with craniofacial synostosis typically have airway obstruction secondary to maxillary hypoplasia in the setting of normal nasopharyngeal and oropharyngeal soft tissue development. As many as 50% of infants with craniofacial anomalies require a tracheostomy at some point in their life.[57]

TREATMENT

Treatment options for nasal obstruction include observation or medical or surgical management, with securing an adequate airway as the first goal of therapy. In newborns, the nasal passages are approximately 50% of the total airway resistance. Over the first 6 months of life, the internal nasal airway doubles in size, often leading to spontaneous resolution of symptoms present at birth.[43,58] In addition to the increased area of the nasal passage, cervical growth and descent of the larynx during the first months of life facilitate mouth breathing.[2]

Conservative management for mild symptoms includes discontinuation of vigorous suctioning and introduction of gentle suctioning with swabbing for mucus removal as needed. Humidification with administration of saline drops may be beneficial. Other medications include nasal steroid drops (dexamethasone ophthalmic solution, beclomethasone, or triamcinolone spray), and application of decongestant drops (phenylephrine 0.125% or oxymetazoline 0.025%) twice daily for a maximum of 3 days.[39,59] Most infants respond quickly to this regimen within 3 to 5 days, and symptoms resolve within 2 to 4 weeks. No response or worsening would require prompt further evaluation. It may be prudent to discharge patients with a cardiopulmonary monitor and instruct parents in airway management and cardiopulmonary resuscitation.

Severe obstruction may necessitate endotracheal intubation or tracheostomy until further surgical intervention depending on the infant's condition and associated anomalies. Respiratory distress may be treated with placement of a nasal trumpet if able to be placed on 1 side, or an oral airway. An endotracheal tube placed transorally into the esophagus opens the mouth, establishes an oral airway, and can be used for feedings. A McGovern nipple (a large nipple with the end cut off) allows infants to mouth breathe between swallows while feeding, and this can be secured as an oropharyngeal airway between feedings.[60] Many infants have associated feeding problems and uncoordinated swallowing efforts, placing them at risk for failure to thrive and recurrent aspiration.[61] These infants require nutritional and speech pathology assessment and support, and may ultimately require gavage feedings.

Surgical intervention is indicated in infants with respiratory distress, unresponsiveness to conservative measures, or failure to thrive.[14] In patients with a stable respiratory status, surgeons may apply the rule of tens and delay surgery until the child is 10 lbs, 10 weeks of age, and has a hemoglobin of 10.[10] Other cases, such as unilateral choanal atresia, may be repaired later in childhood.

SUMMARY

Severity of nasal obstruction in the newborn ranges from being a nuisance to a life-threatening scenario. It is an important clinical entity for pediatricians to recognize, quickly evaluate, and treat. Causality has a broad differential diagnosis and may be multifactorial in nature. Although the most common etiology is inflammation of the nasal mucosa, other possibilities must be considered when evaluating the infant with nasal obstruction, and further evaluation of associated abnormalities may be warranted. Management may be complex and require a multidisciplinary approach including neonatologists, pediatricians, obstetricians, and pediatric subspecialists, including: otolaryngologists, anesthesiologists, neurosurgeons, plastic surgeons, ophthalmologists, gastroenterologists, nutritionists, speech pathologists, and support services.

REFERENCES

1. Miller MJ, Martin RJ, Carlo WA, et al. Oral breathing in newborn infants. J Pediatr 1985;107:465–9.
2. Keller JL, Kacker A. Choanal atresia, CHARGE association, and congenital nasal stenosis. Otolaryngol Clin North Am 2000;33:1343–51.
3. Leonard DS, O'Keefe M, Rowley H, et al. Neonatal respiratory distress secondary to bilateral intranasal dacryocystoceles. Int J Pediatr Otorhinolaryngol 2008; 72:1873–7.
4. Coates H. Nasal obstruction in the neonate and infant. Clin Pediatr 1992;31: 25–9.
5. Engel R, Lussky RC, Cifuentes RF. Assessing nasal patency in neonates. Minn Med 1998;81:4–5.
6. Myer CM III, Cotton RT. Nasal obstruction in the pediatric patient. Pediatrics 1983;72:766–77.
7. Ramsden JD, Campisi P, Forte V. Choanal atresia and choanal stenosis. Otolaryngol Clin North Am 2009;42:339–52.
8. Effat KG. Use of the automatic tympanometer as a screening tool for congenital choanal atresia. J Laryngol Otol 2005;119:125–8.
9. Jaffe BF. Classification and management of anomalies of the nose. Otolaryngol Clin North Am 1981;14:989–1004.
10. Brown OE, Pownell P, Manning SC. Choanal atresia: a new anatomic classification and clinical management applications. Laryngoscope 1996;106:97–101.
11. Carpenter RJ, Neel HB III. Correction of congenital choanal atresia in children and adults. Laryngoscope 1977;87:1304–11.
12. Adil E, Huntley C, Choudhary A, et al. Congenital nasal obstruction: clinic and radiologic review. Eur J Pediatr 2012;171:641–50.
13. Brown O, Myer C, Manning S. Congenital nasal pyriform aperture stenosis. Laryngoscope 1989;99:86–91.
14. Tate JR, Sykes J. Congenital nasal pyriform aperture stenosis. Otolaryngol Clin North Am 2009;42:521–5.
15. Belden CJ, Mancuso AA, Schmalfuss IM. CT features of congenital nasal pyriform aperture stenosis: initial experience. Radiology 1999;213:495–501.
16. Beregszaszi M, Leger J, Garel C, et al. Nasal pyriform aperture stenosis and absence of the anterior pituitary gland: report of two cases. J Pediatr 1996; 25:169–88.
17. Tavin E, Stecker E, Marion R. Nasal pyriform aperture stenosis and the holoprosencephaly spectrum. Int J Pediatr Otorhinolaryngol 1994;28:199–204.

18. Sevel D. Development and congenital abnormalities of the nasal lacrimal apparatus. J Pediatr Ophthalmol Strabismus 1981;18:13–9.
19. Peterson RA, Robb RM. The natural course of congenital obstruction of the nasolacrimal duct. J Pediatr Ophthalmol Strabismus 1978;15:246–50.
20. Roy D, Guevara N, Santini J, et al. Endoscopic marsupialization of congenital nasolacrimal duct cyst with dacryocele. Clin Otolaryngol 2002;27:167–70.
21. Devine RD, Anderson RL, Bumstead RM. Bilateral congenital lacrimal sac mucoceles with nasal extension and drainage. Arch Ophthalmol 1983;101:246–8.
22. Hughes GB, Sharpino G, Hunt W, et al. Management of the congenital midline nasal masses: a review. Head Neck Surg 1980;2:222–33.
23. Hedlund G. Congenital frontonasal masses: developmental anatomy, malformations, and MR imaging. Pediatr Radiol 2006;36:647–62.
24. Denoyelle F, Ducroz V, Roger G, et al. Nasal dermoid sinus cysts in children. Laryngoscope 1997;107:795–800.
25. Anderson PJ, Dobson C, Berry RB. Nasal dermoid cysts in siblings. Int J Pediatr Otorhinolaryngol 1998;44:155–9.
26. Wardinsky TD, Pagon RA, Kropp RJ, et al. Nasal dermoid sinus cysts: association with intracranial extension and multiple malformations. Cleft Palate Craniofac J 1991;28:87–95.
27. Zapata S, Kearns DB. Nasal dermoids. Curr Opin Otolaryngol Head Neck Surg 2006;14:406–11.
28. Rahbar R, Shah P, Mulliken JB, et al. The presentation and management of nasal dermoid. Arch Otolaryngol Head Neck Surg 2003;129:464–71.
29. Blumenfeld R, Skolnik EM. Intranasal encephaloceles. Arch Otolaryngol 1965;82:527–31.
30. Woodward PJ, Sohaey R, Kennedy A. A comprehensive review of fetal tumors with pathologic correlation. Radiographics 2005;25:215–42.
31. Hobson D, Rees E, Viswalingam ND. Chlamydial infections in neonates and older children. Br Med Bull 1983;39:128–32.
32. Goh BT, Forster GE. Sexually transmitted diseases in children: chlamydial oculogenital infection. Genitourin Med 1993;69:213–21.
33. Center for Disease Control and Prevention. Sexually transmitted diseases treatment guidelines. MMWR Recomm Rep 2010;59:36–56.
34. Boot JM, Oranje AP, de Groot R, et al. Congenital syphilis. Int J STD AIDS 1992;3:161–7.
35. Hughes CA, Harley EH, Milmoe G, et al. Birth trauma in the head and neck. Arch Otolaryngol Head Neck Surg 1999;125:193–9.
36. Podoshin L, Gertner R, Radis M, et al. Incidence and treatment of deviation of nasal septum in newborns. Ear Nose Throat J 1991;70:485–7.
37. Tasca I, Compadretti GC. Immediate correction of nasal septum dislocation in newborns: long term results. Am J Rhinol 2004;18:47–51.
38. Jablon JH, Hoffman JF. Birth trauma causing nasal vestibular stenosis. Arch Otolaryngol Head Neck Surg 1997;123:1004–6.
39. Olnes SQ, Schwartz RS, Bahadori RS. Diagnosis and management of the newborn and young infant who have nasal obstruction. Pediatr Rev 2000;21:416–20.
40. Gowdar K, Bull MJ, Schreiner RL, et al. Nasal deformities in neonates. Am J Dis Child 1980;134:954–7.
41. Ingall M, Glaser J, Meltzer R, et al. Allergic rhinitis in early infancy. Pediatrics 1965;35:108–12.

42. Najjar S. Respiratory manifestations in infants with hypothyroidism. Arch Dis Child 1962;37:603–5.
43. Haddad J Jr. Congenital disorders of the nose. In: Kliegman RM, Behrman RE, Jenson HB, et al, editors. Nelson textbook of pediatrics. 19th edition. Philadelphia: Saunders Elsevier; 2011. p. 1742–4.
44. Le Gras M, Seifert B, Casiro O. Neonatal nasal obstruction associated with methyldopa treatment during pregnancy. Am J Dis Child 1990;144:143–4.
45. Barbero P, Ricagni C, Mercado G, et al. Choanal atresia associated with prenatal methimazole exposure: three new patients. Am J Med Genet A 2004;129: 83–6.
46. Osguthorpe J, Shirley R. Neonatal respiratory distress from rhinitis medicamentosa. Laryngoscope 1987;97:829–31.
47. Carr M, Poje C, Ehrig D, et al. Incidence of reflux in young children undergoing adenoidectomy. Laryngoscope 2001;111:2170–2.
48. Yellon R, Goldberg H. Update on gastroesophageal reflux disease in pediatric airway disorders. Am J Med 2001;111(8A):78S–84S.
49. Contencin P, Narcy P. Nasopharyngeal pH monitoring in infants and children with chronic rhinopharyngitis. Int J Pediatr Otorhinolaryngol 1991;22:249–56.
50. Rosbe K, Kenna M, Auerbach A. Extraesophageal reflux in pediatric patients with upper respiratory symptoms. Arch Otolaryngol Head Neck Surg 2003; 129:1213–20.
51. Wang W, Tovar JA, Eizaguirre I, et al. Airway obstruction and gastroesophageal reflux: an experimental study on the pathogenesis of this association. J Pediatr Surg 1993;28:995–8.
52. Beste D, Conley S, Brown C. Gastroesophageal reflux complicating choanal atresia repair. Int J Pediatr Otorhinolaryngol 1994;29:51–8.
53. Sirotnak J, Brodsky L, Pizzuto M. Airway obstruction in the Crouzon syndrome: case report and review of the literature. Int J Pediatr Otorhinolaryngol 1995;31: 235–46.
54. Derkay C, Grundfast K. Airway compromise from nasal obstruction in neonates and infants. Int J Pediatr Otorhinolaryngol 1990;19:241–9.
55. Shott SR, Myer CM, Willis R, et al. Nasal obstruction in the neonate. Rhinology 1989;27:91–6.
56. Usowicz AG, Golabi M, Curry C. Upper airway obstruction in infants with fetal alcohol syndrome. Am J Dis Child 1988;140:1039–41.
57. Boston M, Rutter MJ. Current airway management in craniofacial anomalies. Curr Opin Otolaryngol Head Neck Surg 2003;11:428–32.
58. Stocks J, Godfrey S. Nasal resistance in infancy. Respir Physiol 1978;34: 233–46.
59. Nathan C, Seid A. Neonatal rhinitis. Int J Pediatr Otorhinolaryngol 1997;39: 59–65.
60. Drake AF, Ferguson MO. Controversies in upper airway obstruction. In: Bailey BJ, Johnson JT, Newlands SD, editors. Head and neck surgery otolaryngology. 4th edition. Philadelphia: Lippincott Williams & Wilkins; 2006. p. 803–13.
61. Dinwiddie R. Congenital upper airway obstruction. Paediatr Respir Rev 2004;5: 17–24.

Enlarged Neck Lymph Nodes in Children

Karthik Rajasekaran, MD, Paul Krakovitz, MD*

KEYWORDS

- Enlarged lymph nodes • Lymphadenopathy • Cervical adenopathy
- Pediatric lymph nodes • Neck mass

KEY POINTS

- Cervical lymphadenopathy is a common and usually benign finding.
- A thorough history and physical examination usually are sufficient to establish a diagnosis.
- Most often, cervical lymphadenopathy is self-limited, and treatment is not required.
- Further diagnostic laboratory and imaging studies may be warranted in the event of persistent or worrisome lymphadenopathy.
- Surgery should be reserved for lymphadenopathy that remains undiagnosed or has failed to resolve with medical treatment.

INTRODUCTION

Enlarged cervical lymph nodes are a common finding on physical examination in the pediatric population. Lymph nodes are discrete, ovoid structures that are widely distributed throughout the body. Lymphadenopathy is defined as an abnormality in the size and/or character of the lymph node. In general, lymph nodes larger than 1 cm in diameter are considered enlarged, and defined as cervical lymphadenopathy.[1–3]

Most commonly, lymphadenopathy represents a transient response of lymphatic tissue hyperplasia to a local benign inflammatory process. Up to 90% of children between the ages of 4 and 8 have palpable cervical lymph nodes.[4]

Lymphadenopathy, however, can also represent other more significant pathology, including a neoplastic process. Specifically, about 15% of biopsied cervical lymph nodes in children represent a malignancy.[5,6] It is therefore critical to understand the differential diagnosis to direct an appropriate and timely evaluation (**Fig. 1**).

Head and Neck Institute, A71, Cleveland Clinic, Cleveland, OH 44195, USA
* Corresponding author.
E-mail address: krakovp@ccf.org

Pediatr Clin N Am 60 (2013) 923–936
http://dx.doi.org/10.1016/j.pcl.2013.04.005
0031-3955/13/$ – see front matter © 2013 Elsevier Inc. All rights reserved.
pediatric.theclinics.com

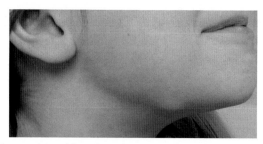

Fig. 1. Patient with an enlarged lymph node.

PATHOPHYSIOLOGY

The lymphatic system is the defense system of the human body, and lymph nodes are the "police headquarters" that aid in this immune defense. When the human body is presented with a pathogen, a local inflammatory reaction occurs, that results in the pathogen being carried to the lymph nodes. Once in the lymph nodes, neutrophils are the initial defense cell that acts on the pathogen. If this does not eradicate the pathogen, macrophages are summoned, which trap, phagocytose, degrade and present the organisms as antigens on the MHC molecules. Other defense mechanisms include the complement system that is activated by proteins in the blood that attach to the pathogen. If the pathogen evades these defense mechanisms and invades the human cell, a stress signal can be released that causes the natural killer T cell to cause the human cell to die, eradicating the pathogen with it. Another method that the body employs to defend itself from pathogens is to use antibodies, which are produced by B cells. These antibodies attach to the pathogen surface proteins, which can activate the complement cascade or interfere with the function of the pathogen itself. Other cells utilized include dendritic cells that can induce helper T cells to release chemicals that enhance B cell function, as well as stimulate macrophages and neutrophils to arrive at the lymph node. Lastly, the cytotoxic T cell can be summoned to the lymph node to directly kill the cell. This entire immune response within the lymph node ultimately leads to its size increase.

ETIOLOGY

The causes of cervical lymphadenopathy can be classified into 6 major categories[2,7]:

1. Infections:
    The most common cause of cervical lymphadenopathy in children is from a viral upper respiratory tract infection.[8] The other viruses listed in **Box 1** have all been associated with cervical lymphadenopathy as well.
    - Group A β-hemolytic streptococci and *Staphylococcus aureus* are the most common causes of bacterial cervical lymphadenitis in children.[9,10]
        ○ Prevalence of methicillin-resistant *S aureus* (MRSA) is increasing; one study reports a rate rising from 15% to 40% in a 3-year period, whereas other studies report much higher rates.[11–13]
    - Anaerobic bacteria from dental caries and periodontal disease are other bacterial causes of cervical lymphadenopathy.
    - Cat scratch disease caused by *Bartonella henselae* is estimated to have an annual incidence of 9.3 per 100,000 with most cases reported from September to January.[14]

Box 1
Viral infections that cause cervical lymphadenopathy

a. Upper Respiratory Tract Infection Viruses

   i. Rhinovirus

   ii. Adenovirus

   iii. Influenza virus

   iv. Parainfluenza virus

   v. Respiratory synctial virus

b. Epstein Bar Virus

c. Cytomegalovirus

d. Togavirus

e. Varicella-zoster virus

f. Herpes Simplex virus

g. Paramyxovirus

h. Coxackievirus A and B

i. Echovirus

j. Enterovirus

k. Human Herpesvirus-6

l. Human Immunodeficiency Virus

- Atypical mycobacteria and mycobacteria are other important causes of sub-acute or chronic cervical lymphadenopathy.[2]
- Fungal infections associated with lymphadenopathy are typically seen in immunocompromised patients.
- Cervical adenopathy caused by parasitic infections other than *Toxoplasma gondii* is uncommon in the United States.

2. Immunologic diseases:
   a. Rheumatoid arthritis
   b. Mixed connective tissue disease
   c. Sjogren syndrome
   d. Graft-versus-host disease
3. Malignancies:

The most common malignancies that are known to cause cervical lymphadenopathy are listed in **Box 2**.

During the first 6 years of life, neuroblastoma and leukemia are the most common tumors associated with cervical lymphadenopathy, followed by rhabdomyosarcoma and non-Hodgkin lymphoma.[2] After 6 years of life, Hodgkin lymphoma is the most common tumor associated with cervical lymphadenopathy, followed by non-Hodgkin lymphoma and rhabdomyosarcoma (**Fig. 2**).[2]

Metastatic disease can also present as cervical lymphadenopathy. The common diseases associated with this are thyroid carcinoma and nasopharyngeal carcinoma (**Fig. 3**).

Box 2
Malignancies that can cause cervical lymphadenopathy

Malignancies

a. Hodgkin Lymphoma

b. Non-Hodgkin lymphoma

c. Neuroblastoma

d. Leukemia

e. Rhabdomyosarcoma

f. Metastatic disease

---

4. Lipid storage diseases:
   a. Gaucher disease
   b. Niemann-Pick disease
5. Endocrine diseases
   a. Hyperthyroid
   b. Adrenal insufficiency
   c. Thyroiditis
6. Miscellaneous:
   Other miscellaneous causes of cervical lymphadenopathy are listed in **Box 3**.
   a. Kawasaki disease: The presence of nonsuppurative cervical lymphadenopathy greater than 1.5 cm is the 1 of the 5 diagnostic criteria.[15]
   b. Serum sickness: an allergic reaction, which can also provoke cervical and generalized lymphadenopathy by forming systemic antigen-antibody complexes after exposure to certain medications. A list of these medications is listed in **Box 3**.
   c. Diphtheria, tetanus, and pertussis (DTP)-induced cervical lymphadenopathy: a rare complication from the vaccination from unknown etiology.
   d. Kikuchi-Fujimoto disease: formerly known as subacute necrotizing histiocytic lymphadenitis, is a rare cause of persistent cervical adenopathy, which is unresponsive to antibiotic therapy. It usually affects young Japanese women with tender lymphadenopathy.

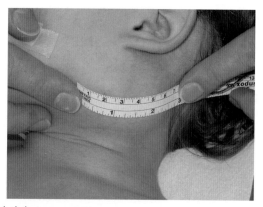

Fig. 2. Child with rhabdomyosarcoma.

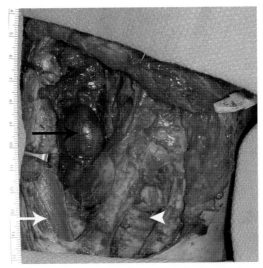

Fig. 3. Intraoperative photograph of metastatic lymphadenopathy from a patient with thyroid cancer (*black arrow* represents the metastatic lymph node, *arrowhead* represents trachea, *white arrow* represents sternocleidomastoid muscle).

CLINICAL EVALUATION

A thorough history of the present illness is paramount in the diagnosis and management of a neck mass. Important details of the history are listed in the following paragraphs.

Box 3
Other causes of cervical lymphadenopathy

Miscellaneous

a. Kawasaki disease

b. Drugs

    i. Phenytoin

    ii. Isoniazid

    iii. Pyrimethamine

    iv. Allopurinol

    v. Phenylbutazone

c. Serum sickness

d. Post vaccination

e. Rosai-Dorfman disease

f. Kikuchi Fujimoto disease

g. Sarcoidosis

Age

The age of the child can sometimes help narrow the list of infectious organisms or disease process

- Staphylococcus aureus is most commonly seen in ages from neonates to 4 years of age.
- Group B streptococcus has a predilection for neonates and infants.
- Streptococcus pyogenes and atypical mycobacteria are more commonly seen in children between the age of 1 and 4.
- Between the ages of 5 and 15, Bartonella Henselae and anaerobic bacteria are the more common infectious causes of cervical lymphadenopathy.

Location and Time Duration of Lymph Nodes

The laterality and chronicity of the lymph nodes vary by the disease processes, as described in **Table 1**. Usually lymphadenopathy of a shorter duration (days to weeks) is associated with a reactive disorder, whereas a longer duration is more concerning for malignancy. However, this is not reliable in separating benign from malignant disease.

Associated Symptoms

The symptoms associated with lymph node enlargement may provide helpful information in determining a cause for lymphadenopathy (**Table 2**).

In general, focal symptoms, such as tenderness, erythema, and swelling usually indicate an acute infection or a rapidly proliferating process with painful expansion of the lymph node capsule. On the other hand, a malignant process more often causes painless, nontender lymph node enlargement, resulting in lymph nodes that may be hard and attached to surrounding tissues or soft because of extensive necrosis. Other symptoms, such as fever and weight loss, may be associated with a malignant lymphoma or systemic inflammatory disorders.

Other Pertinent Details of the History

It is important to inquire about preceding tonsillitis, or recent exposure to an upper respiratory tract infection, tuberculosis, or streptococcal pharyngitis, as it can suggest the corresponding disease. Additionally inquiring about recent exposure to cats or rabbits, periodontal disease, recent vaccinations, and medication use are other important details.

Table 1
Association between length of time and location of lymph nodes with different diseases/organisms

Acute Unilateral Cervical Lymphadenopathy	Acute Bilateral Cervical Lymphadenopathy	Subacute/Chronic Cervical Lymphadenopathy
a. Viral upper respiratory tract infection b. Streptococcal pharyngitis c. Kawasaki disease	a. Streptococcal infection b. Staphylococcal infection	a. Mycobacterial infection b. Cat-scratch disease c. Toxoplasmosis d. Epstein-Barr virus e. Cytomegalovirus f. AIDS

Table 2
Disease processes and their associated clinical symptoms

Diseases/Organisms	Associated Symptoms
Upper respiratory tract infection	• Fever • Sore throat • Cough
Lymphoma/Tuberculosis	• Fever • Night sweats • Weight loss
Infectious mononucleosis	• Fever • Fatigue • Malaise
Cytomegalovirus	• Mild symptoms; patients may have hepatitis
Cat-scratch disease	• Fever in one-third of patients
Group A streptococcal pharyngitis	• Fever • Pharyngeal exudates
Serum sickness	• Fever • Malaise • Arthralgia • Urticaria
Sarcoidosis	• Hilar nodes • Skin lesions • Dyspnea
Tularemia	• Fever • Ulcer at inoculation site
Toxoplasmosis	• Fever • Malaise • Sore throat • Myalgia

PHYSICAL EXAMINATION

A systematic physical examination is the next important aspect of the clinical evaluation. Important details are listed as follows.

General

Overall height, weight, and state of health are important to ascertain. Malnutrition or poor growth can suggest a chronic disease, such as tuberculosis, malignancy, or immunodeficiency.

Characteristics of the Lymph Tissue

All lymph nodes should be thoroughly evaluated. Features to discern are the following:

1. Generalizability of location:
   - Acute posterior cervical lymphadenopathy is typically seen in children with rubella, toxoplasmosis, and infectious mononucleosis.[16]
   - Supraclavicular lymphadenopathy has an increased risk for malignancy.
   - The laterality of cervical lymphadenopathy, as described in **Table 1**, is also important to discern, as this can narrow the differential.

2. Quality:

The qualities of the lymph nodes that should be assessed are tenderness, erythema, warmth, mobility, fluctuance, and consistency (**Figs. 4** and **5, Table 3**).

3. Quantity:

Higher number of peripheral lymphadenopathy at different sites, including those outside the head and neck, correlates with an increased risk of malignancy.[17] Generally, supraclavicular nodes of any size should be regarded with a high index of suspicion.[17–19]

Associated Clinical Features on Physical Examination

A detailed physical examination can yield other key findings that may be useful in identifying the potential disease process (**Table 4**).

DIFFERENTIAL DIAGNOSIS

- 22% of patients who appear to have lymphadenopathy will instead have some other type of head and neck mass (**Fig. 6, Table 5**).[20]

DIAGNOSTIC EVALUATION
Laboratory Testing

Laboratory tests are not particularly required for the evaluation of children with cervical lymphadenopathy. Certain laboratory tests may be helpful in the workup of lymphadenopathy:

1. Complete blood cell count (CBC)
    a. Bacterial lymphadenitis will demonstrate leukocytosis with a left shift.
    b. Leukemia will demonstrate pancytopenia or presence of blast cells.
    c. Infectious mononucleosis will demonstrate atypical lymphocytosis.
2. Erythrocyte sedimentation rate
    a. Bacterial lymphadenitis will demonstrate a significantly elevated erythrocyte sedimentation rate.
3. Rapid streptococcal antigen test can be used to detect a streptococcal infection.
4. Purified protein derivative (PPD) test can be used to detect tuberculosis.

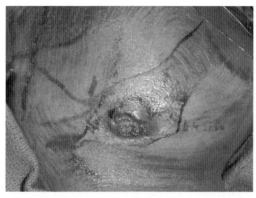

Fig. 4. Child with atypical mycobacteria. Note the skin color change and drainage from the mass. Location around the mandible is common for this pathology.

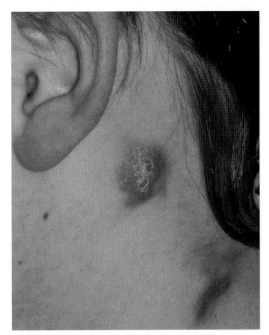

Fig. 5. Child with mycobacterium tuberculosis. Note skin changes.

5. Specific serologic tests:
   a. Epstein-Barr virus
   b. Cytomegalovirus
   c. *Bartonella henselae*
   d. Cytomegalovirus
   e. Infectious mononucleosis
   f. Toxoplasmosis

Table 3
Various disease processes and their associated lymph node qualities

Disease	Lymph Node Qualities
Viral infection	• Soft • Not fixed to underlying structures
Bacterial infection	• Tender • Fluctuant • Not fixed to underlying structures
Acute pyogenic process	• Erythema • Warmth
Abscess formation	• Fluctuance
Malignancy	• No signs of acute inflammation • Hard • Often fixed to underlying tissue
Atypical mycobacterium	• Matted • Skin involvement
Mycobacterium tuberculosis	• Erythema

Table 4
Diseases and their associated clinical features

Disease	Associated Clinical Features
Group A streptococcal infection	• Tonsillar exudate • Absence of cough • Erythematous oropharynx
Epstein-Barr virus	• Hepatosplenomegaly • Pharyngitis • Maculopapular rash
Rubeola	• Cough • Coryza • Conjunctivitis • Koplik spot • Maculopapular rash that spreads from head to toe
Rubella	• Forchheimer spots • Maculopapular rash lasts 3 d • Polyarthritis
Leukemia	• Pallor • Petechiae • Hepatosplenomegaly
Kawasaki disease	• 5 d fever • Bilateral painless conjunctivitis • Polymorphous exanthema • Erythema and infection of lips/oral cavity

Imaging

Imaging studies are ancillary tests that should be tailored based on patient presentation, physical examination, and clinical suspicion. They aid in defining the size, number, location, and composition of enlarged cervical lymph nodes. Imaging modalities that currently play a role in evaluating pediatric lymphadenopathy include ultrasound, computed tomography (CT), and magnetic resonance imaging (MRI).

Ultrasound is advocated for use as the initial imaging modality of choice for palpable neck masses in children to avoid radiation exposure from CT.[21] It is useful in determining whether the lesion is solid or cystic in composition. It can be used to guide biopsies of potentially neoplastic masses or drainage of infectious fluid collections.[22] Color Doppler helps in detection of abnormal vascularity associated with infectious or inflammatory neck disorders. It is also useful for the detection of vascular

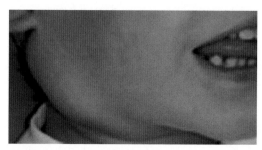

Fig. 6. Child with a neck mass that appears as lymphadenopathy. This patient has a lymphatic malformation.

Table 5 Differential diagnosis of head and neck masses	
Neck Mass	**Features**
Thyroglossal duct cyst	• Midline congenital neck mass • Typically presents after an upper respiratory infection as a painful, erythematous, and tender midline neck mass
Dermoid cyst	• Midline congenital neck mass • Usually attached to the skin • Formed from epithelium entrapped in tissue during embryogenesis
Branchial cyst	• Second most common congenital neck mass • Lateral congenital neck mass • Arises from incomplete obliteration of the pharyngeal pouches and clefts during embryogenesis
Lymphovascular anomaly	• Most common lymphatic malformation • Usually soft and fluctuant
Hemangioma	• Most common vascular tumor • Presents as red or bluish soft multilocular mass

components of tumors and vascular malformations.[23] Other advantages of the ultrasound include lack of radiation exposure, no need for sedation, easy availability, fast interpretations, and lower cost compared with cross-sectional imaging. The disadvantage of ultrasound is that it is dependent on technician experience (**Fig. 7**).

CT and MRI provide additional information and can complement each other. They are particularly useful in evaluating neck masses located within the deep neck, which often cannot be adequately assessed by ultrasound. Advantages of CT over MRI are that CT is more readily available, has lower cost, and has faster scan times, which decreases the likelihood for motion degradation of scan quality or need for sedation. One of the disadvantages of CT over MRI is that it is associated with a relatively high level of ionizing radiation exposure to the thyroid gland (**Fig. 8**).[24,25]

MRI is the imaging modality of choice to evaluate pediatric neck masses with suspected intracranial or intraspinal extension. Advantages of an MRI are that there is a lack of radiation exposure and it can evaluate the lymph nodes with different tissue signal intensities, thereby imparting additional information on the quality and

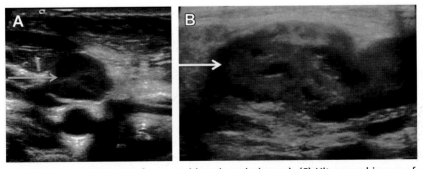

Fig. 7. (A) Ultrasound image of a normal lymph node (*arrow*). (B) Ultrasound image of an enlarged lymph node (*arrow*).

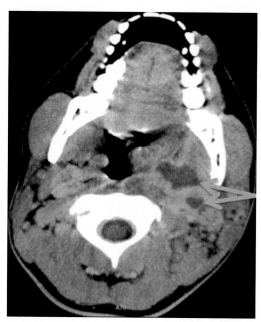

Fig. 8. CT scan of the neck demonstrating a posterior parapharyngeal suppurative lymphadenopathy and abscess (*arrows*).

characteristics of the lymph node. A disadvantage of an MRI is that it usually requires sedation for infants and young children to prevent movement in the scanner.

Diagnostic Biopsy

Biopsies of cervical adenopathy are often required when further diagnostic information is required. A fine needle aspirate (FNA) biopsy is a reliable tool in the evaluation of palpable cervical lymphadenopathy. An FNA represents an accurate, inexpensive, and rapid technique to elucidate the etiology of the cervical adenopathy.

- An FNA is recommended in the following scenarios when other diagnostic evaluation has been unrevealing[26,27]:
  - Supraclavicular lymph nodes that are enlarged.
  - Presence of persistent systemic signs:
    - Fever
    - Weight loss
    - Arthralgia
    - Hepatosplenomegaly
  - Fixation of the node to the skin and deep tissues
  - A persistent node, despite trial of antibiotics
  - An enlarged node that has been increasing in size over 2 weeks
  - A node that has not returned to baseline size after 8 to 12 weeks

Limitations to the FNA are that it can yield an inadequate sample size for analysis and culture,[27] and it is considered accurate only when it yields positive findings.[28]

An excisional biopsy is the gold standard for a tissue diagnosis.[28] The biopsy should be taken of the largest and the firmest node that is palpable.[29] The node should be removed intact with the capsule.[29]

MANAGEMENT

- Management algorithms in cases of generalized lymphadenopathy have been established, but there is still a lack of formal guidelines for persistent cervical lymphadenopathy in the pediatric population.[30]
- If a benign reactive process is suspected, often observation coupled with cultures or serologic identification of the inciting organism and appropriate antimicrobial therapy are sufficient.
- Further workup may be warranted when a malignancy is suspected, or when lymphadenopathy persists despite antibiotics, or if there is failure of lymph node regression after 4 to 6 weeks.

SUMMARY

- Cervical lymphadenopathy is a common and usually benign finding.
- A thorough history and physical examination usually are sufficient to establish a diagnosis.
- Most often, cervical lymphadenopathy is self-limited, and treatment is not required.
- Further diagnostic laboratory and imaging studies may be warranted in the event of persistent lymphadenopathy.
- Biopsy should be considered when the diagnosis is unable to be made by other means or for surgical cure.
- Surgery should be reserved for patients with unresolved lymphadenopathy or lymphadenopathy that has failed to resolve with medical treatment.

ACKNOWLEDGMENTS

We thank Unni Udayasankar, MD, from the Department of Diagnostic Radiology at the Cleveland Clinic for his assistance in acquiring the diagnostic images in this article.

REFERENCES

1. Ferrer R. Lymphadenopathy: differential diagnosis and evaluation. Am Fam Physician 1998;58:1313–20.
2. Leung AK, Robson WL. Childhood cervical lymphadenopathy. J Pediatr Health Care 2004;18:3–7.
3. Nield LS, Kamat D. Lymphadenopathy in children: when and how to evaluate. Clin Pediatr 2004;43:25–33.
4. Park YW. Evaluation of neck masses in children. Am Fam Physician 1995;51: 1904–12.
5. Knight PJ, Hamoudi AB, Vassy LE. The diagnosis and treatment of midline neck masses in children. Surgery 1983;93:603–11.
6. Moussatos GH, Baffes TG. Cervical masses in infants and children. Pediatrics 1963;32:251–6.
7. Parisi E, Glick M. Cervical lymphadenopathy in the dental patient: a review of clinical approach. Quintessence Int 2005;36:423–36.
8. Peters TR, Edwards KM. Cervical lymphadenopathy and adenitis. Pediatr Rev 2000;21:399–405.
9. Barton LL, Feigin RD. Childhood cervical lymphadenitis: a reappraisal. J Pediatr 1974;84:846–52.
10. Dajani AS, Garcia RE, Wolinsky E. Etiology of cervical lymphadenitis in children. N Engl J Med 1963;268:1329–33.

11. Zaoutis TE, Toltzis P, Chu J, et al. Clinical and molecular epidemiology of community-acquired methicillin-resistant *Staphylococcus aureus* infections among children with risk factors for health care-associated infection: 2001-2003. Pediatr Infect Dis J 2006;25:343–8.

12. Braun L, Craft D, Williams R, et al. Increasing clindamycin resistance among methicillin-resistant *Staphylococcus aureus* in 57 northeast United States military treatment facilities. Pediatr Infect Dis J 2005;24:622–6.

13. Chen AE, Goldstein M, Carroll K, et al. Evolving epidemiology of pediatric *Staphylococcus aureus* cutaneous infections in a Baltimore hospital. Pediatr Emerg Care 2006;22:717–23.

14. Jackson LA, Perkins BA, Wenger JD. Cat scratch disease in the United States: an analysis of three national databases. Am J Public Health 1993;83:1707–11.

15. Gersony WM. Diagnosis and management of Kawasaki disease. JAMA 1991;265: 2699–703.

16. Leung AK, Davies HD. Cervical lymphadenitis: etiology, diagnosis, and management. Curr Infect Dis Rep 2009;11:183–9.

17. Soldes OS, Younger JG, Hirschl RB. Predictors of malignancy in childhood peripheral lymphadenopathy. J Pediatr Surg 1999;34:1447–52.

18. Kumral A, Olgun N, Uysal KM, et al. Assessment of peripheral lymphadenopathies: experience at a pediatric hematology-oncology department in Turkey. Pediatr Hematol Oncol 2002;19:211–8.

19. Lake AM, Oski FA. Peripheral lymphadenopathy in childhood. Ten-year experience with excisional biopsy. Am J Dis Child 1978;132:357–9.

20. Yaris N, Cakir M, Sozen E, et al. Analysis of children with peripheral lymphadenopathy. Clin Pediatr 2006;45:544–9.

21. Meuwly JY, Lepori D, Theumann N, et al. Multimodality imaging evaluation of the pediatric neck: techniques and spectrum of findings. Radiographics 2005;25: 931–48.

22. Anne S, Teot LA, Mandell DL. Fine needle aspiration biopsy: role in diagnosis of pediatric head and neck masses. Int J Pediatr Otorhinolaryngol 2008;72: 1547–53.

23. Restrepo R, Oneto J, Lopez K, et al. Head and neck lymph nodes in children: the spectrum from normal to abnormal. Pediatr Radiol 2009;39:836–46.

24. Goske MJ, Applegate KE, Boylan J, et al. The Image Gently campaign: working together to change practice. AJR Am J Roentgenol 2008;190:273–4.

25. Brenner DJ, Hall EJ. Computed tomography—an increasing source of radiation exposure. N Engl J Med 2007;357:2277–84.

26. Knight PJ, Mulne AF, Vassy LE. When is lymph node biopsy indicated in children with enlarged peripheral nodes? Pediatrics 1982;69:391–6.

27. van de Schoot L, Aronson DC, Behrendt H, et al. The role of fine-needle aspiration cytology in children with persistent or suspicious lymphadenopathy. J Pediatr Surg 2001;36:7–11.

28. Moore SW, Schneider JW, Schaaf HS. Diagnostic aspects of cervical lymphadenopathy in children in the developing world: a study of 1,877 surgical specimens. Pediatr Surg Int 2003;19:240–4.

29. Twist CJ, Link MP. Assessment of lymphadenopathy in children. Pediatr Clin North Am 2002;49:1009–25.

30. Umapathy N, De R, Donaldson I. Cervical lymphadenopathy in children. Hosp Med 2003;64:104–7.

Infantile Hemangiomas of the Head and Neck

Kevin C. Huoh, MD[a], Kristina W. Rosbe, MD[b],*

KEYWORDS

- Pediatric hemangioma • Subglottic hemangioma • Head and neck • PHACES
- Propranolol • Glucose transporter 1 (GLUT 1)

KEY POINTS

- Hemangiomas are the most common benign tumor of childhood, and 60% occur in the head and neck.
- Most hemangiomas do not require intervention.
- Patients with complex hemangiomas benefit from a multidisciplinary approach.
- Propranolol is now first-line therapy for many hemangiomas requiring treatment.
- Ongoing multi-institutional clinical trials should help to identify future potential therapies.

INTRODUCTION

Infantile hemangiomas (IHs) are the most common benign tumor in children. They are vascular tumors consisting of immature cells and disorganized blood vessels. IHs are diagnosed in approximately 4% to 10% of children, usually before the age of 1 year.[1] The incidence is higher in premature infants, babies from multiple gestation pregnancies, babies from in vitro fertilization, White race, and females.[2]

Although IHs can be diagnosed on any cutaneous surface, more than 60% of lesions present in the head and neck and may have significant aesthetic and functional consequence (**Fig. 1**).[3] Ulceration during rapid growth and subsequent scar formation can result in permanent cosmetic deformities. High-risk areas include the nasal tip and periorbital region. Subglottic hemangiomas are associated with stridor and airway distress.

Historically, hemangiomas were referred to as stork bites or angel's kisses. They usually are not noticed at birth but present within a few weeks of life. Unlike vascular malformations, IHs undergo 3 distinct phases of growth: a rapid proliferative phase, a quiescent phase, and a slow involutional phase.[3]

[a] Department of Otolaryngology-Head and Neck Surgery, Stanford University School of Medicine, 801 Welch Road, Stanford, CA 94305, USA; [b] Division of Pediatric Otolaryngology, Department of Otolaryngology-Head and Neck Surgery, University of California, San Francisco, 2330 Post Street, Suite 310, San Francisco, CA 94115-0342, USA
* Corresponding author.
E-mail address: krosbe@ohns.ucsf.edu

Pediatr Clin N Am 60 (2013) 937–949
http://dx.doi.org/10.1016/j.pcl.2013.04.003   **pediatric.theclinics.com**

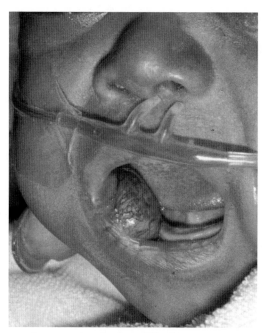

Fig. 1. Intraoral hemangioma causing feeding difficulties.

Most IHs require no intervention and result in minimal cosmetic deformity after involution. Educating parents about the natural history of IH is an important component of care. High-risk features of IH include facial location, segmental distribution, and large size. Management of high-risk IHs is often best performed in the context of a multidisciplinary vascular anomalies center because of the complex therapeutic decisions involved. Specialties most commonly involved in managing and treating IHs of the head and neck include general pediatricians, pediatric dermatologists, plastic and reconstructive surgeons, and pediatric otolaryngologists.

PATHOPHYSIOLOGY

IHs are vascular tumors comprised primarily of endothelial cells. Although the exact molecular mechanisms for the proliferation and involution of IHs are not fully understood, the cellular development of the tumors has been described. Evidence suggests that some may arise from developmental errors occurring as early as 4 to 6 weeks' gestation. IHs are believed to arise from aberrant angiogenesis (formation of blood vessels from preexisting vasculature) and vasculogenesis (formation of new blood vessels from progenitor cells). Several molecular receptor pathways associated with the development of the vascular system have been identified in the lesions. These pathways include the vascular endothelial growth factor (VEGF) pathway and the β-adrenergic receptor pathway.

The VEGF receptor pathway is a common mechanism of angiogenesis in both benign and malignant tumors. Drugs designed to counter the VEGF pathway such as bevacizumab have found success in the treatment of malignancies as well as benign vascular conditions.

Endothelial cells in IHs are derived from hemangioma stem cells. During proliferation, these hemangioma stem cells produce VEGF-A, which binds to VEGF receptors and stimulates angiogenesis and differentiation of stem cells into aberrant endothelial cells.[4] In vitro studies have found that hypoxia and estrogen synergistically enhance hemangioma proliferation.[5]

Most recently, the β-adrenergic receptor pathway has garnered attention in the pathophysiology of IHs because of the serendipitous discovery of propranolol as an effective therapeutic agent. Several hypotheses have been proposed to explain the powerful effects that propranolol has on IHs.

One hypothesis is that propranolol causes β-adrenergic vasoconstriction within the hemangiomas. This vasoconstriction may lead to decreased bulk and flow through the IHs. Recent studies using ultrasonography have shown a decrease in lesion volume and vessel density after initiation of propranolol therapy.[6]

Others have proposed a direct effect on apoptosis in capillary endothelial cells. A recent study published by Chim and colleagues[4] suggests that propranolol induces regression of IHs through a downregulation of VEGF-A and HIF-1-α, a potent master regulator of angiogenesis. In addition, downstream products of the decreased VEGF-A expression may exert a direct cytotoxic effect in the form of decreased endothelial cell migration and apoptosis.

One important distinction between the vasculature found in IHs from normal cutaneous vessels is the presence of glucose transporter 1 (GLUT1). Studies support that 97% of hemangiomas test positive for GLUT1.[7] Normally, GLUT1 is found only in placental blood vessels and vessels at the blood-brain barrier. This has proved to be a reliable diagnostic test to differentiate IHs from other hemangiomalike lesions and has been used to confirm subglottic involvement of IH.[8] Although this discovery has led to several theories of a placental role in the development of IHs, no definitive conclusions have been made.[3] However, there are GLUT1 negative hemangiomas, including noninvoluting congenital hemangiomas and rapidly involuting congenital hemangiomas, but these are rare and do not follow the typical clinical course of IH.

Recent data suggest that the mammalian target of rapamycin (mTOR) (a protein kinase) pathway may also play a role in angiogenesis during IH development. Rapamycin, an mTOR inhibitor, has been found to prevent new blood vessel formation and increase regression of already formed blood vessels.[9] Further research of the molecular triggers of the quiescent and involution phases of the natural history of IH may help identify novel treatment of IHs.

DIAGNOSIS

IHs are best diagnosed from history and thorough physical examination. Imaging is generally not necessary for diagnosis, but if performed, magnetic resonance imaging (MRI) with gadolinium is the study of choice. IHs have a typical appearance on MRI described as a salt and pepper pattern (**Fig. 2**). Clinically, IHs are generally not present at birth; however, an area of cutaneous abnormality can be observed in the form of pallor, duskiness, or telangiectasias. IHs are classified by their depth of penetration and location.

Superficial lesions are characterized by involvement of the upper dermis and were historically described as strawberry red lesions. Deep lesions occupy dermal and subcutaneous tissues. Their appearance is darker and may be more palpable as a soft tissue mass.

IHs can exist as focal lesions or can present as larger, widespread segmental lesions (**Fig. 3**). Localized IHs arise from 1 central focus, whereas segmental lesions involve a developmental segment of the body or a larger anatomic territory. A third category of indeterminate hemangiomas is reserved for lesions that are not clearly

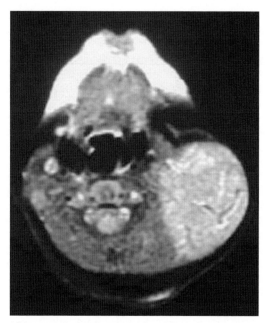

Fig. 2. MRI of parotid hemangioma showing salt and pepper appearance.

either localized or segmental in nature. Patients with multiple localized lesions are classified as having multifocal disease. Extracutaneous hemangiomas, especially intra-abdominal and hepatic hemangiomas, are more commonly found in patients with multifocal disease.[10] Patients identified with 5 or more cutaneous IHs are generally recommended to undergo abdominal MRI because of the high incidence of liver involvement.

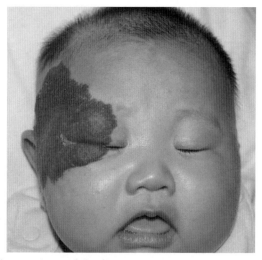

Fig. 3. Segmental hemangioma of the face.

As discussed earlier, IHs distinguish themselves from other vascular lesions in their 3 distinct intervals of development. These intervals comprise proliferative, quiescent, and involutional phases. The proliferative phase usually begins shortly after birth and continues throughout the first year of life. Most lesions achieve 80% of size by 5 months of age.[11] This relatively active proliferative phase is then followed by a period of quiescence.

The involutional phase can take months to years to complete. Superficial lesions change from bright red to a dull red, followed by gray. Topographically, superficial IHs flatten and soften during the involutional phase. Most IHs complete their involution by the age of 10 years. Although most involuted IHs leave imperceptible scar, some patients can be left with dense fibrofatty tissue or cutaneous telangiectasias after involution.

During the proliferative phase, superficial hemangiomas close to the cutaneous surface can ulcerate. Lesions exposed to friction or chronic moist conditions are also more likely to ulcerate. Segmental IHs are also more likely to ulcerate. Ulceration can cause significant discomfort, bleeding, and scarring if not treated expeditiously. Overall, ulceration occurs in approximately 15% of patients, with a median onset of 4 months.[12]

Within the head and neck, IHs that undergo ulceration can cause significant morbidity, with resultant scarring of sensitive structures. In particular, the ear and the nose are at significant risk of cartilage necrosis and loss with deeply ulcerative lesions.

Subglottic Hemangioma

In addition to cosmetic concerns, head and neck IHs may also pose functional concerns with respect to breathing when they occur in the subglottic region. Subglottic hemangiomas can occur in isolation or can present along with cutaneous IHs (**Fig. 4**). Especially at risk are patients with hemangiomas in the segmental beard distribution (**Fig. 5**). The beard pattern describes a segmental hemangioma involving

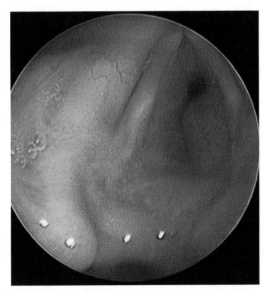

Fig. 4. Bilateral subglottic hemangioma.

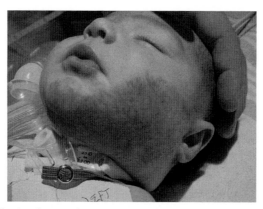

Fig. 5. Beard distribution hemangioma.

the preauricular area, chin, lower lip, and neck. The coexistence of subglottic hemangioma in patients with beard lesions has been described as high as 63%.[13]

Children with subglottic hemangiomas usually present before 6 months of age with biphasic stridor, which can be exacerbated with agitation, crying, or upper respiratory tract infection.[14] They may be initially diagnosed with croup. Any infant with recurrent croup, who is not responding to standard medical treatment, especially with a coexisting cutaneous IH, should undergo an airway evaluation to rule out airway IH. Infants may also present with feeding difficulties or failure to thrive. The most common site for airway IH is the subglottis. Complete airway evaluation involves direct laryngoscopy and bronchoscopy in the operating room with a pediatric anesthesiologist and pediatric otolaryngologist.

PHACES Syndrome

Another special consideration in diagnosis of head and neck IH is PHACES syndrome. First described in 1996, PHACES is an acronym that delineates the characteristic features of the disease: posterior fossa anomalies, hemangioma, arterial lesions, cardiac abnormalities/aortic coarctation, eye abnormalities, and sternal defects.[15] PHACES is commonly associated with large cervicofacial segmental hemangiomas (**Fig. 6**). In the

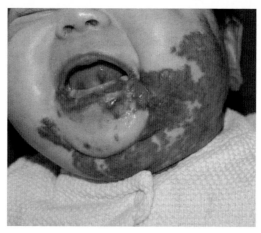

Fig. 6. Infant with PHACES syndrome.

largest series of patients with PHACES evaluated for subglottic hemangiomas, Durr and colleagues[16] found a coexisting incidence of 52%. Although the specific diagnostic criteria for PHACES are beyond the scope of this article, suspicion should be raised for patients with large segmental cervicofacial lesions. These children should undergo brain imaging, echocardiogram, and formal ophthalmologic evaluation to assess for PHACES. In addition, the threshold for referral to a pediatric otolaryngologist should be low for airway endoscopy in this subset of patients with IH.[15]

Parotid Hemangioma

Parotid gland hemangiomas also merit special mention in discussion of cervicofacial IHs (**Fig. 7**). Benign tumors of the parotid gland are uncommon in the pediatric population. Of patients with benign lesions of the parotid, most of these are hemangiomas. Similar to cutaneous IHs, parotid hemangiomas undergo several phases of development. However, parotid hemangiomas tend to have profuse growth, which can be both disfiguring and create significant vascular shunting. The proximity of the gland to the facial nerve also poses therapeutic challenges.[17,18] High-output congestive heart failure has also been reported.[19]

TREATMENT

Because of the natural history of IHs to involve over the duration of childhood, many lesions can simply be observed. However, active nonintervention is perhaps a better term than observation, because lesions should undergo routine examination for developing features that warrant active intervention. Educating parents about the natural history of IHs is an important aspect of care.

Factors that lead to the initiation of treatment include size, location, the presence of ulceration, cosmetic considerations, functional compromise, and psychosocial implications. Once the decision to initiate treatment is made, options include pharmacologic and surgical management. If psychosocial well-being is a factor in the initiation of treatment, the decision should be made before the child starts school.

Pharmacologic Treatment Options

One of the most exciting advances in treatment of IHs has dramatically changed the pharmacologic management of IH. Previously, systemic high-dose corticosteroid therapy was the treatment of choice in IH of all locations, including subglottic and parotid lesions. This regimen was associated with high morbidity. However, the discovery by Leaute-Labreze and colleagues[20] that propranolol was efficacious in the treatment of IHs caused a paradigm shift in contemporary IH management.

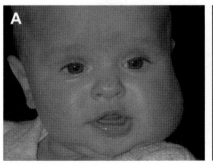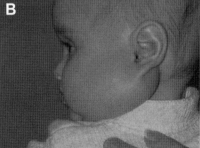

Fig. 7. (*A, B*) Parotid hemangioma.

Until recently, the pharmacologic agent of choice in the treatment of IH has been systemic corticosteroid therapy. Corticosteroids are most effective during the proliferative phase of IH development and can slow or cause cessation of growth. Prednisone is dosed usually at 2 to 3 mg/kg/d for 4 to 8 weeks. Thereafter, the dosage is tapered depending on the age of the child and IH response. Response rates of up to 90% have been reported. However, prolonged use of corticosteroids carries high risk of adverse effects, including behavioral changes, hypertension, immunosuppression, gastrointestinal irritation, adrenal insufficiency, and cushingoid facies.[21]

In the now famous report by Leaute-Labreze and colleagues,[20] 2 patients with large segmental cervicofacial IHs were treated with propranolol when symptoms of high-output cardiac failure occurred. The investigators noted rapid and dramatic regression of the cutaneous lesions as well. Nine additional patients were treated with similar results. Another study reaffirmed the rapid regression with significant IH involution within the first week of treatment initiation.[22]

A randomized control trial has shown that propranolol given at 2 mg/kg/d is superior to placebo in reducing the volume, color, and increase of focal or segmental IHs in children younger than 6 months up to 5 years of age.[23] Although no studies have compared propranolol with corticosteroid therapy prospectively, 2 large retrospective analyses showed propranolol to be superior to corticosteroids in regression of IHs and was also better tolerated.[24,25]

Propranolol therapy has also become the treatment of choice for subglottic hemangiomas. Soon after the initial reports of successful treatment of cutaneous IHs with propranolol, several case series have reported beneficial results also with subglottic hemangiomas.[26,27] In these patients, propranolol was often given in conjunction with corticosteroids. However, with more experience, propranolol is sometimes used now as first-line therapy without corticosteroids for airway hemangioma.[28]

Recently, a consensus statement was published regarding the initiation and use of propranolol for IH.[29] In the statement, the investigators discuss their recommendations concerning dosing and monitoring of therapy (**Table 1**). The target dose for propranolol is 2 mg/kg/d divided in 3 doses with a range between 1 and 3 mg/kg/d. The medication is titrated based on patient tolerance of side effects, notably hypotension, bradycardia, and hypoglycemia. Outpatient titration is appropriate for infants and toddlers older than 8 weeks of gestationally corrected age without significant comorbid conditions. Otherwise, inpatient titration and monitoring are recommended. Education of parents and pediatricians for vigilant monitoring of heart rate and adhering to a frequent feeding schedule (every 3 hours) is crucial when starting propranolol therapy. Parents must also be told that if the infant alters feeding especially in the face of an illness, propranolol dosing may need to be temporarily reduced to minimize the risks of hypoglycemia. Reactive airway disease and significant cardiac disease (cardiogenic shock, heart failure, sinus bradycardia, greater than first-degree heart block, hypotension) are contraindications to instigating propranolol therapy. In addition, it is recommended to monitor blood glucose levels during titration of hospitalized infants and to encourage feedings every 3 to 4 hours for infants younger than 6 months.[26,30] A meta-analysis of 154 patients found an overall adverse event rate of 18% for patients being treated with propranolol.[31]

Although there is no firm consensus on appropriate pretreatment cardiac evaluation or monitoring of symptoms during titration, many practitioners consult cardiology and obtain baseline electrocardiogram and echocardiograms. However, there is consensus that high-risk populations, such as those infants with PHACES, should undergo a more thorough cardiac workup before starting propranolol. Concerns have

Table 1
Initiation and use of propranolol for IHs

Contraindications	Pretreatment Electrocardiography	Hospitalization for Initiation	Cardiovascular Monitoring	Preventing Hypoglycemia
Cardiogenic shock	Heart rate lower than normal for age (<70 for infant <1 mo old or >1 y old; <80 for infants 1–12 mo)	Infants <8 wk old	Baseline HR and BP (BP in infants can be challenging so HR preferred)	Feed every 4 h in infants <6 wk
Sinus bradycardia	Family history of congenital cardiac conditions or arrhythmias	Infants with inadequate social support	HR and BP 1–2 h after initial dose and after dose increase (>0.5 mg/kg/d)	Feed every 5 h in infants 6 wk to 4 mo of age
Hypotension	Family history of maternal connective tissue disease	Infants with comorbid conditions affecting the cardiovascular system	HR and BP once target dose reached	Feed every 6–8 h if >4 mo old
>First-degree heart block	Patient history of arrhythmia or arrhythmia on examination	Infants with comorbid conditions affecting the respiratory system	Hold dose for bradycardia (as described in column 2)	Hold or discontinue during illness resulting in low or no oral intake
Heart failure		Infants with airway hemangioma	Hold dose for systolic BP <57 mm Hg in newborn; <85 mm Hg at 6 mo; <88 mm Hg at 1 y	
Bronchial asthma		Infants with comorbid conditions affecting blood glucose maintenance		
Hypersensitivity to propranolol				

Abbreviations: BP, blood pressure; HR, heart rate.

also been raised in patients with PHACES found to have significant cerebral vascular anomalies that they may be at added risk of stroke if hypotension were to occur during propranolol treatment.

Optimal duration of propranolol treatment remains unknown. Propranolol, in contrast to corticosteroids, is effective in both the proliferative and involutional phases. Average treatment durations are approximately 12 months but rebound growth after 18 months of treatment has been reported.

Despite the overwhelming success of propranolol therapy for IH with response rates of 90%, there are subsets of patients who do not respond. Risk factors for nonresponders include focalized IH, central upper and lower face IH, and IH possessing both superficial and deep components. Topical β-blocker therapy, such as timolol 0.5% solution, has been shown to be effective in some superficial IHs.[32]

Other medications that have been used in the treatment of refractory hemangiomas include vincristine, the antimicrotubule vinca alkaloid, and interferon α, the potent immune modulating drug. In general, these 2 agents are reserved for IHs refractory to other pharmacologic agents and lesions that pose serious life-threatening consequences. Interferon α poses serious neurotoxic side effects, including spastic diplegia. Vincristine is a chemotherapeutic agent also with neurotoxic side effects.

Another modality used to treat IH is laser therapy. The most commonly used type of laser is the pulsed dye laser (PDL) with a wavelength targeted against hemoglobin and thus efficacious for treatment of IHs. Although the role of PDL during ulceration and proliferation of IHs is controversial, PDL is commonly used for diminishing telangiectasias and erythema after the involutional phase.[33]

Surgical Treatment Options

Although propranolol and the other pharmacologic regimens described earlier are highly efficacious in the treatment of IH, some lesions remain refractory to these medications. In this subset of patients, surgical options are available. Risk factors for scarring that may merit early excision include an IH that is very pedunculated, very ulcerated, or has a thick dermal component.

For focal cutaneous lesions, standard elliptical excision of IH is preferred. If natural relaxed skin tension lines are respected, the cosmetic appearance of the excision is usually favorable. For cutaneous changes after surgical excision, laser therapy can be used.

Subglottic hemangiomas that do not respond to propranolol or corticosteroid therapy pose a unique functional challenge because they often cause severe airway narrowing and functional compromise. Previously, tracheotomy was routinely used as a primary treatment of subglottic hemangioma. The tracheotomy remains in place until the subglottic lesion involutes or the child's airway grows and airway symptoms improve. However, given the success of pharmacologic management and other surgical options, tracheotomy is rarely used because of the morbidity and potential mortality of an indwelling tracheotomy tube as well as the additional home care issues related to tracheotomy.[14]

Surgical management of subglottic hemangioma includes endoscopic laser or microdebrider excision, or complete surgical resection through a transcervical laryngofissure approach.[27]

Endoscopic laser resection with a carbon dioxide laser has historically had a high success rate. However, there is a high recurrence rate after these procedures, and repeat excisions are often required. Overly aggressive laser therapy can lead to subglottic scarring and stenosis.[14] This modality is generally contraindicated in those patients with circumferential subglottic IH. There is also a small risk of airway fire. The percentage of inspired oxygen should be kept around 30% and excessive charring avoided to prevent this devastating complication.

Complete surgical resection has the advantage of requiring usually only a single procedure. A transverse neck incision is made to gain access to the laryngeal framework. The inferior thyroid cartilage is divided in the midline and the subglottic hemangioma is carefully excised through a submucosal approach. The laryngeal framework is reapproximated with an interpositional cartilage graft, often harvested from the thyroid cartilage, and the patient is left intubated for several days postoperatively.[34]

Symptomatic parotid hemangiomas refractory to pharmacologic management are surgically excised through a preauricular facelift or modified Blair incision. Intraoperative neurophysiologic facial nerve monitoring is used to aid in the identification of the facial nerve and branches during surgical dissection. Although temporary facial nerve weakness may occur, permanent injury is uncommon.[18]

SUMMARY/DISCUSSION

IHs are a common benign vascular tumor of childhood. Although the natural history of the disease includes a proliferative phase followed by involution, functional and aesthetic considerations play a role in the decision to initiate treatment. In the head and neck, special attention is given to subglottic hemangiomas, which can cause life-threatening airway compromise. Propranolol has now proved to be effective as a first-line therapy for many IHs. However, some patients do not respond to propranolol therapy. Future research into the molecular mechanisms for hemangioma proliferation and involution may identify new therapeutic targets.

REFERENCES

1. Kilcline C, Frieden IJ. Infantile hemangiomas: how common are they? A systematic review of the medical literature. Pediatr Dermatol 2008;25:168–73.
2. Haggstrom AN, Drolet BA, Baselga E, et al. Prospective study of infantile hemangiomas: demographic, prenatal, and perinatal characteristics. J Pediatr 2007; 150:291–4.
3. Hartzell LD, Buckmiller LM. Current management of infantile hemangiomas and their common associated conditions. Otolaryngol Clin North Am 2012;45: 545–56, vii.
4. Chim H, Armijo BS, Miller E, et al. Propranolol induces regression of hemangioma cells through HIF-1alpha-mediated inhibition of VEGF-A. Ann Surg 2012;256: 146–56.
5. Kleinman ME, Greives MR, Churgin SS, et al. Hypoxia-induced mediators of stem/progenitor cell trafficking are increased in children with hemangioma. Arterioscler Thromb Vasc Biol 2007;27:2664–70.
6. Bingham MM, Saltzman B, Vo NJ, et al. Propranolol reduces infantile hemangioma volume and vessel density. Otolaryngol Head Neck Surg 2012;147:338–44.
7. North PE, Waner M, Mizeracki A, et al. A unique microvascular phenotype shared by juvenile hemangiomas and human placenta. Arch Dermatol 2001;137:559–70.
8. Badi AN, Kerschner JE, North PE, et al. Histopathologic and immunophenotypic profile of subglottic hemangioma: multicenter study. Int J Pediatr Otorhinolaryngol 2009;73:1187–91.
9. Greenberger S, Yuan S, Walsh LA, et al. Rapamycin suppresses self-renewal and vasculogenic potential of stem cells isolated from infantile hemangioma. J Invest Dermatol 2011;131:2467–76.

10. Horii KA, Drolet BA, Frieden IJ, et al. Prospective study of the frequency of hepatic hemangiomas in infants with multiple cutaneous infantile hemangiomas. Pediatr Dermatol 2011;28:245–53.
11. Chang LC, Haggstrom AN, Drolet BA, et al. Growth characteristics of infantile hemangiomas: implications for management. Pediatrics 2008;122:360–7.
12. Chamlin SL, Haggstrom AN, Drolet BA, et al. Multicenter prospective study of ulcerated hemangiomas. J Pediatr 2007;151:684–9.
13. Orlow SJ, Isakoff MS, Blei F. Increased risk of symptomatic hemangiomas of the airway in association with cutaneous hemangiomas in a "beard" distribution. J Pediatr 1997;131:643–6.
14. Rahbar R, Nicollas R, Roger G, et al. The biology and management of subglottic hemangioma: past, present, future. Laryngoscope 2004;114:1880–91.
15. Metry D, Heyer G, Hess C, et al. Consensus statement on diagnostic criteria for PHACE syndrome. Pediatrics 2009;124:1447–56.
16. Durr ML, Meyer AK, Huoh KC, et al. Airway hemangiomas in PHACE syndrome. Laryngoscope 2012;122:2323–9.
17. Greene AK, Rogers GF, Mulliken JB. Management of parotid hemangioma in 100 children. Plast Reconstr Surg 2004;113:53–60.
18. Weiss I, O TM, Lipari BA, et al. Current treatment of parotid hemangiomas. Laryngoscope 2011;121:1642–50.
19. Girard C, Bigorre M, Guillot B, et al. PELVIS syndrome. Arch Dermatol 2006;142:884–8.
20. Leaute-Labreze C, Dumas de la Roque E, Hubiche T, et al. Propranolol for severe hemangiomas of infancy. N Engl J Med 2008;358:2649–51.
21. Bennett ML, Fleischer AB Jr, Chamlin SL, et al. Oral corticosteroid use is effective for cutaneous hemangiomas: an evidence-based evaluation. Arch Dermatol 2001;137:1208–13.
22. Katona G, Csakanyi Z, Gacs E, et al. Propranolol for infantile haemangioma: striking effect in the first weeks. Int J Pediatr Otorhinolaryngol 2012;76:1746–50.
23. Hogeling M, Adams S, Wargon O. A randomized controlled trial of propranolol for infantile hemangiomas. Pediatrics 2011;128:e259–66.
24. Bertrand J, McCuaig C, Dubois J, et al. Propranolol versus prednisone in the treatment of infantile hemangiomas: a retrospective comparative study. Pediatr Dermatol 2011;28:649–54.
25. Price CJ, Lattouf C, Baum B, et al. Propranolol vs corticosteroids for infantile hemangiomas: a multicenter retrospective analysis. Arch Dermatol 2011;147:1371–6.
26. Rosbe KW, Suh KY, Meyer AK, et al. Propranolol in the management of airway infantile hemangiomas. Arch Otolaryngol Head Neck Surg 2010;136:658–65.
27. Truong MT, Perkins JA, Messner AH, et al. Propranolol for the treatment of airway hemangiomas: a case series and treatment algorithm. Int J Pediatr Otorhinolaryngol 2010;74:1043–8.
28. Fuchsmann C, Quintal MC, Giguere C, et al. Propranolol as first-line treatment of head and neck hemangiomas. Arch Otolaryngol Head Neck Surg 2011;137:471–8.
29. Drolet BA, Frommelt PC, Chamlin SL, et al. Initiation and use of propranolol for infantile hemangioma: report of a consensus conference. Pediatrics 2013;131:128–40.
30. Javia LR, Zur KB, Jacobs IN. Evolving treatments in the management of laryngotracheal hemangiomas: will propranolol supplant steroids and surgery? Int J Pediatr Otorhinolaryngol 2011;75:1450–4.

31. Menezes MD, McCarter R, Greene EA, et al. Status of propranolol for treatment of infantile hemangioma and description of a randomized clinical trial. Ann Otol Rhinol Laryngol 2011;120:686–95.

32. Chakkittakandiyil A, Phillips R, Frieden IJ, et al. Timolol maleate 0.5% or 0.1% gel-forming solution for infantile hemangiomas: a retrospective, multicenter, cohort study. Pediatr Dermatol 2012;29:28–31.

33. Batta K, Goodyear HM, Moss C, et al. Randomised controlled study of early pulsed dye laser treatment of uncomplicated childhood haemangiomas: results of a 1-year analysis. Lancet 2002;360:521–7.

34. O-Lee TJ, Messner A. Subglottic hemangioma. Otolaryngol Clin North Am 2008; 41:903–11, viii–ix.

Chronic Cough in Children

Johana B. Castro Wagner, MD[a],*, Harold S. Pine, MD[b]

KEYWORDS

- Chronic cough • Specific cough • Chest radiograph • Systematic approach
- Buckwheat honey • Dextromethorphan

KEY POINTS

- Cough not associated with "colds" may be present in up to 28% of boys and 30% of girls.
- Chronic cough in children lasts more than 4 weeks. In 3 to 4 weeks most infectious causes of cough should have resolved.
- Cough can be classified as specific or nonspecific. Specific cough has clinical characteristics or "pointers." The characteristics of the cough point to a possible cause.
- Most common causes behind chronic cough include recurrent respiratory tract infections, postinfectious cough, protracted bacterial bronchitis, gastroesophageal reflux, laryngopharyngeal reflux, asthma and upper airway cough syndrome.
- Over-the-counter cough medicines are not recommended by the American Academy of Pediatrics (AAP). The Food and Drug Administration (2008) did not approve its usage for children younger than 4 years. Codeine and dextromethorphan are efficacious in reducing severity and frequency of chronic cough in adults.
- The AAP recommends treating cough in children with homemade syrup based on buckwheat honey (a dark variety of honey).
- Novel therapies for symptomatic treatment currently being studied are targeting specific channels and receptors involved in the cough reflex pathway (eg, transient receptor potential [TRP] channels).

 Video of cough caused by *Bordetella pertussis* in a child accompanies this article at http://www.pediatric.theclinics.com/

INTRODUCTION

In the United States cough is the most common complaint for medical office visits,[1] accounting for 3% of medical consultations during childhood.[2] Recent community-based surveys have shown that cough not associated with "colds" may be present in up to 28% of boys and 30% of girls.[3]

No relationships to disclose.
[a] Department of Pediatrics, University of Texas Medical Branch, 301 University Boulevard, Galveston, TX 77555, USA; [b] Department of Otolaryngology—Head and Neck Surgery, University of Texas Medical Branch, 7.104 John Sealy Annex, 301 University Boulevard, Galveston, TX 77555, USA
* Corresponding author.
E-mail address: jbcastro@utmb.edu

Pediatr Clin N Am 60 (2013) 951–967
http://dx.doi.org/10.1016/j.pcl.2013.04.004
0031-3955/13/$ – see front matter © 2013 Elsevier Inc. All rights reserved.

Certainly, cough in children is disruptive not only for the child but also for the parents. It impairs the quality of life in both, adding significant stress.[4] It affects the child's sleep, school performance, and playtime. It creates anxiety for parents who fear that their child is ill, and annoys teachers and classmates in the school setting.[3]

An efficient and rational approach to the management of the child with a cough invites the following considerations.

DEFINING COUGH

Cough is a protective reflex. It is part of the normal respiratory physiology of the muco-ciliary system responsible for clearing excessive secretions and airway debris from the respiratory tract.[1] Cough is the key component for the airway's defense mechanism.[5] From the larynx to the segmental bronchi, there are receptors capable of triggering cough.[6] These receptors are stimulated by chemical irritants and mechanical stimuli.[7] The physiology of the cough reflex involves a central and a peripheral pathway. The central pathway is a brainstem reflex associated with the center controlling the breathing function. This center undergoes a differentiation process in children reaching maturation by adolescence. In comparison with adults, children's neurologic characteristics associated with the cough reflex are more sensitive to certain environmental exposures.[8]

NORMAL OR EXPECTED COUGH IN CHILDREN

Healthy school-age children with no respiratory illness may experience approximately 11 cough episodes per day with no other symptoms associated. According to Munyard and Bush,[9] previously healthy children may cough 34 times in a 24-hour period. These "normal" coughing episodes may be worrisome for parents and may be mistaken for other disorders.[8]

WHEN COUGH BECOMES ABNORMAL: CHRONIC COUGH

Chronic cough in children has been defined as a daily cough that lasts more than 4 weeks. There is no clear definition on when cough should be considered acute or chronic among the pediatric population. A period of 1 to 3 weeks allows most infectious causes of cough to have resolved in children.[8] Based on the features associated with cough, for practical reasons it can be classified as specific or nonspecific.[7] Specific cough is when there are clinical characteristics or "pointers" associated with the cough (**Table 1**).[10] Unlike in the adult population, these characteristics are more recognizable in children and point to a possible origin: brassy, croupy, honking, staccato. These pointers permit the early recognition of the cause (eg, the brassy cough associated with tracheomalacia has a sensitivity of 57% and specificity of 81%).[10] Nonspecific cough is a dry chronic cough in an otherwise healthy child, which has no other clinical symptoms associated with it.[3] It has been postulated that the majority of children with a nonspecific cough show an association with increased cough receptor sensitivity and postinfectious cough. Some studies suggest that it may resolve spontaneously.[8]

MOST COMMON CAUSES OF CHRONIC COUGH
Recurrent Respiratory Tract Infections

Recurrent episodes of respiratory infections are the main cause of chronic cough in healthy children,[3] especially among those of preschool age.[11] Parents may appreciate it as a single prolonged episode of upper respiratory infection (URI) associated with cough for several weeks. In reality, after further questioning there is a recognizable period (sometimes very short) of improvement.[5] Moreover, if a child has not fully

Table 1
Clinical pointers

Cough Characteristic	Suggested Underlying Etiology
Wheezing episodes, other atopy (eg, eczema), dry cough worse at nighttime	Asthma, gastroesophageal reflux disease
Clearing throat, allergic salute	Upper airway cough syndrome
Wet or productive cough	Cystic fibrosis, protracted bacterial bronchitis, primary ciliary dyskinesia, immune deficiency
Choking with feeds	Recurrent aspiration
Brassy or barking cough, stridor	Croup, tracheomalacia/bronchomalacia, airway compression
Honking cough, absent during sleep	Psychogenic cough
Progressive with weight loss, fevers	Tuberculosis
Staccato	*Chlamydia*
Paroxysmal (with or without whoop)	Pertussis and parapertussis
Dry cough and restrictive spirometry	Interstitial lung disease

Data from Shields MD, Bush A, Everard ML, et al, British Thoracic Society Cough Guideline Group. BTS guidelines: recommendations for the assessment and management of cough in children. Thorax 2008;63(Suppl 3):iii1–15; and Chang AB, Glomb WB. Guidelines for evaluating chronic cough in pediatrics: ACCP evidence-based clinical practice guidelines. Chest 2006;129(Suppl 1):260S–83S.

recovered from a previous upper respiratory infection and acquires a different virus causing similar symptoms, the cough associated with it may seem prolonged.[10] URIs are episodic, increase in frequency during winter, and are associated with crowded living conditions, exposure to environmental pollution, and attendance at daycare facilities.[3] Monto[12] identified a mean annual incidence for URIs in children younger than 4 years of 5 to 8 episodes, and in children between 10 and 14 years of 2.4 to 5 episodes.

In a 2-year prospective cohort study done in 2003 in the Netherlands by Versteegh and colleagues,[13] the frequency of different respiratory pathogens in children with prolonged coughing was investigated. A single infectious agent was found in 36%, 2 in 26%, and more than 2 in 5% of the children. Among the most frequent pathogens, they identified rhinovirus (32%), pertussis (17%), and respiratory syncytial virus (11%). A very strong seasonal influence on the number on infections, but not on the number of mixed infections, was recognized. The investigators also concluded that there was a high frequency of mixed-pathogen infections regardless of the season, with an increased frequency in older children.[13]

Postinfectious Cough

Postinfectious Cough is a troublesome condition that affects the patient during the day and night, following a respiratory infection.[3] It may last more than 3 weeks, but usually less than 8 weeks.[14] It has been reported that up to 40% of school-age children continue coughing 10 days after a common cold, with 10% of preschool children having a persistent cough after 25 days.[15]

Epithelial disruption and inflammation by neutrophils and lymphocytes are thought to play a main role in the etiology. Inflammation of the mucosa promotes the production of mucus, stimulating the cough receptors and the expectoration or clearance of the airway.[14] Of note, less than 5% of coughs persisting for more than 8 weeks are believed to be postinfectious (other than pertussis).[16] *Mycoplasma* infection should also be considered when the cough presents in school-age children or adolescents.[5]

Bordetella pertussis (Video 1) is a gram-negative bacterium that causes a unique respiratory infection associated with prolonged coughing after resolution of the disease. It is characterized by spasmodic episodes of cough after the initial infection, which resolves slowly over a period of up to 6 months.[3] A prospective study of 64 school-age children with documented *B pertussis* infection, performed in 2006 by Harnden and colleagues,[17] concluded that infected children may continue coughing as long as 2 months after the onset of their illness. Pertussis infection should be suspected in children with a known sick contact even if the child has been immunized, as partial vaccine failure has been reported.[18]

Protracted Bacterial Bronchitis

This term was introduced by Marchant and colleagues[19] and was defined as a chronic wet cough that lasts more than 4 weeks in the absence of underlying respiratory disorders (ie, cystic fibrosis, primary ciliary dyskinesia, immunodeficiencies), and achieves resolution with antibiotic therapy.[20] It is poorly characterized and is misdiagnosed most of the time as asthma.[1] This concept is not readily accepted by the pediatric population, and has been described as an adult illness.[20] Nonetheless, it has been suggested that most children with chronic wet cough have a bacterial infection in the lower respiratory tract.[21] The disease is caused by biofilms of bacteria in the airway associated with an intense neutrophilic airway inflammatory response.[11] The most common organisms associated with protracted bacterial bronchitis are *Streptococcus pneumoniae*, *Haemophilus influenzae*, and *Moraxella catarrhalis*. If avoidance of a diagnostic bronchoscopy is desired, a reasonable approach is a trial with antibiotics.[1]

A prospective study in children with a median age of 2.6 years indicated that the primary cause of cough was a protracted bacterial bronchitis in 40%. Upper airway cough syndrome (UACS), asthma, and gastroesophageal reflux disease (GERD) accounted for less than 10% of cases.[19] Similarly, in 2011 Zgherea and colleagues[20] reviewed 197 charts of children (0–3 years of age) with wet cough, and concluded that 56% of cases had purulent findings on bronchoscopy and, subsequently, 46% had positive bacterial cultures. Among the most common bacteria identified were *H influenzae* (49%), *S pneumoniae* (20%), *M catarrhalis* (17%), *Staphylococcus aureus* (12%), and *Klebsiella pneumoniae* (in 1 patient). The diagnosis is made clinically, and investigation for underlying conditions (cystic fibrosis, immunodeficiencies) must be sought. Physiotherapy and a prolonged course of antibiotic treatment (4–6 weeks) are recommended.[3]

Gastroesophageal Reflux and Laryngopharyngeal Reflux

Gastroesophageal/laryngopharyngeal reflux is a physiologic event that happens in healthy children,[14] and is also present in 40% to 65% of healthy infants.[1] It peaks at 1 to 4 months of age, resolving spontaneously by 12 months.[2] It becomes a disease when it is accompanied by symptoms (apnea, bradycardia, arching back, cough, failure to thrive), mucosal damage, and physical complications.[22] Dysfunction of the lower esophageal sphincter is the major cause, but impaired acid clearance may also play a role.[2] The theory behind the association between GERD and cough is not clear, but one proposed hypothesis involves irritation of the vagal nerve fibers in the esophagus. This event results in parasympathetic response that produces bronchoconstriction, stimulating the cough. Another hypothesis proposes that acidification of the distal portion of the esophagus stimulates cough receptors present in the mucosa.[23,24] For infants and children, a detailed history and physical examination should be sufficient to identify gastroesophageal reflux, and diagnostic testing is not usually necessary.[25] Further evaluation is only indicated when complications resulting from the disease have been identified. Various diagnostic tests are available: barium contrast study (upper gastrointestinal series in fluoroscopic examination), esophageal pH monitoring, esophageal manometry, endoscopy with biopsy, and scintigraphy. Therapy includes lifestyle modifications including volume restriction for feeds, positioning, and adding materials to thicken the feeding, such as rice solids. Pharmacologic therapy includes antacid H2-blockers (eg, ranitidine) and proton-pump inhibitors (eg, omeprazole) for children older than 1 year.[25]

Asthma

Asthma is a chronic airway inflammatory disease associated with bronchial hyperresponsiveness and reversible airway obstruction.[2] It is characterized by cough, wheezing, shortness of breath, and chest tightness.[14] The presence of other atopic features such as allergic rhinitis, eczema, allergic conjunctivitis, and urticaria are helpful in confirming atopy and supporting the diagnosis of asthma.[2] Cough-variant asthma is a variation in which the sole manifestation is cough, with no associated wheezing.[14] A heightened cough reflex sensitivity appears to be the cause in this case. Diagnosis is supported by a strong atopic history, rapid improvement with antiasthma medication, and relapse after such medication is stopped.[3] Diagnosis can be further supported by allergic testing (eg, skin prick) and spirometry.[7] Nocturnal cough has been used frequently as an indicator of asthma in children; nonetheless, Ninan and colleagues[26] reported that only one-third of children who presented with cough during the night (with no associated wheezing or breathing difficulty) had any association with asthma. A cough that wakes up a child from sleep suggests 2 possibilities: underlying reactive airway disease or asthma, and GERD; the latter is exacerbated while the child is lying down.

Upper Airway Cough Syndrome

This new term has been preferred over the well-known postnasal drip syndrome when discussing cough associated with upper airway conditions.[27] The specific abnormalities associated with this syndrome are allergic rhinitis, nonallergic rhinitis, nonallergic rhinitis with eosinophilia, postinfectious rhinitis, bacterial sinusitis, allergic fungal sinusitis, abnormal anatomy, chemical or irritant rhinitis, and rhinitis medicamentosa.[28] Afferent fibers from the vagus nerve are embedded in the posterior pharynx. For this reason, any abnormality affecting this area will trigger cough including the nasal secretions.[14] The latter has inflammatory capacity and direct mechanical stimulation of the cough receptors[2,7]; this is also apparent in children with the common cold who suffer postnasal drip and subsequent cough. Other irritants aside from mucus can trigger the receptors, including changes in temperature or humidity.[14] Diagnosis relies on the history taking and physical examination. Most of the time imaging will be unnecessary. With regard to therapy, patients with postnasal drainage refractory to antihistamine medications may benefit from intranasal corticosteroid and/or anticholinergic nasal spray (ipratropium bromide). This agent may provide the drying effect required with minimal secondary reactions and may be used in children older than 5 years.[14] Nasal steroids are indicated for children older than 2 years.

OTHER LESS COMMON CAUSES
Otogenic Causes: Stimulation of Arnold Nerve

In some cases the auricular branch of the vagus nerve can be stimulated by a foreign body in the ear canal, triggering cough. A similar response will be produced whenever the posterior-inferior wall of the external acoustic meatus is stimulated.[14] There have been cases reported of chronic cough triggered by wax impaction and cholesteatoma.[29] Despite the rarity of this diagnosis in actual practice, physicians should maintain awareness of its possibility when examining the patient.

Inhalation of Foreign Body

Inhalation of a foreign body may be considered at any age, but most commonly in children between 1 and 3 years old.[7] Most of the time, coughing will occur acutely and needs to be addressed promptly (especially with vegetable matter: popcorn and peanuts).[14] A history suggestive of foreign-body aspiration should trigger the appropriate consultation to consider endoscopy. In some cases, a previously missed inhalation of a foreign body can lead to chronic cough (nonvegetable small objects).[30] A missed case can lead to permanent lung damage.[14] Vegetable matter (eg, peanuts and popcorn) are associated not only with obstruction but also with erosion and scarring. Nonvegetable objects (eg, metal, plastic, or other biologically inert material) are not associated with an inflammatory response, and symptoms may be mild, potentially leading to a missed diagnosis.[31]

Functional Respiratory Disorder

Functional respiratory disorder (FRD) has been variably referred to as habit cough, tic cough, and psychogenic cough. It is has been described as a tic-like cough,[3] characterized by sudden, brief, intermittent, involuntary, or semivoluntary movements or sounds. Phonic tics include cough, throat clearing, sniffing, and grunting,[32] occurring most commonly in older children and adolescents.[3] Symptoms may be precipitated by a viral infection and are sometimes associated with secondary gain (school absence).[5] The cough of FRD can be mistakenly attributed to asthma or UACS if the cough is dry.[33] The usual presentation is a harsh, dry, honking, repetitive cough that occurs throughout the day. Affected children often remain unperturbed. The condition improves with activities that distract the child, resolves with sleep,[1] and is often exacerbated by stress.[3] Habit cough is a diagnosis of exclusion and usually responds to behavioral modification techniques rather than pharmacotherapy.[14]

HOW TO APPROACH CHRONIC COUGH IN CHILDREN

Guidelines for the evaluation and treatment of chronic cough have been published by the American College of Chest Physicians (ACCP), the British Thoracic Society (BTS), and the European Respiratory Society, but vary somewhat.[28] The approach to a patient with chronic cough has 2 objectives: (1) to determine whether a diagnosis can be reached clinically or if it will require further investigation; (2) to determine the most appropriate management based on etiology, including behavioral therapy and supportive treatment.[3]

Obtaining a detailed history and a thorough physical examination are absolutely essential for the investigation, and often allow the clinician to avoid unnecessary procedures.[7]

Important Historical Features

- Consider the age of the patient. Younger age suggests anatomic abnormalities of the upper and lower airway and the gastrointestinal tract, or foreign-body aspiration, as the necessary developmental skills are attained (**Table 2**).[1]
- Note other medical conditions and respiratory antecedents such as bronchiolitis, pneumonia, rhinitis, sinusitis, foreign-body aspiration, and surgeries.[7]

Table 2
Most frequent causes according to age

<1 y	1–6 y	>6 y
Gastroesophageal reflux	Respiratory tract infection	Asthma
Congenital malformation	Asthma	Postnasal drip, sinusitis (upper
Congenital heart disease	Gastroesophageal reflux	airway cough syndrome)
Neonatal infection	Foreign-body aspiration	Gastroesophageal reflux
Cystic fibrosis	Immunodeficiencies,	Smoking
Passive smoking	bronchiectasis	Pulmonary tuberculosis
Environmental pollution	Passive smoking	Bronchiectasis
		Psychogenic cough

Data from Urgelles Fajardo E, Barrio Gómez de Agüero MI, Martínez Carrasco MC, et al. Tos persistente. Protocolos diagnósticos y Terapéuticos de la AEP: Neumología. Available at: http://www.aeped.es/sites/default/files/documentos/9_4.pdf. Accessed: January 15, 2013.

- Observe feedings by trained staff.[3] Considerations include aspiration caused by tracheo-esophageal fistula, laryngeal cleft, congenital malformations (tracheobronchomalacia), cystic fibrosis, primary ciliary dyskinesia (especially suspicious when there is chronic rhinitis from birth), lung infection in utero, or perinatal infections (cytomegalovirus, respiratory syncytial virus, *Chlamydia*).[3] Older children and teens have an etiology similar to that in the adult population (GERD, asthma, and postnasal drip).[1]
- Define the time of onset of the cough. Is it truly a chronic cough or is there an identifiable period of improvement?[1,7]
- Differentiation between a wet cough and dry cough provides an important clinical clue. A wet cough is associated with secretions detected on bronchoscopy.[1,20] A recent cross-sectional survey of more than 2000 children aged 11 to 15 years found a 7.2% prevalence of chronic productive cough, and 47% of these children had asthma.[34]
- Signs of serious conditions should not be overlooked on initial evaluation, including neonatal onset, cough with feeding, sudden onset, chronic wet cough with phlegm production, associated night sweats, or weight loss.[3]
- Identify factors that exacerbate (cold air, exercise, feeding, seasonal) or alleviate (bronchodilators, antibiotics) the cough.[3]
- Unlike the adult population, children have limited tools with which to assess quality of life and cough severity (eg, Leicester Questionnaire used in adults). A pediatric cough questionnaire has been developed by the Italian Society of Cough Study (Pediatric Cough Questionnaire), which includes inquiries about type, duration, severity, and frequency of cough, impact on sleep, and disturbances of children, parents, school, and physical activities. These same questions must be reassessed whenever the effectiveness of therapy is evaluated.[8,35]

Important Physical Features

- Assess the general state and nutrition.[7]
- Examine each system, with special focus on the respiratory tract and adjacent anatomic structures. The upper airway examination should include nose examination for pale and swollen turbinates, nasal crease, nasal polyps, allergic shiners, and Dennie-Morgan lines. The pharynx should be assessed for postnasal purulent discharge, and erythematous and cobblestoned posterior pharynx. The ears must be closely inspected for embedded hairs, foreign objects,

and wax impaction.[29] The thorax must be inspected, auscultated, and palpated. Skin should be inspected for dermatitis.[7]

Panelists at a session of the 2012 Annual Meeting of American Academy of Otolaryngology–Head and Neck Surgery addressed the importance of recognizing the respiratory tract as a unified system. Anything that disturbs one part of it will have an effect distally, because of a shared inflammatory process that is occurring across the entire tract.[36] For this reason, a condition identified in the upper airway will inevitably affect the lower airway.

Initial Testing

Clinicians should use the history and the physical findings to guide further diagnostic testing. Previous medical records and testing should be reviewed.[1] Features of important, commonly available testing modalities are discussed here.

Chest Radiograph

A chest radiograph is recommended as the initial investigation for children with chronic cough. It will provide the physician with a good overview of the initial status of the lungs, and clues for further testing.[3] Some identifiable findings associated with chronic cough are shown in **Figs. 1–4**.

Chest computed tomography

High-resolution computed tomography of the chest is currently the gold standard when assessing the small airways. It is more likely than spirometry to detect small airway disease (**Fig. 5**).[10]

Flexible bronchoscopy

Flexible bronchoscopy is indicated when suspecting an anatomic abnormality, a previous identified radiologic abnormality, or a suspected foreign-body aspiration, or for microbiological study of secretions. For these reasons, utility of bronchoscopy will depend on the child's history, physical findings, and available expert evaluation.[10]

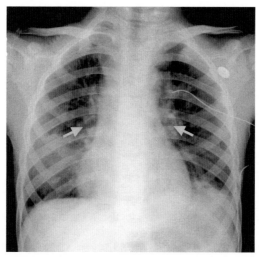

Fig. 1. Chest radiograph demonstrating parahilar peribronchial infiltrates (*arrows*) and partial atelectasis of both lower lobes secondary to mucus plugs, in a patient with asthma. (*Courtesy of* Dr Leonard E. Swischuk, Galveston, TX.)

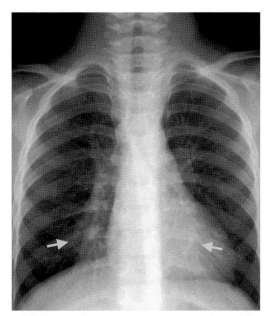

Fig. 2. Chest radiograph demonstrating typical parahilar peribronchial infiltrates (*arrows*) in chronic bronchitis, in a patient with cystic fibrosis. (*Courtesy of* Dr Leonard E. Swischuk, Galveston, TX.)

In cases of suspected foreign-body aspiration, rigid bronchoscopy should also be available (**Fig. 6**).

Spirometry

This test is useful in identifying reversible airway obstruction. Spirometry can be reliable when obtained in children older than 6 years and in some older than 3 years if

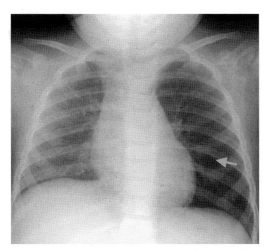

Fig. 3. Chest radiograph demonstrating obstructive emphysema of the left lung (*arrow*) secondary to foreign-body aspiration with popcorn. (*Courtesy of* Dr Leonard E. Swischuk, Galveston, TX.)

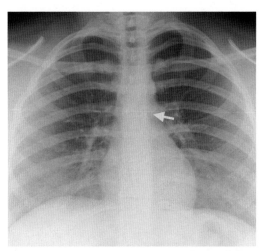

Fig. 4. Chest radiograph demonstrating metal star (*arrow*) at the origin of the left bronchi, in a patient with foreign-body aspiration. (*Courtesy of* Dr Leonard E. Swischuk, Galveston, TX.)

trained staff is available.[10] Spirometry performed before and after administering an inhaled bronchodilator that demonstrates more than 12% improvement in FEV_1 (forced expiratory volume in 1 second) suggests asthma as the cause.[1]

An integrated approach to the evaluation of chronic cough for children is proposed in **Fig. 7**, with consideration of recommendations made by the ACCP.[10] An additional algorithm is proposed for the assessment and management of a child with chronic specific cough (**Fig. 8**).[10]

TREATING NONSPECIFIC CHRONIC COUGH

Cough is merely a symptom and is not a diagnosis. The clinician's primary objective should always be to identify the underlying cause of cough and not just give

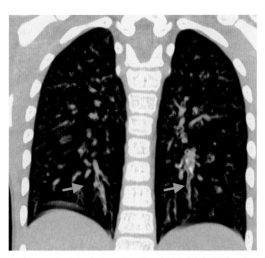

Fig. 5. Chest computed tomograph demonstrating bronchial thickening (*arrows*) in chronic bronchitis, in a patient with cystic fibrosis. (*Courtesy of* Dr Leonard E. Swischuk, Galveston, TX.)

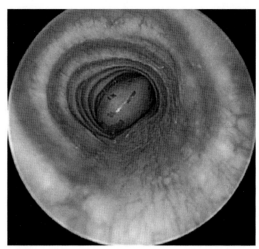

Fig. 6. Rigid bronchoscopy in foreign-body aspiration: a nut found in the distal trachea. (*Courtesy of* Dr Harold S. Pine, Galveston, TX.)

medications to suppress it.[7] However, treatment of chronic nonspecific cough (cough with no specific pointers) remains a challenge for the health care provider.[10] For symptomatic treatment, the authors recommend the following.

Nonprescription or over-the-counter (OTC) cough medicines are not recommended by the American Academy of Pediatrics (AAP), and in 2008 the Food and Drug Administration (FDA) did not approve its use for children younger than 4 years.[37] A systematic review conducted in June 2012 concluded that codeine and dextromethorphan were efficacious in reducing the severity and frequency of chronic cough in adults and the older pediatric population.[38] Nonetheless, the same medications have demonstrated little benefit beyond the placebo effect for symptomatic relief in children.[1,39] Similarly, there are no studies that recommend oral steroid use for symptomatic relief of nonspecific cough in children.[8]

Suppressing cough in many respiratory conditions may be hazardous and contraindicated.[39] The AAP has advised against using dextromethorphan and codeine when treating cough. These medications have been associated with significant side effects on overdosing, both intentional and unintentional.[40,41] Moreover, dosage guidelines for cough are extrapolated from the adult data and are thus imprecise for children.[39] In the same sense, the use of mucokinetic agents (ie, guaifenesin) has not been proved to be beneficial.[14]

The AAP recommends homemade syrup to treat cough, the goal being to reduce irritation of upper airway that triggers it. Based on age, the syrup preparation consists of the ingredients listed in **Table 3**.[37]

Buckwheat honey (a dark variety of honey) has been shown to work better than OTC syrups for coughs.[42] The World Health Organization suggests that demulcents such as honey may soothe the throat, providing antioxidant and potential antimicrobial effects by increasing the release of cytokine.[42]

As another general measure for coughing spasms it is recommended to expose the child to warm mist (eg, foggy bathroom), which relaxes the airway spasm and thins the phlegm. Humidifier usage is also advised because dry air worsens the cough.[37]

As a general environmental measure, it is important to remove children with chronic cough from exposure to airborne irritants such as tobacco smoke.[3] The adolescent

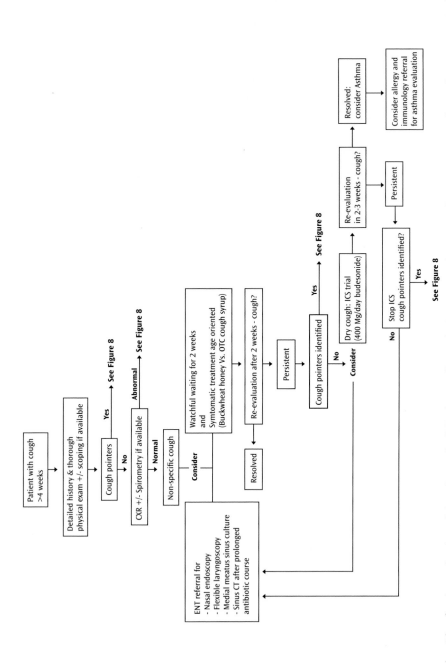

Fig. 7. Algorithm for the evaluation of chronic cough. CXR, chest radiograph; CT, computed tomography; ENT, ear/nose/throat department; ICS, inhaled corticosteroid; OTC, over-the-counter.

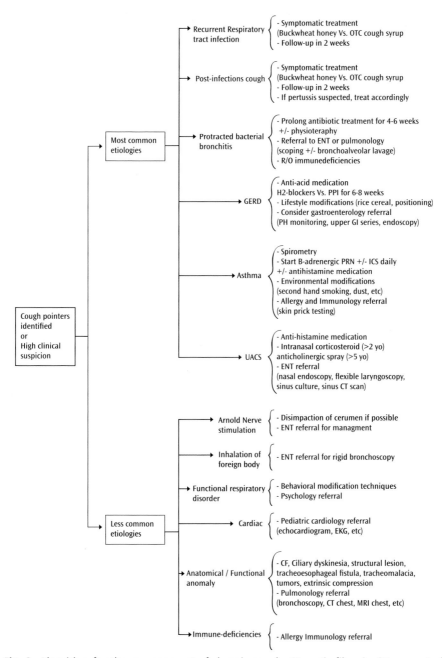

Fig. 8. Algorithm for the management of chronic cough. CF, cystic fibrosis; CT, computed tomography; ENT, ear/nose/throat department; EKG, electrocardiogram; GERD, gastro-esophageal reflux disease; GI, gastrointestinal; MRI, magnetic resonance imaging; OTC over-the-counter; PPI, proton-pump inhibitor; PRN, as required; R/O, rule out; UACS, upper airway cough syndrome.

Table 3		
Recommended preparation of homemade syrup		
3 mo to 1 y	**1–6 y**	**>6 y**
Provide warm clear fluids (eg, water or apple juice). Amount: 1–3 teaspoons (5–15 mL) 4 times a day. Avoid honey for children younger than 1 y	Provide dark honey (or corn syrup) ½ to 1 teaspoon (2–5 mL) as needed for cough. Honey has the capability to thin secretions and loosen the cough	May use cough drops to coat the irritated throat

Data from Schmitt BD. American Academy of Pediatrics: home care advice for cough. Available at: http://www.healthychildren.org/English/health-issues/conditions/ear-nose-throat/Pages/Coughs-and-Colds-Medicines-or-Home-Remedies.aspx. Accessed November 18, 2012.

who develops recurrent or persistent cough should be asked about cigarette smoking[3] or use of other inhaled substances including cannabis, and cessation must be advised.

Some clinical trials have demonstrated levodropropizine and moguisteine (peripherally acting nonopioid antitussive agents) to be efficacious for the symptomatic treatment of a dry nonspecific cough in the pediatric population. Their effect consists in modulating the sensory neuropeptide level within the respiratory tract, with a favorable benefit/risk profile in comparison with central antitussives. Levodropropizine has also been shown to produce less daytime somnolence than dropropizine, a similar antitussive. Nonetheless, these agents are not readily available in the United States as of this time.[43]

Furthermore, there is a growing interest in cough at both the scientific and clinical levels. Recent studies continue to discover a variety of receptors and channels associated with the cough reflex neurologic pathway, including the trigeminal afferents expressing transient receptor potential (TRP) channels. Novel therapies that target these receptors (eg, trigeminal TRPV1) for the symptomatic treatment of cough are being developed, and are proposed as potential modulators of the cough response.[44] Considering the neurologic differences between adults' and children's cough reflex pathway, it is necessary to continue exploring new therapies, with few potential adverse effects, to provide relief in the pediatric population.

An important aspect of treatment is for health care providers to assess the extent of disruption to the child and caregivers caused by this problem. Clinicians must address parental expectations for treatment and take this into consideration when deciding the best intervention for the child.[10]

Acknowledging their concerns and anxieties is necessary when caring for children with chronic cough. Physicians must also recognize that parents navigate the Internet for information about home management of cough in children, and may find inaccurate or misleading advice.[10] Individualized advice and counseling with sensitivity to cultural issues and the parental desire to help the child is important. Providing written information with no discussion proffers little benefit.[10]

SUMMARY

- Chronic cough in children has been defined as a cough that lasts more than 4 weeks. A period of 3 to 4 weeks allows most infectious causes of cough to have resolved.[3]

- Most common causes of chronic cough include recurrent respiratory tract infections, postinfectious cough, protracted bacterial bronchitis, gastroesophageal/laryngopharyngeal reflux, asthma, and UACS.
- The approach to a patient with chronic cough has 2 objectives. (1) Decide if a diagnosis can be easily made clinically or whether it will require further investigation. (2) Decide if there is any effective treatment or whether reassurance, supportive treatment, and follow-up will be needed.[3]
- A detailed history followed by a thorough physical examination is necessary to guide further testing and to avoid unnecessary procedures.[7]
- Identifying clinical pointers (see **Table 1**) in a specific cough will determine an approach different to that taken for a nonspecific cough.
- Nonprescription or OTC cough medicines are not recommended by the AAP, and in 2008 the FDA did not approve their usage in children younger than 4 years.[37] Buckwheat honey (a dark variety of honey) has been shown to work better than OTC syrups for coughs.[42]
- Recent studies continue to discover a variety of receptors and channels associated with the cough reflex neurologic pathway. Novel therapies for the symptomatic treatment of cough are targeting these receptors.[44]

SUPPLEMENTARY DATA

Supplementary data related to this article can be found online at http://dx.doi.org/10.1016/j.pcl.2013.04.004.

REFERENCES

1. Goldsobel A, Chipps B. Cough in the pediatric population. J Pediatr 2010;156(3): 352–358.e1. http://dx.doi.org/10.1016/j.jpeds.2009.12.004.
2. Chow PY, Ng DK. Chronic cough in children. Singapore Med J 2004;45(10):462–8 [quiz: 469].
3. Shields MD, Bush A, Everard ML, et al, British Thoracic Society Cough Guideline Group. BTS guidelines: recommendations for the assessment and management of cough in children. Thorax 2008;63(Suppl 3):iii1–15.
4. Marchant JM, Newcombe PA, Juniper EF, et al. What is the burden of chronic cough for families? Chest 2008;134:303–9.
5. Ewig JM. Chronic cough. Pediatr Rev 1995;16(2):72–3.
6. Chang AB. Cough, cough receptors, and asthma in children. Pediatr Pulmonol 1999; 28:59–70 pii:10.1002/(SICI)1099-0496(199907)28:1<59::AID-PPUL10>3.0.CO;2-Y.
7. Urgelles Fajardo E, Barrio Gómez de Agüero MI, Martínez Carrasco MC, et al. Tos persistente. Protocolos diagnósticos y terapéuticos de la AEP: neumología. Available at: http://www.aeped.es/sites/default/files/documentos/9_4.pdf. Accessed January 15, 2013.
8. Chang AB. Cough: are children really different to adults? Cough 2005;1(1):7.
9. Munyard P, Bush A. How much coughing is normal? Arch Dis Child 1996;74: 531–4.
10. Chang AB, Glomb WB. Guidelines for evaluating chronic cough in pediatrics: ACCP evidence-based clinical practice guidelines. Chest 2006;129(Suppl 1): 260S–83S.
11. Everard ML. 'Recurrent lower respiratory tract infections'—going around in circles, respiratory medicine style. Paediatr Respir Rev 2012;13(3):139–43. http://dx.doi.org/10.1016/j.prrv.2012.03.003.

12. Monto AS. Studies of the community and family: acute respiratory illness and infection. Epidemiol Rev 1994;16(2):351.

13. Versteegh FG, Weverling GJ, Peeters MF, et al. Community-acquired pathogens associated with prolonged coughing in children: a prospective cohort study. Clin Microbiol Infect 2005;11(10):801–7.

14. Ramanuja S, Kelkar PS. The approach to pediatric cough. Ann Allergy Asthma Immunol 2010;105(1):3–8.

15. Hay AD, Wilson A, Fahey T, et al. The duration of acute cough in pre-school children presenting to primary care: a prospective cohort study. Fam Pract 2003; 20(6):696–705.

16. Kwon NH, Oh MJ, Min TH, et al. Causes and clinical features of subacute cough. Chest 2006;129(5):1142–7.

17. Harnden A, Grant C, Harrison T, et al. Whooping cough in school age children with persistent cough: prospective cohort study in primary care. BMJ 2006; 333(7560):174–7.

18. Torvaldsen S, Simpson JM, McIntyre PB. Effectiveness of pertussis vaccination in New South Wales, Australia, 1996-1998. Eur J Epidemiol 2003;18(1):63–9.

19. Marchant JM, Masters IB, Taylor SM, et al. Utility of signs and symptoms of chronic cough in predicting specific cause in children. Thorax 2006;61(8):694–8.

20. Zgherea D, Pagala S, Mendiratta M, et al. Bronchoscopic findings in children with chronic wet cough. Pediatrics 2012;129(2):e364–9.

21. Seear M, Wensley D. Chronic cough and wheeze in children: do they all have asthma? Eur Respir J 1997;10(2):342–5.

22. Kelkar P, Weldon D. Approach to the patient with chronic cough. In: Adkinson NF, Bochner BS, Busse WW, et al, editors. Middleton's allergy principles & practice. 7th edition. Maryland Heights (MO): Elsevier; 2009. p. 1395–404.

23. Marchant JM, Chang AB. Chronic cough in children. In: Redington AE, Morice AH, editors. Acute and chronic cough, lung biology in health and disease. London: Taylor and Francis Group; 2005. p. 401–26.

24. Shannon R, Baekey DM, Morris KF, et al. Ventrolateral medullary respiratory network and a model of cough motor pattern generation. J Appl Phys 1998;84: 2020–35.

25. Sullivan JS, Sundaram SS. Gastroesophageal reflux. Pediatr Rev 2012;33(6): 243–54.

26. Ninan TK, Macdonald L, Russell G. Persistent nocturnal cough in childhood: a population based study. Arch Dis Child 1995;73(5):403–7.

27. Pratter MR. Chronic upper airway cough syndrome secondary to rhinosinus diseases (previously referred to as postnasal drip syndrome): ACCP evidence-based clinical practice guidelines. Chest 2006;129(Suppl 1):63S–71S.

28. Rank MA, Kelkar P, Oppenheimer JJ. Taming chronic cough. Ann Allergy Asthma Immunol 2007;98(4):305.

29. Raman R. Impacted ear wax—a cause for unexplained cough? Arch Otolaryngol Head Neck Surg 1986;112(6):679.

30. Raman TS, Mathew S, Ravikumar, et al. Atelectasis in children. Indian Pediatr 1998;35:429–35.

31. Wei JL, Holinger LD. Management of foreign bodies of the airway. In: Shields T, LoCicero J, Reed CE, et al, editors. General thoracic surgery, vol. 1, 7th edition. Philadelphia: Lippincott Williams & Wilkins; 2009. p. 927–30.

32. Irwin RS, Baumann MH, Bolser DC, et al. Diagnosis and management of cough executive summary: ACCP evidence-based clinical practice guidelines. Chest 2006;129(Suppl 1):1S–23S.

33. Weinberger M, Abu-Hasan M. Pseudo-asthma: when cough, wheezing, and dyspnea are not asthma. Pediatrics 2007;120(4):855–64.
34. Carter ER, Debley JS, Redding GR. Chronic productive cough in school children: prevalence and associations with asthma and environmental tobacco smoke exposure. Cough 2006;2(11):10–4.
35. De Blasio F, Dicpinigaitis PV, Rubin BK, et al. An observational study on cough in children: epidemiology, impact on quality of sleep and treatment outcome. Cough 2012;8(1):1.
36. Collins T. Opportunity knocks. Otolaryngologist can play bigger role in treating chronic cough. ENT Today 2012;7(10):1, 24–5.
37. Schmitt BD. American Academy of Pediatrics: home care advice for cough. Available at: http://www.healthychildren.org/English/health-issues/conditions/ear-nose-throat/Pages/Coughs-and-Colds-Medicines-or-Home-Remedies.aspx. Accessed November 18, 2012.
38. McCrory DC, Coeytaux RR, Yancy WS Jr, et al. Assessment and management of chronic cough [internet]. Rockville (MD): Agency for Healthcare Research and Quality (US); 2013 (Comparative Effectiveness Reviews, No. 100). Available at: http://www.ncbi.nlm.nih.gov/books/NBK116707/. Accessed December 5, 2012.
39. Use of codeine- and dextromethorphan-containing cough remedies in children. American Academy of Pediatrics. Committee on drugs. Pediatrics 1997;99(6): 918–20. http://dx.doi.org/10.1542/peds.99.6.918.
40. Lokker N, Sanders L, Perrin EM, et al. Parental misinterpretations of over-the-counter pediatric cough and cold medication labels. Pediatrics 2009;123(6): 1464–71.
41. Schaefer MK, Shehab N, Cohen AL, et al. Adverse events from cough and cold medications in children. Pediatrics 2008;121(4):783–7.
42. Paul IM, Beiler J, McMonagle A, et al. Effect of honey, dextromethorphan, and no treatment on nocturnal cough and sleep quality for coughing children and their parents. Arch Pediatr Adolesc Med 2007;161(12):1140.
43. De Blasio F, Virchow JC, Polverino M, et al. Cough management: a practical approach. Cough 2011;7(1):7.
44. Haque RA, Chung KF. Cough: meeting the needs of a growing field. Cough 2005; 1(1):1.

Pediatric Dysphagia

Kedar Kakodkar, MD, James W. Schroeder Jr, MD*

KEYWORDS

- Swallowing disorders • Feeding disorders • Dysphagia

KEY POINTS

- Feeding and swallowing disorders in the pediatric population are becoming more common, particularly in infants born prematurely and in children with chronic medical conditions.
- The normal swallowing mechanism is divided into 4 stages: the preparatory, the oral, the pharyngeal, and the esophageal phases.
- Feeding disorders have multiple causes; medical, nutritional, behavioral, psychological, and environmental factors can all contribute.
- Pathologic conditions involving any of the anatomic sites associated with the phases of swallowing can negatively impact the coordination of these phases and lead to symptoms of dysphagia and feeding intolerance.
- The most common examinations used to evaluate children with feeding disorders include bedside swallow evaluation, upper gastrointestinal series, videofluoroscopic swallow study, flexible endoscopic evaluation of swallowing, and flexible endoscopic evaluation of swallowing plus sensory testing.
- A multidisciplinary team armed with the knowledge of the complexity of the swallowing mechanism, an awareness of the pathologic conditions that can affect swallowing, and an understanding of the different clinical and instrumental testing options available is imperative when treating children with dysphagia.

INTRODUCTION

Feeding and swallowing disorders in the pediatric population are becoming more common, particularly in infants born prematurely and in children with chronic medical conditions.[1] A multidisciplinary approach to the workup of these patients is imperative to facilitate the early recognition of feeding problems, to identify the underlying conditions that may be contributing to the feeding problem, and to determine the most appropriate intervention necessary to achieve the best outcome for the child and the family. The multispecialty team should include the pediatrician, otolaryngologist, speech and language pathologist, occupational therapist, radiologist, dietician, and social worker, among others.

Division of Pediatric Otolaryngology, Ann & Robert H. Lurie Children's Hospital of Chicago, 225 East Chicago Avenue, Box 25, Chicago, IL 60611-2605, USA
* Corresponding author.
E-mail address: jschroeder@luriechidrens.org

Pediatr Clin N Am 60 (2013) 969–977
http://dx.doi.org/10.1016/j.pcl.2013.04.010
0031-3955/13/$ – see front matter © 2013 Elsevier Inc. All rights reserved.

The normal swallowing mechanism is divided into 4 stages: the preparatory, the oral, the pharyngeal, and the esophageal phases. The first 2 phases are under voluntary control, except in the newborn period, when the sucking reflex is regulated at the level of the brain stem.[2] The first phase is the preparatory phase, also known as the oral preparatory phase. In this phase food is taken into the oral cavity, chewed and moistened with saliva, and prepared into a bolus, which is held between the hard palate and oral tongue. This process first becomes evident at approximately 6 months of age. It is at this time that solids can be consumed. Before this age, the preparatory phase is limited to sucking from a nipple.

The second phase is the oral phase, during which food is moved from the mouth to the pharynx. Through highly coordinated movements, the soft palate elevates to prevent regurgitation into the nasopharynx and tongue movement propels food into the oropharynx.

The pharyngeal phase follows the oral phase. It begins as the bolus passes the tonsillar pillars and moves into the hypopharynx en route to the esophagus. During this phase, the palate elevates and approximates the pharyngeal musculature, cessation of breathing occurs, the larynx rises, the vocal folds adduct, and the base of tongue and pharyngeal muscles propel the bolus through a relaxed upper esophageal sphincter. The act of swallowing results in mechanical closure of the airway and transient cessation of breathing. The esophageal phase begins when the bolus enters the esophagus and ends when it passes into the stomach.

The act of swallowing is a complex act involving coordination between neural reflexes and voluntary effort that matures with development. An abnormality in neural or anatomic development can lead to swallowing dysfunction or dysphagia. Congenital or acquired structural or anatomic anomalies may cause airway and swallowing defects. This article provides an overview of the anatomic sites involved with feeding and swallowing, associated pathologic condition, clinical and instrumental evaluation, as well as treatment options.

EPIDEMIOLOGY

The overall incidence of dysphagia in children is increasing. A major contributor to this increase is the improved ability to care for infants born prematurely (<37 weeks' gestation). Survival rates for preterm infants have improved and the percentage of infants born prematurely has increased 20% since 1990.[3,4] Early gestational age, low birth weight, and especially very low birth weight (<500 g or 1 lb, 2 oz) are strong predictors of infant mortality, morbidity, and cerebral palsy (CP).[5,6] In premature children the neurologic ability necessary to achieve a coordinated, functional swallow has not developed, hence the high incidence of feeding issues in these patients.

The rising incidence of pediatric feeding issues can also be attributed to the increased life expectancy of infants with comorbidities, such as chronic lung disease and congenital abnormalities. The treatment of these conditions can involve repeated, persistent, or prolonged orotracheal or oroesophageal instrumentation, which can inhibit the development of a normal swallow.

CAUSES OF DYSPHAGIA

Feeding disorders have multiple causes; medical, nutritional, behavioral, psychological, and environmental factors can all contribute.[7,8] The medical causes of dysphagia can be organized into diagnostic categories that include neuromuscular disorders, aerodigestive tract anatomic abnormalities, genetic abnormalities, mucosal and esophageal pathologic abnormality, and other conditions affecting suck/swallow/

breathing coordination.[9] Rommel and colleagues[10] categorized feeding problems as either medical, oral, or behavioral, stating that adequate management of medical and oral feeding disorders is beneficial because the stress induced by the feeding problem burdens the child's mental and psychologic development. The cause of the dysphagia may be due to a combination of causes further complicating the workup.[11]

Neuromuscular Disorders

Neuromuscular disorders encompass many diseases that impair the functioning of the muscles, either directly, being pathologic conditions of the muscle, or indirectly, being pathologic conditions of nerves or neuromuscular junctions. A disorder of this type can potentially cause low muscle tone and poor coordination of the swallowing mechanism, which can result in respiratory compromise, aspiration, and poor weight gain. As initially proposed by Ramsay and colleagues,[12] the origin of a feeding-skills disorder is more likely to be neurophysiologic than experiential or environmental. This concept was illustrated by a study conducted by Rommel and colleagues that assessed feeding among 700 infants and young children with dysphagia and demonstrated a significant correlation between prematurity and feeding disorders. This study also noted that children with feeding disorders had a significantly lower birth weight for gestational age, which implies that feeding problems could be related to intrauterine growth retardation. More specifically, 38% of infants in this group needing assisted ventilation had an underlying neurologic condition. Preterm infants, who often have associated comorbidities, have been shown to be at risk for neuromuscular disorders, in addition to respiratory and developmental issues with subsequent dysphagia. A gestational age of 34 weeks is considered critical for the development of feeding efficiency and tolerance.[13,14] The correlation between oral feeding disorders and a history of ventilation, aspiration, and nasogastric tube feeding indicates that medical intervention may influence oral feeding skills. These findings are strengthened by the work of Blaymore-Bier and colleagues,[15] who demonstrated that premature low-birth-weight infants with prolonged intubation had significantly poorer sucking abilities at term and at age 3 months.

Central nervous system conditions are also associated with dysphagia. These conditions include CP, Arnold-Chiari malformations, and cerebral vascular accident. CP, in particular, is the most common neurogenic condition associated with dysphagia in children. Over the past 20 years, the life expectancy of children with CP has been increasing, and some think this is a contributing factor to the rising incidence of pediatric swallowing disorders. CP has been reported in 20% of infants born between 24 and 26 weeks' gestation and in 4% of infants born at 32 weeks' gestation.[5] In a study by Selley and colleagues[16] approximately 30% of children who had CP and were referred to a feeding program had histories of preterm birth. Children with other developmental abnormalities are also noted to have increased life expectancy as well. Increased awareness and detection have led to an increase in prevalence of pediatric dysphagia among children with neuromuscular abnormalities.

Anatomic Abnormalities of the Aerodigestive Tract

The 4 phases of swallowing are a coordinated effort designed to produce a bolus of food and direct that bolus to the stomach with simultaneous airway protection. The anatomic sites associated with the phases of swallowing include the nasal cavity, nasopharynx, oral cavity, oropharynx, hypopharynx, larynx, and esophagus. Pathologic conditions involving any of these anatomic sites can negatively impact the coordination of the phases of swallowing and lead to symptoms of dysphagia and feeding intolerance.

Nasal cavity and nasopharynx

Nasal and nasopharyngeal obstruction can impair breathing, which in turn negatively impacts the coordination of the oral and the pharyngeal phases of swallowing, leading to dysphagia, especially in newborn infants, who are obligate nasal breathers. Nasal obstruction can be caused by allergic rhinitis, adenoid or turbinate hypertrophy, choanal atresia, pyriform aperture stenosis, or congenital mass (encephalocele, dermoid, glioma). Bilateral nasal obstruction presents early in life, whereas unilateral obstruction may not present until much later with symptoms of nasal congestion and rhinorrhea. Bilateral choanal atresia is a severe form of nasal obstruction and usually presents as cyclical cyanosis in infancy relieved with crying.

Oral cavity and oropharynx

Mouthing and sucking movements have been observed by ultrasonography in fetus at 13 weeks' gestation. In the severely preterm infant, mouthing patterns persist until approximately 32 weeks' gestational age, when these disordered patterns of sucking bursts and pauses are replaced with identifiable rhythmic sucking and swallowing that more closely resemble a normal swallow.[17] At approximately 3 to 4 months of age, the infant develops lateral tongue movements that allow some bolus manipulation, and by 6 months of age, infants can remove soft-textured food from a spoon. At 12 months, the sucking becomes less prominent and children transition to drinking from a cup. The ability to produce and propel a bolus of food continues to improve by 18 to 24 months of age.[17–21] Development of the oral and pharyngeal phases of swallowing requires normal anatomy. Children with anatomic abnormalities of the oral cavity and oropharynx often present with poor feeding skills in infancy.[22] Anatomic abnormalities include cleft lip/palate, genetic conditions such as CHARGE syndrome (coloboma, heart anomalies, chaonal atresia, retardation of growth and development, and genital abnormalities), Treacher-Collins syndrome, Stickler syndrome, and Pierre-Robin sequence (retrognathia, glossoptosis, and cleft palate). Macroglossia can be associated with genetic conditions as well, such as Down and Beckwith-Wiedemann syndromes.

Hypopharynx and larynx

The pharyngeal phase of swallowing involves laryngeal elevation, transient cessation of breathing, and airway protection. Anatomic abnormalities that can contribute to dysphagia in infancy include laryngomalacia, vocal fold paralysis, vallecular cysts, posterior laryngeal cleft, and laryngeal webs.

Laryngomalacia is the most common cause of stridor in infants, accounting for approximately 70% of cases. Infants with laryngomalacia present with inspiratory stridor caused by the dynamic collapse of supraglottic tissue that occurs during inspiration. Laryngomalacia can be quite severe and can be accompanied by increased work of breathing, subcostal retraction, cyanosis, feeding difficulties, and subsequent failure to thrive. The respiratory distress can lead to a disorganized and poorly coordinated suck-swallow-breathe sequence. If the child takes a breath too soon in the sequence, they may aspirate before the bolus has had a chance to pass the larynx. Clinical findings are confirmed by flexible fiberoptic laryngoscopy performed by an otolaryngologist. More than 90% of infants with laryngomalacia do not require intervention because the symptoms are mild and typically resolve by age 6 months to 2 years of age. Almost all cases of laryngomalacia have signs of associated gastroesophageal reflux disorder (GERD).[23] GERD has been associated with laryngeal edema and decreased laryngeal sensation, which can lead to laryngeal residue or laryngeal penetration that does not initiate a cough response and may be aspirated.[24] Medical and behavioral treatment of GERD can improve the symptoms of laryngomalacia and the associated dysphagia.[23] Severe or refractory laryngomalacia can be treated surgically by performing a supraglottoplasty, during which the posterior supraglottic tissues are trimmed and the aryepiglottic folds are cut, releasing a posteriorly displaced epiglottis.

Esophagus and trachea

The pharyngeal and esophageal phase of swallowing may be negatively impacted by pathologic conditions involving the esophagus and trachea, more specifically, tracheoesophageal fistula and inflammatory conditions, such as GERD and eosinophilic esophagitis.

Conditions Affecting the Suck-swallow-breathing Coordination

A coordinated suck-swallow-breathe sequence depends on the infant's ability to suck efficiently and swallow rapidly as the bolus is formed to minimize the duration of airflow interruption.[25] Preterm infants have a difficult time coordinating these activities and therefore have a high incidence of feeding difficulty. Lau and colleagues prospectively studied a group of full-term and premature infants and examined the relationship between suck-swallow and swallow-breathe. The preterm infants were found to swallow preferentially at different phases of respiration than those of their full-term counterparts. As feeding performance improved, sucking and swallowing frequency, bolus size, and suction amplitude increased. It is speculated that feeding difficulties in preterm infants are more likely to result from inappropriate swallow-respiration interfacing than suck-swallow interaction.

The anatomy of the oral cavity and the mandible changes with development. In the infant, the act of sucking is facilitated by the relatively small mandible and oral cavity with respect to the tongue. Sucking occurs when the infant's lips close around the breast or nipple, and the tongue seals against the pharynx, creating a closed system. The preterm infant generates lower suction pressures, with a smaller amount of milk received per sucking interval.[26] Preterm infants and those with conditions such as choanal atresia, laryngomalacia, bronchopulmonary dysplasia, and cardiac disease also may have a difficult time generating sufficient suction pressure and therefore fail to achieve an appropriate suck-swallow-breathe pattern, which leads to poor feeding skills in infancy.[22]

EVALUATION TECHNIQUES

The evaluation of a child with a feeding disorder begins with a thorough history and physical examination by a physician, which is supplemented by a clinical swallow assessment performed by a qualified feeding specialist. Detailed information regarding the structure and function of the oral, pharyngeal, laryngeal, and upper esophageal swallow complex is collected. An assessment of the potential benefits of compensatory and treatment strategies is also determined. The most common examinations include bedside swallow evaluation, upper gastrointestinal series (UGI), videofluoroscopic swallow study (VFSS), flexible endoscopic evaluation of swallowing (FEES), and FEES plus sensory testing (FEES-ST).[2,9] Other diagnostic testing that may be needed in assessing the cause of a swallowing dysfunction include computed tomographic imaging, pulmonary function testing, esophagoscopy, and bronchoscopy.

Bedside Swallow Examination

A bedside swallow evaluation is performed by a speech pathologist to gain a preliminary understanding of the clinical signs of dysphagia that a patient has. By introducing oral feeding material, which includes foods of different consistency and color, the examination may help determine the cause of the dysphagia, the readiness of the patient to accept oral intake, and the ability of the patient to comply with subsequent radiographic studies. This information is invaluable to the rest of the multidisciplinary team with regard to further testing and selection of optimal swallowing instructions.

Upper Gastrointestinal Series

The UGI is a radiologic examination of the upper gastrointestinal tract and consists of a series of radiographic images delineating the esophagus, stomach, and duodenum. In the setting of dysphagia, a UGI can be helpful by noting anatomic and functional abnormalities, obstructions, as well as physiology of the oropharyngeal structures and UGI system.[2,9]

Videofluoroscopic Swallow Study

The VFSS, also known as a modified barium swallow, is the most commonly used study to examine dysphagia and is particularly useful in assessing oropharyngeal dysphagia. Barium-impregnated liquid and solids are ingested, which images the structures of the oral cavity, pharynx, and cervical esophagus during swallowing. VFSS may also screen structures distal to the cervical esophagus.[9,11] The main objectives of the VFSS are to provide information about the anatomy and possible structural pathologic abnormality that may be present, to investigate the movement and coordination of these structures with respect to bolus passage, and to define strategies to aid with safe and efficient feeding. It is also important to note that children must be able and willing to participate in this examination for it to be of any benefit.

It is also important to note the difference between a barium swallow and a modified barium swallow, or VFSS. A barium swallow is performed by a radiologist and radiology technician to evaluate esophageal swallowing from the cricopharyngeus to the gastroesophageal junction, useful in detecting mucosal abnormalities and signs of dysmotility. A modified barium swallow, or VFSS, on the other hand, is performed by a speech pathologist and a radiologist and evaluates oropharyngeal swallowing and all the anatomic structures involved,[9] which allows the detection of aspiration and also for the administration of controlled volumes of a variety of consistencies containing barium.

In addition to UGI, barium swallow, and VFSS, other radiologic testing includes manometric testing, ultrasound, and nuclear scintigraphy. Manometric testing is beneficial in the assessment of the upper pharynx and esophageal motility. Although technically challenging in the pediatric population, manometric testing can also be used to investigate findings performed on barium swallow further by evaluating pathologic condition, such as GERD and stricture. Ultrasound allows a dynamic view of the movement of the tongue, oral cavity, hyoid, and larynx. Aspiration cannot be directly observed and the field-of-view may be limited because bony structures do not allow transmission of sound waves. Nuclear medicine scintigraphy may be used when assessing gastric emptying and GERD. This test is limited in its ability to determine aspiration amount and tends to underestimate reflux events.[27,28]

Flexible Endoscopic Evaluation of Swallowing with or Without Sensory Testing

Otolaryngologists, in coordination with a speech pathologist, perform an FEES to evaluate the structure and function of the nasopharynx, oropharynx, and larynx during phonation and deglutition with and without liquids and solids. For pediatric patients, FEES is particularly helpful with patients who display an inability to handle secretions or cooperate with VFSS and have vocal fold dysfunction. FEES also has the advantage of being able to be performed on a baby while they are breast-feeding from their mother. FEES-ST uses pulses of air that are administered during flexible endoscopy.[9,27] Intact sensory feedback during a well-coordinated swallowing mechanism is necessary to prevent signs and symptoms of dysphagia. Sensory testing is useful in assessing patients preoperatively for airway reconstruction as well as patients with GERD or neurologic disorders who may have heightened sensory thresholds.

TREATMENT OPTIONS

Improvement of a feeding problem in a pediatric patient is most likely to occur when the underlying cause is determined and corrected. Outcomes data for the treatment of dysphagia are limited,[9] in part because dysphagia is often secondary to multiple associated comorbidities or syndromes that in and of themselves have no definitive treatment. Premature infants and/or those infants with comorbidities may benefit from interventions that facilitate the development of oral motor skills, lessen the swallowing dysfunction, or provide supplemental nutrition, frequently requiring ongoing intervention and assessments by the speech pathologist and interdisciplinary team as the child matures. Compensatory swallowing therapies have been shown to improve safety and efficiency among infants and children with dysphagia. These strategies may involve positional adaptations, texture variations, bottle or nipple changes, and instructions to the feeder regarding modifications of the feeding technique such as pacing. It is important to communicate and work with the caregiver to ensure appropriate intervention and feeding exercises are followed.[29–31]

Despite compensatory therapies, alternative feeding methods such as nasogastric and gastric tube feeding are required on either a short-term or a long-term basis.[9,27,32–34] Children require tube feedings because they are at increased risk of aspiration, require nutritional supplementation, experience dysphagia for a prolonged duration, have associated comorbidities, or have significant gastroesophageal reflux leading to aspiration of gastric contents.

SUMMARY

The incidence of dysphagia in children continues to increase, largely because of the improved survival of premature infants and children with chronic medical conditions. The ability to obtain objective outcomes data remains difficult because the cause of feeding problems is often multifactorial. A multidisciplinary team armed with the knowledge of the complexity of the swallowing mechanism, an awareness of the pathologic conditions that can affect swallowing, and an understanding of the different clinical and instrumental testing options available is imperative when treating children with dysphagia.

REFERENCES

1. Hawdon JM. Identification of neonates at risk of developing feeding problems in infancy. Dev Med Child Neurol 2000;2:235–9.
2. Bailey BJ, Johnson JT, Newlands SD, et al. Head & Neck Surgery-Otolaryngology. 4th edition. Lippincott William & Wilkins; 2006.
3. Martin JA, Hamilton BE, Sutton PD, et al. Births: final data for 2003. Natl Vital Stat Rep 2005;54:1–116.
4. Hamilton BE, Minino AM, Martin JA, et al. Annual summary of vital statistics: 2005. Pediatrics 2007;119:345–60.

5. Ancel PY, Livinec F, Larroque B, et al. Cerebral palsy among very preterm children in relation to gestational age and neonatal ultrasound abnormalities: the EPI-PAGE cohort study. Pediatrics 2006;117:828–35.

6. Mathews TJ, MacDorman MF. Infant mortality statistics from the 2003 period linked birth/infant death data set. Natl Vital Stat Rep 2006;54:1–29.

7. Riordan MM, Iwata BA, Wohl KM, et al. Behavioral treatment of food refusal and selectivity in developmentally disabled children. Appl Res Ment Retard 1980;1: 95–112.

8. Babbitt RL, Hoch TA, Coe DA, et al. Behavioral assessment and treatment of pediatric feeding disorders. J Dev Behav Pediatr 1994;15:278–91.

9. Lefton-Greif MA. Pediatric dysphagia. Phys Med Rehabil Clin N Am 2008;19: 837–51.

10. Rommel N, De Meyer AM, Feenstra L, et al. The complexity of feeding problems in 700 infants and young children presenting to a tertiary care institution. J Pediatr Gastroenterol Nutr 2003;37:75–84.

11. Jones P, Altschuler S. Dysphagia teams: a specific approach to a non-specific problem. Dysphagia 1987;2:200–5.

12. Ramsay M, Gisel EG, Bountry M. Nonorganic failure to thrive: growth failure secondary to feeding skills disorder. Dev Med Child Neuol 1993;35(4):285–97.

13. Milla P, Fenton T. Small intestinal motility patterns in the perinatal period. J Pediatr Gastroenterol Nutr 1983;2(Suppl 1):S141–4.

14. Daniels H, Casaer P, Devlieger H, et al. Mechanisms of feeding efficiency in preterm infants. J Pediatr Gastroenterol Nutr 1986;5:593–6.

15. Blaymore-Bier J, Ferguson A, Cho C, et al. Ther oral motor development of low-birth-weight infants who underwent orotracheal intubation during the neonatal period. Am J Dis Child 1993;147:858–62.

16. Selley WG, Parrott LC, Lethbridge PC, et al. Objective measures of dysphagia complexity in children related to suckle feeding histories, gestational ages, and classification of their cerebral palsy. Dysphagia 2001;16:200–7.

17. Bu'Lock F, Woolridge MW, Baum JD. Development of co-ordination of sucking, swallowing and breathing: Ultrasound study of term and preterm infants. Dev Med Child Neurol 1990;32:669–78.

18. Gisel EG. Chewing cycles in 2- to 8-year-old normal children: a developmental profile. Am J Occup Ther 1988;42:40–6.

19. Gisel EG. Development of oral side preference during chewing and its relation to had preference in normal 2- to 8-year-old children. Am J Occup Ther 1988;42:378–83.

20. Sheppard JJ, Mysak ED. Ontogeny of infantile oral reflexes and emerging chewing. Child Dev 1984;55:831–43.

21. Stolovitz P, Gisel EG. Circumoral movements in response to three different food textures in children 6 months to 2 years of age. Dysphagia 1991;6:17–25.

22. Sullivan PB, et al. Prevalence and severity of feeding and nutritional problems in children with neurological impairment: Oxford Feeding Study. Dev Med Child Neurol 2000;42:674–80.

23. Thompson D. Abnormal sensorimotor integrative function of the larynx in congenital laryngomalacia: a new theory of etiology. Laryngoscope 2007; 117(Suppl 114):1–33.

24. Link DT, Willging JP, Miller CK, et al. Pediatric laryngopharyngeal sensory testing during flexible endoscopic evaluation of swallowing: feasible and correlative. Ann Otol Rhinol Laryngol 2000;109:899–905.

25. Lau C, Smith EO, Schanler RJ. Coordination of suck-swallow and swallow respiration in preterm infants. Acta Paediatr 2003;92:721–7.

26. Mathew OP. Science of bottle feeding. J Pediatr 1991;119:511–9.
27. Willging JP, Miller CK, Link DT, et al. Use of FEES to assess and manage pediatric patients. In: Langmore SE, editor. Endoscopic treatment and evaluation of swallowing disorders. 1st edition. New York: Thieme; 2001. p. 213–34.
28. Lefton-Greif MA, Carroll JL, Loughlin GM. Long-term follow-up of oropharyngeal dysphagia in children without apparent risk factors. Pediatr Pulmonol 2006;41:1040–8.
29. Lifschitz CH. Feeding problems in infants and children. Curr Treat Options Gastroenterol 2001;4:451–7.
30. Thach BT. Maturation and transformation of reflexes that protect the laryngeal airway from liquid aspiration from fetal to adult life. Am J Med 2001;111(Suppl 8A):69S–77S.
31. Rudolph CD, Link DT. Feeding disorders in infants and children. Pediatr Clin North Am 2002;49:97–112.
32. Cummings CW, Flint PW, Haughey BH, et al, editors. Cummings: Otolaryngology: Head & Neck Surgery. 4th edition. St. Louis: Elsevier Mosby; 2005.
33. Goldfield EC, Buonomo C, Fletcher K, et al. Premature infant swallowing: patterns of tongue-soft palate coordination based upon videofluoroscopy. Infant Behav Dev 2010;33(2):209–18.
34. Slattery J, Morgan A, Douglas J. Early sucking and swallowing problems as predictors of neurodevelopmental outcome in children with neonatal brain injury. Dev Med Child Neurol 2012;54(9):796–806. http://dx.doi.org/10.1111/j.1469-8749.2012.04318.x.

Chronic Rhinosinusitis in Children

Austin S. Rose, MD*, Brian D. Thorp, MD, Adam M. Zanation, MD,
Charles S. Ebert Jr, MD, MPH

KEYWORDS

- Pediatric sinusitis • Chronic rhinosinusitis • Treatment • Management • Surgery

KEY POINTS

- Chronic rhinosinusitis (CRS) represents a heterogeneous spectrum of diseases.
- The definition of CRS has largely been accepted as the persistence of characteristic signs and symptoms beyond 12 weeks.
- Few randomized, placebo-controlled trials or systematic reviews of the literature exist with recommendations for treatment of CRS in children.
- The medical management of CRS has traditionally included combinations of antihistamines, decongestants, nasal saline irrigation, topical nasal steroids, and oral antibiotics.
- When prolonged efforts at medical therapy have failed, children with persistent CRS should be referred to an otolaryngologist for further evaluation and possible surgical intervention.

CLASSIFICATION OF CRS

Rhinosinusitis can be considered a spectrum of disease characterized by concurrent inflammatory and infectious processes that affect the nasal passages and the contiguous paranasal sinuses.[1–3] Diagnosis and management are aided by the classification of this diverse condition into categories based primarily on the duration of symptoms. In addition, pediatric rhinosinusitis, whether acute or chronic, should be considered a unique conditions because of the differences in predisposing factors and the anatomy of the sinuses seen between children and adults.

Because common viral upper respiratory infections (URI) and acute sinusitis can be difficult to distinguish clinically, acute episodes of sinusitis have traditionally been defined as the persistence of signs and symptoms beyond 10 days, or the concomitant occurrence of related complications, such as orbital abscess or meningitis. Other classifications described in the literature include recurrent acute sinusitis, subacute

Financial Disclosures/Conflict of Interest: The authors have nothing to disclose.
Department of Otolaryngology - Head & Neck Surgery, University of North Carolina School of Medicine, CB #7070, Chapel Hill, NC 27599-7070, USA
* Corresponding author.
E-mail address: austin_rose@med.unc.edu

sinusitis, eosinophilic sinusitis, sinusitis with and without nasal polyps, and relatively distinct disease processes, including invasive and allergic fungal sinusitis.

The definition of CRS has largely been accepted as the persistence of characteristic signs and symptoms beyond 12 weeks. This extended period of chronic symptoms may also be punctuated by episodes of acute exacerbations.

PATHOPHYSIOLOGY

Along with the nasal passages, the paranasal sinuses filter, warm, and humidify inspired air. They are also key in reducing the overall weight of the human skull. Sinuses grow in size and shape throughout childhood, although this progression may be affected by various disease processes, such as cystic fibrosis (CF).[4] The result is an underdeveloped or hypoplastic sinus. The frontal sinuses are the last to fully develop, and generally reach adult size by puberty.

The mucosa of the paranasal sinuses is composed of a ciliated, pseudostratified, columnar epithelium with goblet cells for mucous production, and is similar to that found in the remainder of the tracheobronchial passages. Normal function of the sinuses depends on patent ostia, including the important common pathway of drainage and aeration known as the *osteomeatal complex* (OMC) (**Fig. 1**), and on normal mucous secretion and normal ciliary function. The primary common factor in the pathophysiology of sinus disease is thought to be obstruction of the sinus ostium, either through mechanical means or mucosal inflammation and edema, rather than initial bacterial infection. Obstruction leads to retained secretions and blocks the normal exchange of air, resulting in hypoxia of the sinus mucosa. This process leads to a cycle of mucosal dysfunction characterized by impaired cilia, further retention of secretions, and secondary infection.

Traditionally, normal sinuses, unlike other areas of the upper aerodigestive tract, have been thought to be sterile and without a normal and possibly protective microbial

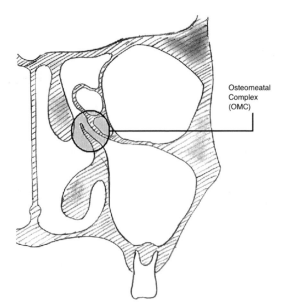

Osteomeatal
Complex
(OMC)

Fig. 1. Diagram of the OMC.

population, although some recent studies suggest otherwise. Abreu and colleagues[5] describe a reduced diversity of sinus microbes in patients with CRS compared with healthy controls. They also used a murine model of CRS to demonstrate the possible protective effects of one organism in particular: *Lactobacillus sakei*. Although many questions remain, these findings may support a new paradigm in which the disturbance of normal sinus microbial populations proves to be an important factor in the pathogenesis of CRS in children. Given their overuse in routine URIs, antibiotics are certainly one factor that might be expected to disrupt normal sinus flora and therefore could potentially be more causative than curative in CRS.

A host of other innate and environmental factors also contribute to the common pathophysiologic pathways in CRS (**Table 1**). Local or anatomic factors include direct sinus obstruction caused by anatomic abnormalities, such as the presence of concha bullosa, septal deviation, nasal polyposis, trauma, and foreign bodies. Conditions contributing to mucosal inflammation and secondary obstruction include URI, bacterial infection, allergy, and gastroesophageal reflux disease (GERD). GERD in particular is known to be prevalent in children with CRS[6] and, in a retrospective study, Bothwell and colleagues[7] demonstrated a significant decrease in the need for sinus surgery among children on antireflux therapy. In addition to allergens, environmental irritants such as air pollutants or tobacco smoke may occasionally play a role in chronic mucosal inflammation.

Bacterial infection has long been considered a key component of CRS, and the pathogens found in children are generally similar to those in adults. The common isolates associated with CRS include those found in acute sinusitis (*Streptococcus pneumoniae, Moraxella catarrhalis*, and nontypeable *Haemophilus influenzae*) and *Staphylococcus aureus, Pseudomonas*, and anaerobes. The possible role of relatively ubiquitous fungi in the CRS inflammatory response has also been proposed, although this remains controversial.[8]

Recent evidence has also supported the role of bacterial exotoxins and biofilm formation in the pathogenesis of CRS. Exotoxins are released by bacteria and may contribute to a symptomatic immune response. In particular, Wang and colleagues[9] demonstrated the presence of staphylococcal exotoxin and its effect on T cells in patients with CRS with nasal polyps. Biofilms form when bacteria aggregate on surfaces within an external matrix of polysaccharides, nucleic acids, and proteins. In CRS, biofilm formation may decrease the efficacy of antimicrobials by as much as 100 fold, allowing bacteria to thrive for a prolonged period within the nose and sinus cavities. In 2005, Sanclement and colleagues[10] used electron microscopy to demonstrate the presence of biofilms in sinus biopsies from 80% of patients undergoing functional endoscopic sinus surgery (FESS) for CRS, whereas none were seen in healthy controls. Other studies have reported the presence of biofilms in adenoid tissue from patients with chronic infectious disease of the upper airways, including

Table 1		
Contributing factors in CRS		
Local	**Inflammatory**	**Systemic**
Sinus obstruction	URI	CF
Septal deviation	Bacterial infection	Primary ciliary dyskinesia
Nasal polyps	Allergy	Immune deficiencies
Trauma	Gastroesophageal reflux disease	
Foreign body	Tobacco smoke	

CRS.[11] The literature suggests that both exotoxins and biofilms may be important factors in the role of bacterial infection in CRS.

When evaluating a child with symptoms of CRS, one should always consider the possibility of underlying disease as a contributing factor. Diseases impacting normal sinonasal function include CF, primary ciliary dyskinesia (PCD), and a variety of immune deficiencies, including the still-developing immature immunity of normal young children.

DIAGNOSIS

Careful history and physical examination is clearly important in the evaluation of this heterogeneous and multifactorial disease. The symptoms of CRS in children are different than in adult patients and include persistent cough, and prolonged anterior and posterior nasal drainage, congestion, low-grade fever, irritability, and behavioral difficulties (**Box 1**). Headache, especially in the frontal area, is a less common complaint among children than adults. Parents may report a history of frequent URI or recurrent acute episodes of sinusitis requiring treatment. Additional history should focus on identification of any potential underlying diseases or contributing environmental factors. The diagnosis of CRS is rarely made in isolation, and commonly associated findings include allergy, asthma, dental disease, CF, PCD, and immunodeficiency syndromes. A nasal foreign body should be considered in children with a history of prolonged unilateral rhinorrhea and a foul odor reported by parents.

Physical examination includes a complete head and neck evaluation with careful attention to the middle ear, because otitis media with effusion (OME) is another common comorbidity. Anterior rhinoscopy (**Fig. 2**) should be performed with a nasal speculum or otoscope using a large ear speculum. Characteristic findings are summarized in **Table 2** and include mucosal erythema and irritation, thickened nasal mucous, polyps, and frank purulent drainage. Periorbital allergic shiners or a pronounced nasal crease may indicate adenoid enlargement or disease. Otolaryngologists will usually include fiberoptic sinonasal endoscopy as part of their examination when possible, allowing improved visualization of the middle meatus, a common site of polyps or purulent drainage from the maxillary and ethmoid sinuses. Endoscopy is also useful for visualizing the posterior nasal cavity, nasopharynx, and adenoid tissue.

The radiologic evaluation of children with suspected CRS is generally reserved for those with disease refractory to medical management. Plain films, computed tomography (CT), and magnetic resonance imaging have all been used in the evaluation of chronic sinusitis; however, CT scanning is generally considered the preferred study

---

Box 1
CRS symptoms

Nasal congestion

Purulent rhinorrhea

Chronic cough

Postnasal drainage

Low-grade fevers

Irritability

Behavioral issues

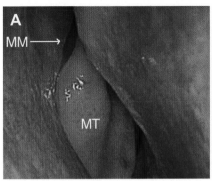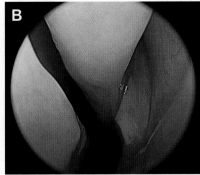

Fig. 2. (*A*) Normal anterior rhinoscopy with view of the middle turbinate (MT) and middle meatus (MM). (*B*) Anterior rhinoscopy demonstrating purulent drainage from the middle meatus.

(**Fig. 3**). CT provides a much higher resolution of bone and soft tissue without the interference of overlying structures compared with plain radiography.[12]

Recent literature has supported restraint in the use of CT scanning in children because of concerns of excess radiation exposure.[13] In evaluating CRS, most otolaryngologists advocate CT scans of the sinuses only when deciding on surgical intervention. In most cases, these scans can also be used intraoperatively, without additional radiation exposure, for image guidance to help reduce the risk of complications during sinus surgery. In a 2012, clinical consensus statement for the American Academy of Otolaryngology-Head and Neck Surgery Foundation, Setzen and colleagues[14] reported a strong consensus (>75% of the panel) for the statement "CT imaging is indicated in pediatric patients for chronic sinusitis when medical management and/or adenoidectomy have failed to control symptoms."

FURTHER EVALUATION

Beyond history-taking and physical examination, the further workup and evaluation of children with suspected chronic sinusitis should include steps to identify or eliminate associated or causative factors (**Box 2**).

- Allergy testing, including total IgE and either serum radioallergosorbent testing or skin end point titration testing can be used to identify children with underlying allergies. Ultimately, immunotherapy may prove beneficial in appropriate patients.
- Bacterial cultures can evaluate for specific pathogens and help guide antimicrobial treatment. Sinus aspirates for culture-directed treatment can be obtained via sinus trephination or intraoperatively. Cultures from the middle meatus are

Table 2
CRS physical findings

Nasal Examination	Head & Neck Examination
Nasal congestion	OME
Purulent drainage	Allergic shiners
Mucosal erythema	Nasal crease
Increased mucous	Sinus tenderness
Nasal polyps	Reduced transillumination

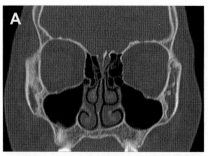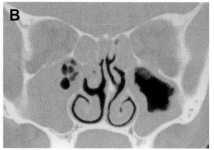

Fig. 3. (*A*) A normal coronal CT scan of the sinuses. (*B*) A coronal CT scan of the sinuses demonstrating bilateral ethmoid sinus opacification, maxillary sinusitis on the right and mucosal thickening within the maxillary sinus on the left.

generally easier to obtain in most cases, and have a high predictive value in the diagnosis of bacterial sinusitis.[15]

- Immunologic testing can diagnose immunodeficiencies and usually includes levels of IgG with subclasses, IgA, and postvaccination titers.
- Sweat chloride or CF genetic testing can be used to rule out CF.
- A nasal or tracheobronchial ciliary biopsy can be obtained to evaluate ciliary function and rule out PCD. Usually, both light microscopy and electron microscopy are performed.
- An otolaryngology referral is recommended for children with suspected CRS refractory to medical management and can facilitate further evaluation and treatment, including fiberoptic nasal endoscopy and surgical intervention, such as adenoidectomy and, if necessary, endoscopic sinus surgery.
- Other consultations that may be of significant help in a multidisciplinary approach to CRS include pediatric allergy and immunology and pediatric pulmonary medicine.

MEDICAL TREATMENT

Evidence suggests that CRS can resolve spontaneously in children and that complications are rare.[16] Still, the various contributing factors in the pathogenesis of CRS

Box 2
CRS workup and evaluation

Allergy testing

Sinus aspirate or middle meatus cultures

Immunologic testing

Sweat chloride or genetic testing for CF

Ciliary biopsy to rule out PCD

Possible consultations:

    Pediatric allergy and immunology

    Pediatric pulmonary medicine

    Otolaryngology

afford several potential targets in treatment when necessary for persistent disease. However, few randomized controlled trials or systematic reviews of the literature exist with recommendations for treatment of this complex disease in children. Much of what is known, therefore, about the efficacy of therapies for CRS is based on findings in adult populations or studies of acute sinusitis. For example, a recent review of the Cochrane and PubMed databases by Makary and Ramadan[17] revealed no randomized controlled studies comparing medical treatment with FESS, or other surgical procedures, for CRS in children.

The medical management of CRS has traditionally included combinations of antihistamines, decongestants, nasal saline irrigation, topical nasal steroids, and oral antibiotics. In a survey of pediatric otolaryngologists in 2005, Sobol and colleagues[18] reported that 95% of respondents used antibiotics in the treatment of CRS, whereas 90% prescribed topical steroids and 68% recommended nasal saline spray. Antihistamines and decongestants are commonly used in suspected sinusitis because of their role in reducing mucosal edema, and to treat any component of underlying allergy. However, in a recent Cochrane systematic review of acute sinusitis, no significant evidence was found to support the use of antihistamines or decongestants.[19]

Nasal saline sprays, or irrigations when tolerated, are also used in the treatment of CRS, and are thought to help primarily in the clearance of sinonasal secretions, pathogens, and debris. Although the Cochrane review could not support any recommendations regarding nasal saline irrigation either, several studies have shown some degree of efficacy in CRS. In a prospective study of 40 children, Wei and colleagues[20] showed a significant improvement in both quality of life and CT scan Lund-Mackay scores after 6 weeks of once-daily nasal saline irrigation. Other reviews of the literature also support a clinical benefit from the use of topical nasal saline.[21] For the most part, the use of regular nasal saline sprays or irrigation is well tolerated in children, with minimal side effects.

Topical nasal steroids suppress mucosal inflammation and are also therefore widely used in the treatment of CRS in children. Examples include fluticasone propionate, which is widely available in generic form, and mometasone furoate, which is indicated for use in nasal congestion because of allergic rhinitis for children 2 years of age and older. Evidence is limited but supports the use of both intranasal and systemic corticosteroids in the treatment of sinusitis, either alone or in combination with antibiotic therapy.[22,23] The use of topical nasal steroids is generally preferred for children with CRS because of their low systemic bioavailability. Systemic side effects are therefore rare, with minor epistaxis the most commonly reported complication.[24] The duration of treatment generally coincides with the longer courses of antibiotics used in CRS, typically 3 to 6 weeks, although long-term prophylactic use seems safe and may help suppress chronic symptoms and recurrent disease. Although controversial, nasal steroids may also have a role in combination with surgery as part of a postoperative and preventive medical regimen along with nasal saline. Although Dijkstra and colleagues[25] found no effect on the recurrence of CRS symptoms or nasal polyps after FESS, others have shown a decreased need for revision surgery in patients with CRS treated with topical nasal steroids postoperatively.[26]

The use of antibiotics in treating acute sinusitis is generally accepted. In choosing a particular agent, however, one should consider the likely offending pathogens and any information on local patterns of antibiotic resistance. Recent guidelines from the Infectious Diseases Society of America include prompt treatment for children with suspected acute bacterial sinusitis.[27] Amoxicillin/clavulanate, or levofloxacin for children with type I hypersensitivity reactions to penicillin, for 10 to 14 days was recommended as first-line treatment.

In CRS, available evidence suggests that longer courses of antibiotic treatment (3–12 weeks) are necessary to achieve any significant benefit.[28] In the absence of culture data, amoxicillin/clavulanate remains a good choice for first-line treatment, although antibiotic choices should also reflect the differences in possible pathogens in CRS, including *S aureus, Pseudomonas*, and anaerobes. Long-term macrolide treatment (12 weeks) may also be of benefit in patients with CRS with low IgE levels.[29]

Although oral and sometimes intravenous are the most frequently used routes of antibiotic administration in CRS, the potential for topical antibiotic therapy has also gained recent attention.[8] The theory is that topical treatment, via spray, nebulizer or irrigation, should serve to deliver a high concentration of antibiotic directly to the sino-nasal mucosa while minimizing systemic side effects. Although recent reviews have not supported the use of topical antibiotics for CRS, several studies have reported symptomatic improvement.[30,31] Uren and colleagues[32] treated 16 patients with surgically recalcitrant CRS and endoscopic cultures positive for *S aureus.* After 3 weeks of twice-daily topical mupirocin, 12 patients were improved symptomatically, with 15 demonstrating an improvement in endoscopic findings and negative cultures.

So far little evidence has shown that topical antibiotics are effective in reducing biofilm formation, although, perhaps surprisingly, regression of biofilms has been reported in patients with CRS after 8 weeks of treatment with oral clarithromycin.[33] Although topical antibiotic treatment is not currently recommended in most cases of CRS, initial findings do seem to warrant further study. Questions regarding dosage, length of therapy, optimal method of delivery, and the potential for combination with other treatments remain to be answered. In summary, topical nasal steroids, nasal saline, and systemic antibiotics when necessary remain the preferred medical treatments for CRS in children based on the best evidence to date.

SURGICAL TREATMENT

When prolonged efforts at medical therapy have failed, children with persistent CRS should be referred to an otolaryngologist for further evaluation and possible surgical intervention. Adenoidectomy is the first line of surgical treatment and is often performed even before radiologic imaging with CT. Large adenoids may physically disrupt the normal mucociliary clearance of the nasal cavity and sinuses, although adenoid tissue of any size is thought to act as a reservoir for bacteria. Evidence also suggests frequent biofilm formation on adenoid tissue in children with CRS.[34] A 2008 meta-analysis of adenoidectomy in children with rhinosinusitis found an overall rate of clinical improvement of approximately 70%, consistent with prior studies.[35] In teenage children, adenoid tissue may tend to recede and become less clinically relevant. For this age group, endoscopic sinus surgery, either with or without treatment of adenoid tissue, may be considered more frequently as an acceptable initial surgical procedure.[36]

The goal of sinus surgery beyond adenoidectomy is generally to enlarge the natural opening of the sinuses, while preserving normal sinus mucosa, in an effort to reestablish sinus aeration and normal mucociliary function. Surgical intervention may also include the removal of any obstructive or diseased tissue, such as nasal polyps. A CT scan is often obtained at this point to demonstrate persistent sinus disease despite maximal medical therapy, and for a careful review of sinonasal anatomy for preoperative planning.

In recent years, the refinement of fiberoptic endoscopes has allowed for most sinus surgery to be performed endoscopically. In children, the most common procedure is limited FESS and involves widening of the natural ostium of the maxillary sinus along with a limited or anterior ethmoidectomy. Some surgeons, however, recommend a complete removal of the anterior and posterior ethmoid cells, resulting in a larger, better-aerated, and well-mucosalized ethmoid cavity. More recently, balloon dilation of sinus ostia known as *balloon catheter sinuplasty* (BCS) has been reported as an alternative to conventional FESS. In children, this is primarily used for treatment of the maxillary sinus and has been described both alone and in combination with other procedures, such as adenoidectomy and ethmoidectomy.

Although surgery is clearly indicated for complications of acute sinusitis or underlying disease such as allergic fungal sinusitis, its role in CRS is less clear. Sinus surgery in CRS is probably best thought of as an adjuvant treatment to medical therapy, with the goal of improving sinus function. Parents should be counseled about reasonable expectations for symptomatic improvement, because children will remain prone to URIs, allergies, and other underlying factors. A reduction in the frequency and severity of symptoms is a reasonable goal, and many children will benefit from continued medical management, including topical nasal steroids and saline postoperatively. In fact, the enlargement of sinus ostia achieved through sinus surgery may also improve the delivery and efficacy of topical treatments such as nasal steroid sprays and saline irrigations.

In terms of the efficacy of FESS in children, most studies are retrospective, although they demonstrate significant clinical improvement for CRS refractory to medical treatment and adenoidectomy. In 2009, Siedek and colleagues[37] reported a 76% rate of improvement in both CRS symptoms and overall quality of life. In a review of 11 studies, Makary and Ramadan[17] found a success rate for pediatric FESS ranging from 82% to 100%. In a study of adults aged 18 years and older, a recent prospective trial found a greater improvement for patients with CRS treated with FESS compared with those managed medically. After 12 months of follow-up, the surgical patients also reported significantly less use of oral antibiotics and steroids and fewer missed days of work or school.[38] Results also seem to be lasting, with one study showing the symptomatic benefits of FESS over medical therapy as far out as 10 years.[39]

Although BCS is appealing as a potentially less invasive technique, its role in children with CRS seems limited to treatment of the maxillary sinuses (**Fig. 4**). Most children lack full development of the frontal sinuses, and dilation is not a particularly effective method for ethmoidectomy. Still, Ramadan and colleagues[40] showed safety of the procedure and an improvement in symptoms for children undergoing BCS, both by itself and with concurrent adenoidectomy. A subsequent prospective

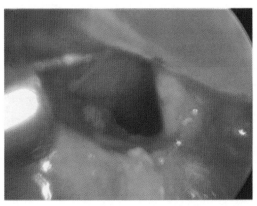

Fig. 4. Dilated maxillary sinus ostium immediately after balloon catheter sinuplasty.

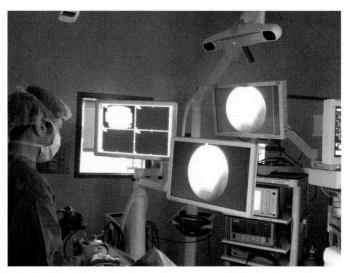

Fig. 5. Endoscopic sinus surgery with use of intraoperative CT image guidance.

review suggested that BCS may be even more effective than adenoidectomy in the treatment of pediatric CRS.[41] In addition, a 2012 review found BCS combined with traditional endoscopic ethmoidectomy comparable to FESS in terms of clinical improvement. The BCS/ethmoidectomy group also required fewer antibiotics postoperatively over 4 months of follow-up.[42] A recent Cochrane review, however, found insufficient evidence to recommend BCS over FESS for the treatment of chronic sinusitis.[43]

Although safe, the potential complications of endoscopic sinus surgery include bleeding, infection, recurrent disease, cerebrospinal fluid leak, and orbital injury, including hematoma and loss of vision. Makary and Ramadan[17] estimated an overall complication rate of 1.4%. In this study, no cases of cerebrospinal fluid leak or major orbital injury such as hematoma or blindness were reported, supporting the relative safety of FESS. Further reducing the risk of complications, the intraoperative use of CT image guidance has quickly become a routine part of endoscopic sinus surgery, and may also facilitate more complete removal of diseased tissue (**Fig. 5**).

SUMMARY

CRS in children is a multifactorial disease, and the evidence seems to support combined approaches to treatment, including medical and, when necessary, surgical options (**Table 3**). As the pathogenesis becomes clearer through ongoing basic

Table 3
Evidence-based treatment in CRS

Medical	Surgical
Watchful waiting	Adenoidectomy
Nasal saline spray/irrigation	Limited FESS
Topical nasal steroids	Balloon catheter sinuplasty
Antibiotics	

science research, the ability to treat CRS effectively and safely in children should continue to improve. The potential roles of protective sinonasal flora and biofilm formation are important areas for further investigation, as are the possible benefits of topical antimicrobial therapy. Regardless of future developments, careful history, physical examination, and workup will remain vital in the diagnosis and management of this disease, as will close communication and cooperation between pediatricians and their colleagues in pediatric allergy and immunology, pediatric pulmonary medicine, and otolaryngology.

REFERENCES

1. Anand VK. Epidemiology and economic impact of rhinosinusitis. Ann Otol Rhinol Laryngol Suppl 2004;193:3–5.
2. Lusk R. Pediatric chronic rhinosinusitis. Curr Opin Otolaryngol Head Neck Surg 2006;14:393–6.
3. Benninger MS, Ferguson BJ, Hadley JA, et al. Adult chronic rhinosinusitis: definitions, diagnosis, epidemiology, and pathophysiology. Otolaryngol Head Neck Surg 2003;129(Suppl 3):S1–32.
4. Woodworth BA, Ahn C, Flume PA, et al. The delta F508 mutation in cystic fibrosis and impact on sinus development. Am J Rhinol 2007;21(1):122–7.
5. Abreu NA, Nagalingam NA, Song Y, et al. Sinus microbiome diversity depletion and Cornybactrium tuberculostearicum enrichment mediates rhinosinusitis. Sci Transl Med 2012;4(151):151ra124.
6. Phipps CD, Wood E, Gibson WS, et al. Gastroesophageal reflux contributing to chronic sinus disease in children. Arch Otolaryngol Head Neck Surg 2000;126: 831–6.
7. Bothwell MR, Parsons DS, Talbot A, et al. Outcome of reflux therapy on pediatric chronic sinusitis. Otolaryngol Head Neck Surg 1999;121(3):255–62.
8. Comstock RH, Lam K, Mikula S. Topical antibiotic therapy of chronic rhinosinusitis. Curr Infect Dis Rep 2010;12:88–95.
9. Wang M, Shi P, Chen B, et al. The role of superantigens in chronic rhinosinusitis with nasal polyps. ORL J Otorhinolaryngol Relat Spec 2008;70(2):97–103.
10. Sanclement JA, Webster P, Thomas J, et al. Bacterial biofilms in surgical specimens of patients with chronic rhinosinusitis. Laryngoscope 2005;115(4):578–82.
11. CalÒ L, Passali GC, Galli J, et al. Role of biofilms in chronic inflammatory diseases of the upper airways. Adv Otorhinolaryngol 2011;72:93–6.
12. Leo G, Triulzi F, Incorvaia C. Sinus imaging for diagnosis of chronic rhinosinusitis in children. Curr Allergy Asthma Rep 2012;12(2):136–43.
13. Brenner DJ, Hall EJ. Computed tomography: an increasing source of radiation exposure. N Engl J Med 2007;357:2277–84.
14. Setzen G, Ferguson BJ, Han JK, et al. Clinical consensus statement: appropriate use of computed tomography for paranasal sinus disease. Otolaryngol Head Neck Surg 2012;147(5):808–16.
15. Elwany S, Helmy SA, El-Reweny EM, et al. Endoscopically directed middle meatal cultures vs computed tomography scans in the diagnosis of bacterial sinusitis in intensive care units. J Crit Care 2012;27(3):315.e1–5.
16. Thomas M, Yawn B, Price D, et al. EPOS primary care guidelines: European position paper on the primary care diagnosis and management of rhinosinusitis and nasal polyps 200—a summary. Prim Care Respir J 2008;17(2):79–89.
17. Makary CA, Ramadan HH. The role of sinus surgery in children. Laryngoscope 2013. [Epub ahead of print].

18. Sobol SE, Samadi DS, Kazahaya K, et al. Trends in the management of pediatric chronic sinusitis: survey of the American Society of Pediatric Otolaryngology. Laryngoscope 2005;115:78–80.

19. Shaikh N, Wald ER, Pi M. Decongestants, antihistamines and nasal irrigation for acute sinusitis in children. Cochrane Database Syst Rev 2012;(9):CD007909.

20. Wei JL, Sykes KJ, Johnson P, et al. Safety and efficacy of once-daily nasal irrigation for the treatment of pediatric chronic rhinosinusitis. Laryngoscope 2011; 121(9):1989–2000.

21. Khianey R, Oppenheimer J. Is nasal saline irrigation all it is cracked up to be? Ann Allergy Asthma Immunol 2012;109(1):20–8.

22. Zalmanovici A, Yaphe J. Intranasal steroids for acute sinusitis. Cochrane Database Syst Rev 2009;(4):CD005149.

23. Venekamp RP, Thompson MJ, Hayward G, et al. Systemic corticosteroids for acute sinusitis. Cochrane Database Syst Rev 2011;(12):CD008115.

24. Skoner D. Update of growth effects of inhaled and intranasal corticosteroids. Curr Opin Allergy Clin Immunol 2003;26(12):863–93.

25. Dijkstra MD, Ebbens FA, Poublon RM, et al. Fluticasone propionate aqueous nasal spray does not influence the recurrence rate of chronic rhinosinusitis and nasal polyps 1 year after functional endoscopic sinus surgery. Clin Exp Allergy 2004;34(9):1395–400.

26. Aukema AA, Mulder PG, Fokkens WJ. Treatment of nasal polyposis and chronic rhinosinusitis with fluticasone propionate nasal drops reduces need for sinus surgery. J Allergy Clin Immunol 2005;115(5):1017–23.

27. Chow AW, Benninger MS, Brook I, et al. IDSA clinical practice guideline for acute bacterial rhinosinusitis in children and adults. Clin Infect Dis 2012;54(8): e72–112.

28. Fokkens WJ, Lund VJ, Mullol J, et al. European position paper on rhinosinusitis and nasal polyps 2012. Rhinology 2012;50:225–6.

29. Adelson RT, Adappa ND. What is the proper role of oral antibiotics in the treatment of patients with chronic sinusitis? Curr Opin Otolaryngol Head Neck Surg 2013;21(1):61–8.

30. Scheinberg PA, Otsuji A. Nebulized antibiotics for the treatment of acute exacerbations of chronic rhinosinusitis. Ear Nose Throat J 2002;81:648–52.

31. Vaughan WC, Carvalho G. Use of nebulized antibiotics for acute infections in chronic sinusitis. Otolaryngol Head Neck Surg 2002;127:558–68.

32. Uren B, Psaltis A, Wormald PJ. Nasal lavage with mupirocin for the treatment of surgically recalcitrant chronic rhinosinusitis. Laryngoscope 2008;118: 1677–80.

33. Tatar EC, Tatar I, Ocal B, et al. Prevalence of biofilms and their response to medical treatment in chronic rhinosinusitis without polyps. Otolaryngol Head Neck Surg 2012;146(4):669–75.

34. Coticchia J, Zuliani G, Coleman C, et al. Biofilm surface area in the pediatric nasopharynx: chronic rhinosinusitis vs obstructive sleep apnea. Arch Otolaryngol Head Neck Surg 2007;133(2):110–4.

35. Brietzke SE, Brigger MT. Adenoidectomy outcomes in pediatric rhinosinusitis: a meta-analysis. Int J Pediatr Otorhinolaryngol 2008;72(10):1541–5.

36. Ramadan HH. Surgical management of chronic sinusitis in children. Laryngoscope 2004;114(12):2103–9.

37. Siedek V, Stelter K, Betz CS, et al. Functional endoscopic sinus surgery – a retrospective analysis of 115 children and adolescents with chronic rhinosinusitis. Int J Pediatr Otorhinolaryngol 2009;73:741–5.

38. Smith TL, Kern R, Palmer JN, et al. Medical therapy vs surgery for chronic rhinosinusitis: a prospective, multi-institutional study with 1-year follow-up. Int Forum Allergy Rhinol 2013;3(1):4–9.

39. Lusk RP, Bothwell MR, Piccirillo J. Long-term follow-up for children treated with surgical intervention for chronic rhinosinusitis. Laryngoscope 2006;116: 2099–107.

40. Ramadan HH, McLaughlin K, Josephson G, et al. Balloon catheter sinuplasty in young children. Am J Rhinol Allergy 2010;24:e54–6.

41. Ramadan HH, Terrell AM. Balloon catheter sinuplasty and adenoidectomy in children with chronic rhinosinusitis. Ann Otol Rhinol Laryngol 2010;119(9): 578–82.

42. Thottam PJ, Haupert M, Saraiya S, et al. Functional endoscopic sinus surgery (FESS) alone versus balloon catheter sinuplasty (BCS) and ethmoidectomy: a comparative outcome analysis in pediatric chronic rhinosinusitis. Int J Pediatr Otorhinolaryngol 2012;76:1355–60.

43. Ahmed J, Pal S, Hopkins C, et al. Functional endoscopic balloon dilation of sinus ostia for chronic rhinosinusitis. Cochrane Database Syst Rev 2011;(7):CD008515.

Training: Simulating Pediatric Airway

Oren Cavel, MD[a],*, Chantal Giguere, MD[a],
Annie Lapointe, MD, MPH[a], Arielle Levy, MD, MEd[b],
Francoise Yung, MD[c], Chantal Hickey, MD[c],
Patrick Froehlich, MD, PhD[a]

KEYWORDS

- Simulation • Pediatric airway • Bronchoscopy • Education • Team work

KEY POINTS

- Simulation is a powerful educational mean already integrated into the curriculum of pediatric, emergency medicine, and anesthesiology programs. The recognition of its value in ENT programs is rising.
- The use of a high-fidelity baby mannequin provides real-time measurable respiratory and cardiovascular responses to the trainee's actions, as well as airway anatomic resemblance sufficient for endoscopy.
- A joint ENT-anesthesiology team can use laryngo-bronchoscopy equipment and a ventilator to create an OR environment and practice the management of genuine cases in the SimLab.
- Simulation scripts can be adapted to match the level of the trainee: from a junior resident learning the basic psychomotor skills, to an ENT specialist desiring to maintain his or her competence in handling complex pediatric airway cases.
- The more SimLabs are created within hospitals, the more medical teams will be encouraged to participate in simulation-based training and further develop it.

 Video of simulated pediatric airway performance accompanies this article at http://www.pediatric.theclinics.com/

[a] Sainte-Justine Pediatric Airway Simulation Group, Department of Otorhinolaryngology, Sainte-Justine Mother and Child University Hospital, University of Montreal, 3175 Cote Sainte-Catherine, Montreal, Quebec H3T 1C5, Canada; [b] Sainte-Justine Pediatric Airway Simulation Group, Department of Emergency Medicine, Sainte-Justine Mother and Child University Hospital, University of Montreal, 3175 Cote Sainte-Catherine, Montreal, Quebec H3T 1C5, Canada; [c] Sainte-Justine Pediatric Airway Simulation Group, Department of Anesthesia, Sainte-Justine Mother and Child University Hospital, University of Montreal, 3175 Cote Sainte-Catherine, Montreal, Quebec H3T 1C5, Canada
* Corresponding author. Department of Otorhinolaryngology, CHU Sainte Justine, 3175 Cote Sainte-Catherine, Montreal, Quebec H3T 1C5, Canada.
E-mail address: orencavel@gmail.com

Pediatr Clin N Am 60 (2013) 993–1003
http://dx.doi.org/10.1016/j.pcl.2013.04.002
pediatric.theclinics.com

INTRODUCTION

The successful management of a pediatric airway case in the operating room (OR) relies on many qualities of intervening team members. The ear, nose, and throat (ENT) specialist should have medical knowledge and the ability to grasp the clinical picture, psychomotor dexterity for the manipulation of the instruments, and familiarity with the assembly of the equipment, as well as teamworking and leadership aptitudes. The anesthesiologist has to deal with a nonsecured and often problematic airway that is being manipulated. The nurse can be required to quickly assemble and provide composite instruments. Acquiring that expertise during residency has so far been limited by the paucity and irregularity of cases, as well as by the fragility of the child's airway, forcing the senior ENT to take over when ventilation is compromised. Similarly, maintaining competence is not always trivial for specialists who work predominantly in the adult milieu, and have to deal with pediatric emergencies occasionally. Hence, the need for an alternative teaching and practicing method is obvious.

Simulation first appeared in the 1920s in aeronautics and quickly became an essential part of learning to fly. In medicine, where the life of some also depends on the ability of others and in situ practice bares risks, the first simulation mannequin, named Resusci Annie,[1] was introduced in the 1960s. Emergency medicine, and later anesthesiology, greatly adopted and developed the mannequin, integrating it into the curriculum of pregraduate and postgraduate years. These disciplines also led the way in research, including an ongoing effort to validate the benefits of simulation and develop sophisticated teaching methods, as well as regularly publishing comprehensive case scenarios in the leading literature.[2] In recent years, the importance of simulation in medical education is being recognized by many additional specialties as providing interactive and safe training conditions, and a variety of dedicated mannequins and accessories have become available.

SIMULATION IN PEDIATRIC ENT

Some ENT centers have joined the progress, focusing mainly on the teaching of anatomy and surgical technique with the use of simulators for temporal bone dissection, flexible bronchoscopy, and endoscopic sinus surgery.[3] In some centers, simulation mannequins were used to teach crisis resource management,[4] generating great enthusiasm among the trained residents. Still, the adhesion rate has only lately started to rise in ENT, as the spread of simulation-based education depends on, among other things, the availability of simulation laboratories. In particular, pure pediatric simulation centers are rare, and pediatric training is generally done in university or adult hospital-affiliated facilities.

The difficulties in teaching pediatric airway endoscopy, which involves high-risk and often low-frequency cases, have brought up the necessity of using an artificial environment to practice technique and case management.

The Simulation Laboratory (SimLab)

The practice of bronchoscopy and esophagoscopy and exercising foreign body (FB) retrieval was initially described by Deutsch and colleagues[5] in 2007, on a high-fidelity, computerized baby mannequin, originally designed for training of emergency medicine cases. As the mannequin's realistic anatomy allowed the performance of endoscopy, it has started assuming a new promising role in ENT training. Studies evaluating this tool have since started to appear, showing improved performance after training[6] and a contribution to ENT residents' confidence when facing situations originally encountered in simulation.[7]

Practice in the SimLab typically involves a homogeneous group of teachers and trainees. Therefore, when simulating a case, an ENT resident or a simulation assistant is usually playing the role of the other team members, as the anesthetist, the emergency physician, or the nurse, which limits the credibility of the resulting situations.

In Situ Simulation in the Operating Room

That difficulty was bypassed by Volk and colleagues,[4] who developed an in situ medical course taking place in the actual OR and the intensive care unit (ICU) and involving ENTs, anesthesiologists, and nurses practicing crisis management with a SimMan (Laerdal Medical, Stavanger, Norway) high-fidelity mannequin. The ensuing improved realism and team dynamics brought about an instructive experience for the trainees and exposed systemic problems within the hospital environment itself.

Reproducing the OR in the SimLab

It is possible to use the same principle of multidisciplinary team training, but this time to practice pediatric airway endoscopy and airway management on a high-fidelity baby mannequin. Hence, by exporting both OR settings and team to the SimLab, authentic OR scenarios can be executed.

In this article, we describe the technical process of setting up the pediatric airway simulation, demonstrating application of an OR scenario in the laboratory, and discussing the immediate and potential benefits, as well as the limitations of such a simulation.

STEPS IN CREATING PEDIATRIC AIRWAY SIMULATION

Establishing the appropriate environment for training in settings that resemble those of an airway case performed in the OR requires the following:

- Using a SimLab
- Gathering the equipment
- Assembling the team
- Defining the learning objectives and case scenarios

The SimLab is ideally located within the pediatric hospital, easily accessible to both residents and staff from the different disciplines, whose schedule is by definition very busy. Alternatively, an adult simulation center can be used if adapted with proper equipment, namely a high-fidelity baby mannequin (Video 1).

The high-fidelity baby mannequin has the size and shape of a 10-month old baby. It is connected to a monitor and possesses basic anatomic as well as computer-controlled dynamic features, allowing the trainee to perform a physical examination and observe an immediate response to certain therapeutic maneuvers. These include a chest wall that moves according to unilateral/bilateral breathing, audible breath sounds, cardiac and vocal sounds, palpable pulses, venous access, and measurable parameters, such as O_2 saturation, CO_2, blood pressure, and so on. Airway wise, it has a vallecula, an epiglottis, arytenoids, and the posterior two-thirds of the vocal cords. The larynx can be shifted anteriorly to make the endotracheal intubation very difficult, and the cords can adduct to mimic a laryngospasm. Below the vocal cords, the trachea presents with a narrower ring in its proximal part that can be considered to be a grade 1 subglottic stenosis, a carina distally leading to the 2 main stem bronchi and their first subdivisions. Far from being perfect, the mannequin's anatomy sufficiently resembles human anatomy to allow the user to recognize the anatomic location of the area he or she is manipulating.

Team

Both an ENT and anesthesiologist attending devoted to simulation-based teaching are essential for multidisciplinary credible training. Preferably, a third physician, who masters the training software can be the simulation manager, responding "on the fly" to critical actions by participants in the scenario's branching points (**Table 1**).

Objective-Based Script

The objectives set for each session should encompass both medical knowledge and team-working skills, and represent the basis for designing the script. The script is built on a predesigned sequence of events that can be modified according to the participants' actions in predefined branching points (named "critical actions"). As much as all the parameters, including cardiac and respiratory rates, O2 saturation, expired CO2 levels, blood pressure, sound effects, vocal cord and larynx position, lung ventilation, and others are defined ahead for every step in the scenario, programing the software and executing the script become easier. In addition, variations to each script can be made according to the participant who is defined as the trainee during the session (**Tables 2–4**).

The Debriefing

Following the execution of the script, the debriefing is an essential part of the training. It can be partially planned in advance, using prepared questions to facilitate the outlining of key teaching points. The rest of it should include factual feedback, focused on performance rather than individuals, with an effort to solicit the trainee's perception of how he or she did and make them reflect about the process they went through when in action.

EXAMPLE OF RUNNING A SCRIPT

The creation of OR setting in the simulation center makes it possible to practice actual surgical cases inspired from common practice, and the clinical experience of the anesthesiologists and the ENTs.

Table 1
Example of team participation in a simulation session

Team Member	Role
Participants	
ENT resident/fellow	Trainee/figure
ENT attending	Active or passive figure
Anesthesia resident/fellow	Trainee/figure
Respiratory technician	Figure
Surgical nurse	Figure
Behind the scene	
Pediatric anesthesia attending	Simulation medical manager
Pediatric emergency medicine staff physician, at the software control	Scenario programing, "on-the-fly" response according to updates provided by the simulation manager
SimLab technician	Equipment and camera setting, possibly software programming

Abbreviation: ENT, ear, nose, and throat.

Table 2
Example of running a script. Presented case: "David, a 5-month-old boy who was extubated 8 days ago after have being intubated for 5 days for acute bronchiolitis. Since discharge from the intensive care unit a week ago, the patient developed progressive dyspnea and stridor at rest. We are suspecting laryngeal or tracheal stenosis, and are about to perform a rigid endoscopic examination to evaluate the airway. After a mask induction, an intravenous (IV) line has been placed and used exclusively to deliver the anesthesia (total IV anesthesia [TIVA]); the patient is spontaneously breathing."

Script Execution	Monitor
ENT resident performs a direct laryngoscopy, sprays the vocal cords with xylocaine, and hands back the patient to the anesthesia team, which bags him. ENT resident checks with nurse that the telescope and camera are ready, performs a laryngoscopy, and installs the laryngeal suspension.	Sinus rhythm, 120/min SpO2 98% Temperature = 36.5°C Insp O2 99%, ET O2 = 85% Insp Ag 5.5%, ET Ag 2.6%
ENT resident introduces the telescope, identifies the subglottic stenosis, and finds it difficult to pass to the trachea. ENT attending suggests release of tension from suspension, ENT resident manipulates the suspension and manages to pass with the telescope.	ET O2 45% Insp Ag 0, ET Ag 0
Telescope advancing along the trachea, up to the carina. Patient coughs, ENT attending advices the to "stay central, don't touch the walls." Anesthesiologist asks to pause the examination to deepen the IV anesthesia.	↓SpO2 85% ↓SpO2 80% Vocal sound: cough
ENT resident removes the telescope, leaves the laryngoscope in place and hands the patient back to the anesthesiologist. Anesthesiologist injects propofol, waits for the saturation to climb and hands back the patient.	↑SpO2 85% ↑SpO2 98%
ENT resident inserts the telescope, tries to demonstrate the main bronchi. Anesthesiologist warns the ENT resident that the patient is apneic and desaturates.	Respiratory rate 0 ↓Spo2 75% ↓Heart rate 100/min
ENT resident asks for an endotracheal tube size 3.5 with a stylet, but fails to intubate the patient through the laryngoscope because of excessive edema. ENT resident asks for a rigid bronchoscope, but discovers none was prepared. ENT resident asks for an endotracheal tube size 2.5 with a stylet, and manages to intubate.	Close vocal cords ↓SpO2 50% ↓Heart rate 70/min
Anesthesiologist auscultates, finds no air entry on the left.	↑SpO2 86% ↑Heart rate 125/min CO2 curve, CO2 60 Selective right lung ventilation
ENT resident pulls back on the tube. Auscultation correct.	↑SpO2 99%

Abbreviations: Ag, inhaled anesthetic agent; ENT, ear, nose, and throat; ET, end tidal; Insp, inspired; SpO2, oxygen saturation.

Table 3
Script: ENT as the trainee

Objectives:
1. Medical: understand the aim of the procedure, recognize the subglottic finding, appropriate choice of instruments, and technical skills in their use.
2. Teamwork: continuous communication with the anesthesiologist, takes the lead for securing the airway.

Programming of the Baby Mannequin	Script: Expected Actions	Consequences of Failure to Perform Expected Action (Branching Points)
Sinus rhythm, 120/min SpO2 = 98% Temperature = 36.5°C Insp O2 99%, ET O2 85% Insp Ag 5.5%, ET Ag 2.6%	Preendoscopy Applies local anesthesia to vocal cords	Cough, at beginning of laryngoscopy. If still does not apply xylocaine, laryngospasm and desaturation
	Performs equipment check	Camera control unit powered off, takes time to connect, anesthesiologist complaining "the patient is waiting"

SpO 98% - T 36.0°C
O2 99% O2 45%
Ag = 0
	Endoscopy – a
	  Identifies the subglottic stenosis
	  Adjusts suspension to navigate along trachea
		Mention at the debriefing: lack of expertise
		Remark from ENT staff: release tension from suspension

↓SpO2 85%
↓SpO2 80%
Vocal sound: cough
	Endoscopy – b
	  Continues endoscopic examination in an attempt to demonstrate the carina and the beginning of the main bronchi
	  Communicates with the anesthesiologist when the patient coughs
	  Obeys immediately to anesthesiologist request to pause the endoscopy for deepening the anesthesia
		If stops after identification of the subglottic stenosis, remark from EA: you are supposed to show the beginning of the 2 bronchi
		Mention at the debriefing
		
		Desaturation, bronchospasm

↑SpO2 85% ↑SpO2 98%	Pause in endoscopy	
Respiratory rate 0 ↓SpO2 75% ↓Heart rate 100/min	Second endoscopy Notices that the saturation is decreasing and proceeds to intubation or proposes to the anesthesiologist to bag him	Rapid desaturation, warning by anesthesiologist and demand to intubate the patient

(continued on next page)

Table 3 *(continued)*		
Programming of the Baby Mannequin	**Script: Expected Actions**	**Consequences of Failure to Perform Expected Action (Branching Points)**

Close vocal cords
↓SpO2 50%
↓Heart rate 70/min
Vocal cord opening
	Intubation
	  Leaves the suspension in place while tries to intubate
	  Uses a small endotracheal tube with a stylet
	  If does not manage to intubate, asks the anesthesiologist to take the lead, calls for help (remark from ENT attending: "try again with a 2.5 with a stylet, do not accept the switch to bag ventilation")
		Unable to visualize the larynx, anterior movement of the larynx
		Bradycardia

↑SpO2 86% ↑Heart rate 125/min CO2 curve, CO2 55 ↑SpO2 99%	After intubation Confirms tube localization with the anesthesiologist	Selective right lung ventilation

Abbreviations: Ag, inhaled anesthetic agent; ENT, ear, nose, and throat; ET, end tidal; Insp, inspired; SpO2, oxygen saturation.

In the example provided in this article, an 8-min script was run, filmed (see Video 1), and analyzed. A fellow in pediatric ENT and a fellow in pediatric anesthesia, both familiar with the script, were asked to perform as junior residents, with the ENT "resident" defined as the primary trainee. The rest of the active participants were the ENT attending assuming her genuine role, as well as the role of the OR nurse, and an respiratory technician (RT). The anesthesia attending was supervising the sequence of events, and communicated via a microphonic headset with the emergency physician, behind the 1-way mirror, who was running the software for on-the-fly adjustments at the branching points.

The case presented in the script was that of a baby with postextubation dyspnea, in which the ENT resident was asked to perform a bronchoscopy to rule out a stenosis. During the procedure, the correct level of anesthesia was difficult to maintain, so that the endoscopy had to be interrupted and later completely stopped to secure the airway. The anesthesiologist warned the ENT when the ventilation was inadequate, and the ENT assumed the leading role in intubating the patient.

The resulting session (see **Table 2**) ended with a debriefing, in which the ENT resident had a chance to watch his recorded performance, identify his own mistakes, and discuss key points with the ENT attending, the anesthesiologist, and the rest of the team.

By applying a few changes to the script, the resident in anesthesia can be considered as the principal trainee (see **Table 4**), and practice a genuine interaction with the surgeon during actual manipulations of the mannequin's airway.

LEARNING OBJECTIVES

So far, the interface of pediatric ENT with simulation involved mainly dealing with emergency room situations, or practicing the technical aspects of bronchoscopy.

Table 4
Script: anesthesiologist as the trainee

Objectives:
1. Medical: understand the aim of the procedure performed by the ENT, understand the limits of spontaneous ventilation versus apnea.
2. Teamwork: continuous communication with the ENT, urges to take appropriate measures to secure the airway, takes over the lead if the ENT does not assume the role of leader

Programming of the Baby Mannequin	Script: Expected Actions	Consequences of Failure to Perform Expected Action (Branching Points)
Sinus rhythm, 120/min SpO2 = 98% Temperature = 36.5°C Insp O2 99%, ET O2 85% Insp Ag 5.5%, ET Ag 2.6%	Pre endoscopy 　Applies local anesthesia to vocal cords or asks the ENT to do so	Cough, at beginning of laryngoscopy. If still doesn't apply xylocaine, laryngospasm and desaturation
	Verifies that ENT is ready before handing him the patient	Camera control unit powered off, takes time to connect, patient not oxygenated for a long time
ET O2 45% Insp Ag 0, ET Ag 0	Beginning of endoscopy	
↓SpO2 85% ↓SpO2 80% Vocal sound: cough	Endoscopy (near the carina) 　Reminds the ENT that the trachea is not anesthetized, communicates with ENT when the patient coughs	Increase coughing, mention at the debriefing
	Request the ENT to pause the endoscopy for deepening the anesthesia	Desaturation, bronchospasm
↑SpO2 85% ↑SpO2 98%	Pause in endoscopy 　Injects propofol 　Can ask ENT to remove the laryngoscope to bag the patient	
	Waits until saturation is 98% before allowing endoscopy to be resumed	Rapid desaturation
Respiratory rate 0 ↓SpO2 75% ↓Heart rate 100/min	Second endoscopy 　Notices desaturation and apnea 　Urges ENT to intubate or proposes to bag the patient	In any case, rapid desaturation and bradycardia

(continued on next page)

Table 4 (continued)		
Programming of the Baby Mannequin	Script: Expected Actions	Consequences of Failure to Perform Expected Action (Branching Points)
Close vocal cords ↓SpO2 50% ↓Heart rate 70/min	Intubation If ENT does not manage to intubate, the trainee is expected to try bag ventilation, then try to intubate	Unable to visualize the larynx, anterior movement of the larynx
	Calls for help	Respiratory technician offers to call for help
	Communicates with ENT, suggests to have tracheotomy set ready (remark by simulation medical manager: "all is ready, but try again to intubate")	
↑SpO2 86% ↑Heart rate 125/min CO2 curve, CO2 55 ↑SpO2 99%	After intubation Confirms tube localization	Selective right lung ventilation, saturation not rising

Abbreviations: Ag, inhaled anesthetic agent; ET, end tidal; Insp, inspired; SpO2, oxygen saturation.

Using a high-fidelity baby mannequin and reproducing the OR settings in the laboratory, we are now getting to the core of airway simulation. The logistic effort might be heavier, particularly regarding the gathering of a multidisciplinary team and the equipment's cost, but still, the teaching content's possible sophistication is worth the effort.

With OR simulation, it is possible today for a multidisciplinary team to practice performing a realistic scenario of pediatric airway management. This represents a learning experience that is as close as possible so far to reality, while still enjoying the benefits of a safe and reproducible environment. On a technical level, the ENT resident, who was the principal trainee in the aforementioned scenario, had to select and prepare the equipment, perform a tracheo-bronchoscopy with laryngeal suspension, identify the subglottic stenosis, respond to tracheal reactivity, and perform a difficult intubation. In other scripts, the technical features could vary and encompass other airway challenges. At the same time, the resident had to understand the procedure, complete the examination despite the difficulties in maintaining an adequate anesthesia, respond to constraints offered by a real anesthesiologist, communicate and coordinate his actions with the rest of the team, and take the lead when necessary. The debriefing conducted at the end of the session reviewed the critical parts of the session and focused on the stages that proved to be problematic for the trainee who was put under pressure.

The learning objectives and accordingly the simulation session's configuration can progress from basic to advanced levels, to fit the needs of any trainee from junior residents[7] to fellows[6] or even specialists. Schematically:

1. Basic level
   - Objectives: learning manual gestures, familiarity with the equipment.
   - Means: introduction to the endoscopy cart, assembling the equipment, practicing laryngoscopy on various airway mannequins.

2. Intermediate level
   - Objectives: medical knowledge (anatomy, pathologies), correct choice of equipment.
   - Means: flexible bronchoscopy simulator, practicing tracheal and esophageal rigid endoscopy on high-fidelity mannequins, retrieval of bronchial FBs, execution of simple scripts by a team composed solely of ENT residents.
3. Advanced level
   - Objectives: case management, teamwork.
   - Means: execution of OR complex scripts by a multidisciplinary team on a high-fidelity mannequin.

To allow the trainee to fully benefit from the simulation-based lessons, the amount of new knowledge the trainee has to assimilate in each practice should be limited. For example, the advantages of teaching bronchoscopy by deconstructing it into sub-tasks were shown by Jabbour and colleagues,[6] who created a half-day simulation course composed of 4 independent teaching modules, including pulmonary anatomy, performance of laryngoscopy, performance of rigid bronchoscopy, and retrieval of an airway FB.

When the focus is to teach clinical reasoning and team leadership by practicing a scenario in an OR setting, this can only be done with trainees who already master the basic and intermediate simulation knowledge.

Competence Maintaining for ENT Specialists

Many ENT specialists who are not routinely performing bronchoscopies end up finding themselves uncomfortable with the procedure as well as its associated risks, and need to be backed up during their duties. Simulation-based OR-like sessions could serve as a means to refresh the memory and practice the required abilities. The scenario's theme and degree of difficulty can be set accordingly to correspond to emergency cases.

Simulation bares 2 additional interests. The first is the ability to assess the technical and clinical skills of an examinee in a standardized setting.[8] The second is the opportunity to test new equipment and practice its handling.

The Downsides of Simulation

The downsides of simulation are few. First, the investment in time and money, especially in the beginning of a development of a simulation program, is considerable. Second, the degree of resemblance of the mannequin's airway to that of a human, both in appearance and in feeling during its manipulation, is limited. Last, residents' self-confidence could be altered when practicing in an artificially stressful situation and facing the team's criticism; a proper debriefing session is essential for that reason.

FUTURE CHALLENGES

There are numerous ways to implement simulation in its various forms in medical education,[9] and the validation of its value in ENT training is an ongoing process taking place in a number of universities, whose relevant publications have started to appear and are likely to do so in the next years. Since the benefits seem obvious and the risk nil, an example should be taken either from the industry[1] or other medical disciplines that embraced it without waiting for the unequivocal proof.

Two factors will further determine the rate of adhesion to simulation programs. One is the creation of simulation laboratories within medical centers that are regularly dealing with pediatric airway, and whose teams will most benefit from training. The second is the ability of the medical community and the manufacturers to collaborate in the development of a mannequin that has both a more authentic anatomy designed specifically for bronchoscopies and a set of laryngeal pathologies whose treatment could be practiced. The incorporation of computerized virtual reality will probably enhance the experience.

SUPPLEMENTARY DATA

Supplementary data related to this article can be found at http://dx.doi.org/10.1016/j.pcl.2013.04.002.

REFERENCES

1. Rosen KR. The history of medical simulation. J Crit Care 2008;23(2):157–66.
2. Sampathi V, Lerman J. Case scenario: perioperative latex allergy in children. Anesthesiology 2011;114(3):673–80.
3. Abou-Elhamd KE, Al-Sultan AI, Rashad UM. Simulation in ENT medical education. J Laryngol Otol 2010;124(3):237–41.
4. Volk MS, Ward J, Irias N, et al. Using medical simulation to teach crisis resource management and decision-making skills to otolaryngology housestaff. Otolaryngol Head Neck Surg 2011;145(1):35–42.
5. Deutsch ES, Dixit D, Curry J, et al. Management of aerodigestive tract foreign bodies: innovative teaching concepts. Ann Otol Rhinol Laryngol 2007;116(5):319–23.
6. Jabbour N, Reihsen T, Sweet RM, et al. Psychomotor skills training in pediatric airway endoscopy simulation. Otolaryngol Head Neck Surg 2011;145(1):43–50.
7. Malekzadeh S, Malloy KM, Chu EE, et al. ORL emergencies boot camp: using simulation to onboard residents. Laryngoscope 2011;121(10):2114–21.
8. Jabbour N, Sidman J. Assessing instrument handling and operative consequences simultaneously: a simple method for creating synced multicamera videos for endosurgical or microsurgical skills assessments. Simul Healthc 2011;6(5):299–303.
9. Deutsch ES. Simulation in otolaryngology: smart dummies and more. Otolaryngol Head Neck Surg 2011;145(6):899–903.

Index

Note: Page numbers of article titles are in **boldface** type.

A

Academic performance
    after cochlear implantation, 852–853
    in obstructive sleep apnea, 828–829
Adenotonsillectomy, **793–807**
    anatomy of, 794
    complications of, 802–804
    for chronic rhinosinusitis, 986
    for obstructive sleep apnea, 832–833
    immunology of, 794–795
    indications for, 795–799
    morbidity in, 833
    polysomnography before, 798–801
    sleep-disordered breathing and, 798–801
    statistics on, 793
    techniques for, 801–802
Airway simulation, **993–1003**
    creation of, 995–996
    downsides of, 1002
    for maintaining competence, 1002
    future challenges in, 1002–1003
    history of, 994
    learning objectives of, 999, 1001–1002
    script for, 996–1000
    simulation laboratory for, 994–995
Allergy testing, for chronic rhinosinusitis, 983
Amoxicillin/clavulanate, for chronic rhinosinusitis, 985–986
Anatomic theory, of laryngomalacia, 896–897
Anesthesiology, simulation training for, **993–1003**
Angel's kisses (hemangiomas), **937–949**
Angiogenesis, aberrant, infantile hemangiomas in, 938–939
Antibiotics
    for chronic rhinosinusitis, 985–986
    for otitis media, 817–818
Antihistamines, for chronic rhinosinusitis, 985
Apert syndrome, otitis media in, 815
Apnea
    obstructive. *See* Obstructive sleep apnea.
    sleep-disordered breathing and, 800–801
Apnea-hypopnea index, in obstructive sleep apnea, 830
Apoptosis, defects of, infantile hemangiomas in, 939
Arnold nerve stimulation, cough in, 955–956

Aryepiglottoplasty, for laryngomalacia, 898–899
Aspiration, in laryngopharyngeal reflux, 867–868
Asthma
    cough in, 955
    in laryngopharyngeal reflux, 870
Atlantoaxial subluxation, after adenotonsillectomy, 804
Audiometric evaluation, for otitis media, 817
Auditory neuropathy spectrum disorder, 842–843

B

Baby mannequin, for airway simulation training, **993–1003**
Bacterial cultures, for chronic rhinosinusitis, 983–984
Balloon catheter sinuplasty, 987–988
Barium swallow, for dysphagia, 973
Bedside swallow examination, for dysphagia, 973–974
Behavioral problems, in obstructive sleep apnea, 828–829
Beta-adrenergic receptor pathway, defects of, infantile hemangiomas in, 939
Biofilms, in chronic rhinosinusitis, 981–982, 986
Biopsy
    for cervical lymphadenopathy, 934
    for chronic rhinosinusitis, 984
Birth trauma, nasal obstruction in, 917
Bordetella pertussis infections, cough in, 954
Breast-feeding, otitis media and, 816
Brodsky grading scale, 795
Bronchitis, cough in, 954
Bronchoscopy
    for chronic cough, 958–959
    for laryngomalacia, 896
    simulation training for, **993–1003**

C

Cancer, cervical lymphadenopathy in, 925
Cardiovascular morbidity, in obstructive sleep apnea, 830
Cartilaginous theory, of laryngomalacia, 897
Cat scratch disease, cervical lymphadenopathy in, 924
Catheters
    balloon, for sinuplasty, 987–988
    nasal, for obstruction evaluation, 905
Cerebral palsy, dysphagia in, 972
Cerebrospinal fluid leak, after cochlear implantation, 856
Cervical lymphadenopathy, **923–936**
    acute, 928
    biopsy for, 934
    chronic, 928
    definition of, 923
    differential diagnosis of, 930
    etiology of, 924–926
    evaluation of, 927–934

imaging for, 932–934
laboratory tests for, 930–931
location of, 929
management algorithms for, 935
pathophysiology of, 924
quality and quantity of nodes in, 930
symptom associated with, 928
CHARGE syndrome, dysphagia in, 972
Chlamydial infections, nasal obstruction in, 915–917
Choanal atresia, 906–907
Chronic rhinosinusitis, **979–991**
classification of, 979–980
definition of, 980
diagnosis of, 982–984
pathophysiology of, 980–982
symptoms of, 982
treatment of, 984–988
versus acute rhinosinusitis, 979–980
Ciliary dysmotility, otitis media in, 814–815
Coblation, for adenotonsillectomy, 802
Cochlear implantation, **841–863**
background of, 842
bilateral, 857–858
candidates for, 845–846
device components and, 843–844
for partial deafness, 858–859
mechanism of action of, 842–843
medical considerations in, 846–847, 857
outcomes of, 847–854
revision, 855
risks of, 854–857
surgical considerations in, 846–847, 857
technique for, 844–845
Cold dissection technique, for adenotonsillectomy, 801
Computed tomography
for cervical lymphadenopathy, 932–933
for chronic cough, 958
for chronic rhinosinusitis, 982–983
for nasal obstruction, 905
Congenital disorders
dysphagia, **969–977**
hearing loss, cochlear implantation for, **841–863**
infantile hemangiomas, **937–949**
laryngomalacia, **893–902**
laryngopharyngeal reflux, **865–878,** 897
nasal obstruction, **903–922**
Continuous positive airway pressure, for obstructive sleep apnea, 833
Cor pulmonale, in obstructive sleep apnea, 830
Corticosteroids
for chronic rhinosinusitis, 985
for infantile hemangiomas, 943–944

Cough
    chronic, **951–967**
        approach to, 956–960, 962
        cause of, 952–956
        definition of, 952
        dry, 957
        incidence of, 951–952
        nonspecific, 952, 960–964
        postinfectious, 953–954
        specific, 952
        treatment of, 960–964
        wet, 957
    definition of, 952
    in laryngomalacia, 894
    in laryngopharyngeal reflux, 871
    normal, 952
Cough syrups, homemade, 962
Craniofacial abnormalities
    nasal obstruction in, 919
    obstructive sleep apnea in, 834–835
    otitis media in, 814–815
C-reactive protein, in obstructive sleep apnea, 830
Cyst(s)
    nasolacrimal duct, 909–910, 912
    vocal, 884–885

    D

Dacryocystitis, 915–917
Dacryocystocele, 910, 912
Deafness, cochlear implantation for, **841–863**
Decongestants
    for chronic rhinosinusitis, 985
    for nasal obstruction, 919
Dermoid, nasal, 911, 913
Drug-induced sleep endoscopy, for obstructive sleep apnea, 834
Dysphagia, **969–977**
    causes of, 970–973
    epidemiology of, 970
    evaluation of, 973–975
    physiology of, 970
    treatment of, 975
Dysphonia. *See* Voice disorders.

    E

Ear
    cochlear implantation in, **841–863**
    infections of. *See* Otitis media.
Edema, after adenotonsillectomy, 803
Electrocautery, for adenotonsillectomy, 801–802

Electrode array, of cochlear implant, 843–844
Electromyography
    laryngeal, 884
    sleep-disordered breathing and, 799–801
Electrooculography, sleep-disordered breathing and, 799–801
Employment benefits, after cochlear implantation, 853
Encephalocele, nasal obstruction in, 911, 914
Encephalography, sleep-disordered breathing and, 799–801
Endoscopy
    airway, simulation training for, **993–1003**
    for chronic rhinosinusitis, 982
    for dysphagia, 973–974
    for laryngopharyngeal reflux, 867–868
    for nasal obstruction evaluation, 905
    for obstructive sleep apnea, 834
Environmental factors
    in chronic rhinosinusitis, 981
    in otitis media, 815–816
Eosinophilic otitis media, 814
Epworth Sleepiness Scale, in obstructive sleep apnea, 828
Esophageal disorders, dysphagia in, 973
Esophagoscopy, simulation training for, **993–1003**
Ethmoidectomy, for chronic rhinosinusitis, 987
Eustachian tube, otitis media and, 810–811, 813–815
Ex utero intrapartum treatment (EXIT) procedure, for nasal obstruction, 915
Exercise, laryngomalacia in, 900
EXIT (ex utero intrapartum treatment) procedure, for nasal obstruction, 915
Exotoxins, in chronic rhinosinusitis, 981
External processor, of cochlear implant, 843–844

F

Facial nerve injury, after cochlear implantation, 856
Facial nerve stimulation, after cochlear implantation, 856
Failure to thrive, in obstructive sleep apnea, 829
Feeding difficulties. *See also* Dysphagia.
    chronic cough in, 957
    in laryngomalacia, 894
Flexible endoscopic evaluation of swallowing, 973–974
Fluticasone, for chronic rhinosinusitis, 985
Foreign body inhalation, cough in, 956
Frontonasal masses, nasal obstruction in, 911
Functional endoscopic sinus surgery, for chronic rhinosinusitis, 986–987
Functional respiratory disorder, cough in, 956
Functional voice disorders, 885
Furstenberg's test, 914

G

Gastroesophageal reflux
    cough in, 954–955

Gastroesophageal (*continued*)
    dysphagia in, 972–973
    extra-esophageal manifestations of. *See* Laryngopharyngeal reflux.
    laryngomalacia and, 897–898
    nasal obstruction in, 918–919
Genetic disorders
    dysphagia in, 972
    otitis media in, 814–815
Gliomas, nasal obstruction from, 911, 914
Glucose transporter 1, in infantile hemangiomas, 939
Gonorrhea, nasal obstruction in, 915–917
Grisel syndrome, 804
Growth failure, in obstructive sleep apnea, 829

H

Hearing
    after cochlear implantation, 847–849
    assessment of, in voice disorders, 882–883
Hearing loss
    causes of, 842–843
    cochlear implantation for, **841–863**
    in otitis media, 817, 820
    incidence of, 842
Heart failure, in obstructive sleep apnea, 830
Hemangiomas, infantile, **937–949**
Hematomas, septal, obstruction from, 917
Hemorrhage, after adenotonsillectomy, 803
Histamine-2 receptor antagonists
    for laryngomalacia, 898
    for laryngopharyngeal reflux, 872
Hoarseness
    in laryngopharyngeal reflux, 870–871
    in vocal nodules, 884–885
    in voice disorders, 882
Holoprosencephaly, nasal obstruction in, 908–909
Honey, for cough, 962
Host factors, in otitis media, 813–815
Humidification
    for cough, 962
    for nasal obstruction, 919
Hypernasal speech, after adenotonsillectomy, 804
Hypertension, in obstructive sleep apnea, 830
Hypopharynx, anatomic abnormalities of, dysphagia in, 972–973
Hypopnea, in obstructive sleep apnea, 830

I

Immune response
    adenoids and tonsils in, 794–795
    cervical lymph nodes in, 924

Immunodeficiency, otitis media in, 813–815
Infantile hemangiomas, **937–949**
    cosmetic and functional significance of, 937–938
    diagnosis of, 939–943
    in PHACES syndrome, 942–943
    indeterminate, 939–940
    locations of, 937, 939–941
    multifocal, 940
    parotid, 943, 947
    pathophysiology of, 938–939
    phases of, 941
    segmental, 939–940
    subglottic, 941–942, 946–947
    superficial, 939
    treatment of, 943–947
Infant-Toddler Meaningful Auditory Integration Scale, 848
Infections
    cervical lymphadenopathy in, 924–925, 928–931
    ear. *See* Otitis media.
    in cochlear implantation, 855–856
    nasal obstruction from, 915–917
    sinusitis. *See* Chronic rhinosinusitis.
    tonsillitis, 796–798
Injections, for vocal fold paralysis, 887
Intubation
    for nasal obstruction, 919
    simulation training for, **993–1003**
    voice disorders in, 886

K

Kartagener syndrome, otitis media in, 814–815
Kawasaki disease, cervical lymphadenopathy in, 926
Kikuchi-Fujimoto disease, cervical lymphadenopathy in, 926

L

Lamina propria, repair of, for voice disorders, 889–890
Language development, after cochlear implantation, 850–852
Laryngomalacia, **893–902**
    anatomic considerations in, 894
    classification of, 896
    clinical presentation of, 894
    dysphagia in, 972–973
    etiology of, 896–897
    in laryngopharyngeal reflux, 868–869
    incidence of, **893**
    late-onset, 899–900
    state-dependent, 899–900
    treatment of, 897–899
    work-up for, 895–896

Laryngopharyngeal reflux, **865–878,** 897
    aspiration with, 867–868
    asthma with, 870
    cough in, 871, 954–955
    definition of, 866
    diagnosis of, 871–873
    hoarseness with, 870–871
    laryngomalacia with, 868–869
    prevalence of, 865–866
    recurrent respiratory papillomatosis with, 869
    subglottic stenosis with, 869
    swallowing impairment with, 867–868
    symptoms of, 866–867
    treatment of, 873–874
    voice disorders in, 884
Laryngoscopy
    for voice disorders, 883–884
    in laryngomalacia, 895–896
Larynx
    anatomy of, 894, 972–973
    development of, 880–881
    disorders of. *See* Voice disorders.
    transplantation of, 889
Laser therapy, for infantile hemangiomas, 946–947
Learning problems, in obstructive sleep apnea, 828–829
Leukemia, cervical lymphadenopathy in, 925
Levodropropizine, for cough, 964
Levofloxacin, for chronic rhinosinusitis, 985–986
Lifestyle modifications
    for laryngomalacia, 897–898
    for laryngopharyngeal reflux, 872
Lipid storage diseases, cervical lymphadenopathy in, 926
Lymphadenopathy, cervical, **923–936**
Lymphomas, cervical lymphadenopathy in, 925

M

Magnetic resonance imaging
    for cervical lymphadenopathy, 932–934
    for infantile hemangiomas, 939
    for nasal obstruction, 905
MGovern nipple, for nasal obstruction, 919
Malignancy, cervical lymphadenopathy in, 925
Mammalian target of rapamycin, in infantile hemangiomas, 939
Manometric testing, for dysphagia, 973
Maxillary expansion, for obstructive sleep apnea, 834
Medialization thyroplasty, for vocal fold paralysis, 887
Meningitis, cochlear implantation and, 847, 856–857
Metastasis, to cervical lymph nodes, 925
Microdebrider technique, for adenotonsillectomy, 802
Moguisteine, for cough, 964

Mometasone, for chronic rhinosinusitis, 985
Myringotomy tube insertion, for otitis media, 816–821

N

Nasal cavity, anatomic abnormalities of, dysphagia in, 972
Nasal obstruction
   dysphagia in, 972
   in newborns, **903–922**
      differential diagnosis of, 905–919
      evaluation of, 903–905
      importance of, **903**
      syndromic associations of, 919
      treatment of, 919
   in obstructive sleep apnea, 833–834
Nasal pyriform aperture stenosis, congenital, 907–909
Nasal septum, deviated, obstruction in, 917
Nasal vestibular stenosis, 917
Nasolacrimal duct cysts, 909–910, 912
Nasopharyngeal stenosis, after adenotonsillectomy, 804
Nasopharynx, anatomic abnormalities of, dysphagia in, 972
Neck, lymphadenopathy of, **923–936**
Neoplasia
   cervical lymphadenopathy in, 925
   infantile hemangiomas, **937–949**
   nasal obstruction from, 915
Neuroblastomas, cervical lymphadenopathy in, 925
Neurologic theory, of laryngomalacia, 897
Neuromuscular disorders, dysphagia in, 972
Newborns, nasal obstruction in, **903–922**
Nissen fundoplication, for laryngopharyngeal reflux, 872
Nodules, vocal, 884–885
Nuclear scintigraphy, for dysphagia, 973

O

Obesity, adenotonsillectomy and, 796
Obstructive sleep apnea, **827–840**
   adenotonsillectomy for, 795
   diagnosis of, 830–832
   morbidity in, 828–830
   persistent, 836–837
   prevalence of, 828
   terminology of, 827–828
   treatment of, 795, 832–835
Oral cavity, anatomic abnormalities of, dysphagia in, 972
Oropharynx, anatomic abnormalities of, dysphagia in, 972
Osteomeatal complex, 980
Otitis media, **809–826**
   acute, clinical manifestations of, 811
   after cochlear implantation, 857

Otitis (*continued*)
  anatomic considerations in, 810–811
  causes of, 812–816
  clinical manifestations of, 811–812
  developmental considerations in, 810–811
  incidence of, 810
  myringotomy tube insertion for, 816–821
  pathogens causing, 815
  practice model for, 819
  rhinosinusitis in, 982
  tympanic membrane retractions in, 812
  with effusion, clinical manifestations of, 811–812
Otogenic causes, of cough, 955–956
Otorrhea, after myringotomy tube insertion, 820–821

P

Pain, after adenotonsillectomy, 803
Palatal surgery, for obstructive sleep apnea, 834
Papillomatosis, recurrent respiratory, 869, 885–886
Paradise criteria, 796–798
Paralysis, vocal fold, 887–889
Parotid hemangiomas, 943, 947
Pediatric Cough Questionnaire, 957
Perilymph gusher, after cochlear implantation, 856
Pertussis, cough in, 954
PHACES syndrome, 942–943
Pierre-Robin sequence, otitis media in, 815
Polysomnography
  for obstructive sleep apnea, 828, 830–832
  sleep-disordered breathing and, 798–801
Postinfectious cough, 953–954
Postnasal drip (upper airway cough syndrome), 955
Premature infants, dysphagia in, 970–971
Propranolol, for infantile hemangiomas, 939, 943–946
Proton pump inhibitors
  for laryngomalacia, 898
  for laryngopharyngeal reflux, 871–872
Psychological factors, in voice disorders, 885
Puberphonia, 885
Pulsed dye laser therapy, for infantile hemangiomas, 946

Q

Quality of life, after cochlear implantation, 853

R

Radiofrequency technique, for adenotonsillectomy, 802
Radiography, for chronic cough, 958
Receiver-stimulator, of cochlear implant, 844–844

Recurrent respiratory papillomatosis, 869, 885–886

Reflux

gastroesophageal. *See* Gastroesophageal reflux.

laryngopharyngeal, **865–878**

Reinnervation, for vocal fold paralysis, 887, 889

Resection, for infantile hemangiomas, 946–947

Respiratory distress, in nasal obstruction, 904

Respiratory disturbance index, in obstructive sleep apnea, 830

Respiratory infections, cough in, 952–954

Reynell Developmental Language Scales, 851

Rhabdomyosarcomas, cervical lymphadenopathy in, 925

Rhinitis, obstruction from, 917–918

Rhinoscopy, for nasal obstruction, 904–905

Rhinosinusitis, chronic, **979–991**

S

Saline irrigation, for chronic rhinosinusitis, 985

Serum sickness, cervical lymphadenopathy in, 926

Simulation, of pediatric airway, for training, **993–1003**

Sinusitis, chronic. *See* Chronic rhinosinusitis.

Sleep apnea

laryngomalacia and, 899–900

obstructive. *See* Obstructive sleep apnea.

Sleep endoscopy, drug-induced, 834

Sleep-disordered breathing. *See also* Obstructive sleep apnea.

adenotonsillectomy for, 795

polysomnography for, 798–801

terminology of, 828

Sleepiness, daytime, in obstructive sleep apnea, 828

Smoking, parental, otitis media in, 815–816

Snoring, in obstructive sleep apnea, 828

Societal benefits, after cochlear implantation, 854

Speech, hypernasal, after adenotonsillectomy, 804

Speech perception, after cochlear implantation, 847–849

Speech production, after cochlear implantation, 850–852

Speech therapy, for laryngopharyngeal reflux, 870–871

Spirometry, 959–960

Staphylococcus aureus infections, cervical lymphadenopathy in, 924

Stork bites (hemangiomas), **937–949**

Streptococcal infections, cervical lymphadenopathy in, 924

Stridor

in laryngomalacia, 894

in subglottic hemangiomas, 942

Subacute necrotizing histiocytic lymphadenitis, 926

Subglottic infantile hemangiomas, 941–942, 946–947

Subglottic stenosis

in intubation, 886

in laryngopharyngeal reflux, 869

Suck-swallow-breathing coordination, dysphagia and, 973

Suctioning, for nasal obstruction, 919

Supraglottoplasty, for laryngomalacia, 898–899
Swallowing
    impaired, 867–868, **969–977**
    physiology of, 970
Syphilis, nasal obstruction in, 917

T

Taste disturbance, in cochlear implantation, 855
Telephone usage, after cochlear implantation, 849
Teratomas, nasal obstruction from, 915
Thyroplasty, medialization, for vocal fold paralysis, 887
Tonsillectomy. *See* Adenotonsillectomy.
Tonsillitis, adenotonsillectomy for, 796–798
Tracheal disorders, dysphagia in, 973
Tracheostomy
    for laryngomalacia, 898–899
    for subglottic hemangiomas, 946
    for vocal fold paralysis, 887
    voice disorders in, 889
Training, airway simulation, **993–1003**
Transplantation, laryngeal, 889
Treacher-Collins syndrome, otitis media in, 815
Tube feedings, for dysphagia, 974
Tympanic membrane
    anatomy of, 810–811
    retractions of, 812
Tympanostomy tube insertion, for otitis media, 816–821

U

Ulceration, in infantile hemangiomas, 941
Ultrasonography
    for cervical lymphadenopathy, 932–933
    for dysphagia, 973
Upper airway cough syndrome, 955
Upper airway resistance syndrome, 828
Upper gastrointestinal series, for dysphagia, 973
Uvulopalatopharyngoplasty, for obstructive sleep apnea, 834

V

Vaccination, DTP, cervical lymphadenopathy in, 926
Vascular endothelial growth factor, defects of, infantile hemangiomas in, 938–939
Velopharyngeal insufficiency, after adenotonsillectomy, 804
Vertigo, after cochlear implantation, 857
Videofluoroscopy
    for dysphagia, 973
    for laryngopharyngeal reflux, 867
Videostroboscopy, in voice disorders, 882–883
Vincristine, for infantile hemangiomas, 946

Viral infections, cervical lymphadenopathy in, 924
Vocabulary development, after cochlear implantation, 852
Vocal fold
    development and structure of, 881
    paralysis of, 887–889
Voice disorders, **879–892**
    adult *versus* pediatric, 879–880
    assessment of, 881–884
    epidemiology of, 880
    future treatments for, 889–890
    laryngeal development and, 880–881
    types of, 884–889
Voice therapy, for vocal nodules, 884–885

    W

Waldeyer ring, 794
Weight loss, for obstructive sleep apnea, 833
Wound complications, in cochlear implantation, 855–856

Moving?

Make sure your subscription moves with you!

To notify us of your new address, find your **Clinics Account Number** (located on your mailing label above your name), and contact customer service at:

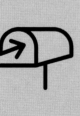

Email: journalscustomerservice-usa@elsevier.com

800-654-2452 (subscribers in the U.S. & Canada)
314-447-8871 (subscribers outside of the U.S. & Canada)

Fax number: 314-447-8029

Elsevier Health Sciences Division
Subscription Customer Service
3251 Riverport Lane
Maryland Heights, MO 63043

*To ensure uninterrupted delivery of your subscription, please notify us at least 4 weeks in advance of move.

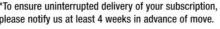